Preface

The field of bariatric surgery has grown exponentially since 1998. Today there are more procedures performed for morbid obesity than for gastroesophageal reflux disease. To meet the public demand for bariatric surgery, more surgeons are taking steps to incorporate bariatric surgery into their surgical practice. Some surgeons have decided to solely dedicate their practice to bariatric surgery while others are performing bariatric surgery as part of their general surgical practice. The American Society for Bariatric Surgery has documented that the number of surgeons performing bariatric surgery has more than quadrupled between 1998 and 2003.

The growth in bariatric surgery in the United States has not come without criticism by the public and third-party payors. One of these concerns relates to the variability in bariatric surgery outcomes and that the surgery is sometimes being performed by inexperienced surgeons at facilities that are not equipped to care for the morbidly obese. This textbook was written with a focus on the comprehensive management of the morbidly obese patient and includes presentations on the preoperative work-up by a multidisciplinary team, essentials of a bariatric program, and perioperative care of the morbidly obese. Several chapters discuss technical details and outcomes of four commonly performed bariatric procedures including vertical banded gastroplasty, laparoscopic adjustable gastric banding, Roux-en-Y gastric bypass and the duodenal switch. Detailed management of perioperative and late complications are discussed. In addition, postoperative nutritional management is emphasized.

In a time when bariatric surgery is coming under scrutiny, this book can be used as a concise reference guide for surgeons and those interested in the care of the morbidly obese. We hope you will enjoy your learning experience, and this book will help in the ongoing efforts to improve the quality of surgical care for these challenging patients.

Harvey J. Sugerman, MD, FACS
Ninh T. Nguyen, MD, FACS

Contents

Preface . . . . *iii*
Contributors . . . . *xi*

1. Obesity: Pathogenetic Mechanisms *1*
John G. Kral
Introduction 1
Detection and Evaluation of Food 2
Processing of Nutrients 2
Nutrient Sensing 3
Hunger and Motivation 4
Surgical Treatment of Overeating 5
Conclusion 7
References 7

2. Epidemiology and Comorbidities of Morbid Obesity *9*
Crystal T. Schlösser and Sayeed Ikramuddin
Epidemiology 9
Social Consequences of Obesity 11
Comorbid Conditions 11
Neoplasia 12
Cardiovascular 12
Pulmonary 14
Endocrine 15
Gastrointestinal 16
Genitourinary 17
Musculoskeletal 18
Hematologic 19
Renal 20
Neurologic 20
Infectious/Immunologic 21
Dermatologic 21
Psychiatric 22
Social/Economic 22

Summary 23
References 23

3. **Treating the Morbidly Obese Patient: A Lifestyle Approach
   to a Chronic Condition** *33*
   *Jennifer E. Taylor, Sara A. Pyle, Walker S. Carlos Poston, and
   John P. Foreyt*
   Introduction 33
   Lifestyle Modification 34
   Dietary Changes 37
   Physical Activity 39
   Combining Behavior Modification and Pharmacotherapy 40
   Surgery 42
   Summary and Conclusions 43
   References 43

4. **Preoperative Evaluation and Intraoperative Care of the Obese** *49*
   *Rodrigo Gonzalez, Scott F. Gallagher, Lisa Saff Koche, and
   Michel M. Murr*
   Introduction 49
   Preoperative Evaluation 49
   Revisional Bariatric Surgery 55
   Intraoperative Care 56
   Conclusion 57
   References 58

5. **Essentials of a Bariatric Surgery Program** *61*
   Samer G. Mattar and Tomasz Rogula
   Introduction 61
   Overview of Etiology and Epidemiology of Morbid
     Obesity 61
   Criteria for Selection of Patients for Bariatric Surgery 62
   Components of a Bariatric Surgery Program 63
   Hospital Requirements 71
   Bariatric Surgery Database 72
   Bariatric Surgery Program Web Site 72
   Conclusion 73
   References 73

6. **Nutrition and Roux-en-Y Gastric Bypass Surgery** *75*
   Jeanne Blankenship and Bruce Wolfe
   Introduction 75
   Pre-Surgical Nutrition Assessment and Management 75
   Pre-Surgical Nutrition Education 78
   Postoperative Diet Guidelines 79
   Nutrient Absorption and Deficiency 80

Malabsorptive Procedures 80
Roux-en-Y (RYGB) 81
Post-surgical Nutrition Assessment 84
Nutrition and Surgical Complications 85
Conclusion 86
References 86

7. **Laparoscopic Vertical Banded Gastroplasty** *91*
   J. K. Champion and Michael Williams
   Introduction 91
   Methods 93
   Results 97
   Discussion 98
   References 100

8. **Physiology of Laparoscopy in the Morbidly Obese** *101*
   David Magner and Ninh T. Nguyen
   Effects of Carbon Dioxide Absorption During
       Pneumoperitoneum 102
   Effects of Increased Intra-Abdominal Pressure During
       Pneumoperitoneum 102
   Conclusions 105
   References 105

9. **The Pathophysiology of Severe Obesity and the Effects of Surgically
   Induced Weight Loss** *109*
   Harvey J. Sugerman
   Introduction 109
   Central (Android) vs. Peripheral (Gynoid) Fat
       Distribution 113
   Hypertension 114
   Cardiac Dysfunction and Dyslipidemia 114
   Pulmonary Dysfunction 115
   Diabetes 116
   Venous Stasis Disease 117
   Degenerative Joint Disease 118
   Gastroesophageal Reflux and Asthma 118
   Urinary Incontinence 118
   Female Sexual Hormone Dysfunction 119
   Pseudotumor Cerebri 119
   Malignancy Risk with Obesity 120
   Hernia Risk with Obesity 120
   Infectious Problems Associated with Morbid Obesity 120
   NALD/NASH 121
   Quality of Life 121
   Mortality 121

Conclusions 122
References 122

10. **Techniques of Laparoscopic Gastric Bypass** *129*
    Benjamin E. Schneider, Ninh T. Nguyen, and Daniel B. Jones
    Introduction 129
    Materials and Methods: Laparoscopic Gastric Bypass
       Technique 129
    Discussion 136
    References 136

11. **Outcome of Laparoscopic Gastric Bypass** *139*
    Corrigan L. McBride, Harvey J. Sugerman, and Eric J. DeMaria
    Introduction 139
    Literature Review—Case Series 139
    Literature Review—Prospective, Randomized Clinical
       Trials 143
    Discussion 145
    References 150

12. **Changing Intestinal Absorption for Treating Obesity** *153*
    *Picard Marceau, Simon Biron, Frédéric Simon Hould, Stéfane Lebel, and
    Simon Marceau*
    Introduction 153
    Development of Bariatric Surgery 154
    Biliopancreatic Diversion 156
    Beneficial Effects of Biliopancreatic Diversion 158
    Detrimental Effect of Biliopancreatic Diversion 162
    Conclusion 164
    References 164

13. **Laparoscopic Adjustable Silicone Gastric Banding** *167*
    Jeff W. Allen and Christine J. Ren
    Introduction 167
    Patient Selection 168
    Operative Technique 169
    Postoperative Management 170
    Complications 173
    Results 176
    Conclusions 178
    References 178

14. **Outcomes of Laparoscopic Adjustable Gastric Banding** *181*
    Paul E. O'Brienz
    Introduction 181
    Laparoscopic Adjustable Gastric Banding 183

Discussion 188
Conclusions 189
References 189

15. **Part II of Debate: Laparoscopic Roux-en-Y Gastric Bypass** *191*
Eric J. DeMaria
Introduction 191
Roux-en-Y Gastric Bypass 191
Laparoscopic Adjustable Gastric Banding (LAGB) 194
Conclusion 203
References 203

16. **Complications of Laparoscopic Bariatric Surgery** *207*
Daniel M. Herron
Introduction 207
Leaks 208
Intestinal Obstruction from Internal Hernia 209
Bleeding 210
Stricture Formation 211
Pulmonary Embolism 212
Cholelithiasis 212
Marginal Ulcer 213
Incisional Hernia 214
Pressure-Related Complications: Rhabdomyolysis and Compartment
    Syndrome 214
Laparoscopic vs. Open Bariatric Surgery 214
Conclusion 215
References 216

17. **Postoperative Follow-Up and Nutritional Management** *219*
Scott A. Shikora and Margaret M. Furtado
Introduction 219
Commonly Performed Bariatric Procedures 219
The Significance of Long-Term Follow-Up 220
Nutritional Deficiencies 221
Protein-Calorie Malnutrition 221
Dehydration 222
Nausea and Vomiting 223
Vitamin Deficiencies 223
Gastrointestinal Issues 226
Conclusions 229
References 230

Index *233*

Contributors

Jeff W. Allen   Department of Surgery and the Center for Advanced Surgical Technologies, University of Louisville School of Medicine, Louisville, Kentucky, U.S.A.

Simon Biron   Department of Surgery, Laval Hospital, Laval University, Quebec, Canada

Jeanne Blankenship   Department of Surgery, University of California Davis School of Medicine, Sacramento, California, U.S.A.

J. K. Champion   Mercer University School of Medicine and Emory-Dunwoody Medical Center, Atlanta, Georgia, U.S.A.

Eric J. DeMaria   Department of Surgery, Duke University, Durham, North Carolina, U.S.A.

John P. Foreyt   Baylor College of Medicine, Houston, Texas, U.S.A.

Margaret M. Furtado   Obesity Consult Center, Center for Minimally Invasive Obesity Surgery, Tufts-New England Medical Center, Boston, Massachusetts, U.S.A.

Scott F. Gallagher   Interdisciplinary Obesity Treatment Group, Department of Surgery, University of South Florida Health Sciences Center, Tampa, Florida, U.S.A.

Rodrigo Gonzalez   Interdisciplinary Obesity Treatment Group, Department of Surgery, University of South Florida Health Sciences Center, Tampa, Florida, U.S.A.

Daniel M. Herron   Section of Bariatric Surgery, Department of Surgery, Mount Sinai School of Medicine, New York, New York, U.S.A.

Frédéric Simon Hould   Department of Surgery, Laval Hospital, Laval University, Quebec, Canada

Sayeed Ikramuddin   Center for Minimally Invasive Surgery, Department of Surgery, University of Minnesota, Minneapolis, Minnesota, U.S.A.

Daniel B. Jones   Harvard Medical School, Beth Israel Deaconess Medical Center, Boston, Massachusetts, U.S.A.

Lisa Saff Koche   Interdisciplinary Obesity Treatment Group, Department of Surgery, University of South Florida Health Sciences Center, Tampa, Florida, U.S.A.

John G. Kral   Department of Surgery, SUNY Downstate Medical Center, Brooklyn, New York, U.S.A.

Stéfane Lebel   Department of Surgery, Laval Hospital, Laval University, Quebec, Canada

David Magner   Department of Surgery, University of California Irvine Medical Center, Orange, California, U.S.A.

Picard Marceau   Department of Surgery, Laval Hospital, Laval University, Quebec, Canada

Simon Marceau   Department of Surgery, Laval Hospital, Laval University, Quebec, Canada

Samer G. Mattar   Department of Surgery, University of Pittsburgh Medical Center, Pittsburgh, Pennsylvania, U.S.A.

Corrigan L. McBride   Department of Surgery, University of Nebraska Medical Center, Omaha, Nebraska, U.S.A.

Michel M. Murr   Interdisciplinary Obesity Treatment Group, Department of Surgery, University of South Florida Health Sciences Center, Tampa, Florida, U.S.A.

Ninh T. Nguyen   Department of Surgery, University of California Irvine Medical Center, Orange, California, U.S.A.

Paul E. O'Brien   The Centre for Obesity Research and Education (CORE), Monash University, Melbourne, Victoria, Australia

Walker S. Carlos Poston   University of Missouri-Kansas City and Mid America Heart Institute, Kansas City, Missouri, U.S.A.

Sara A. Pyle   University of Missouri-Kansas City and Mid America Heart Institute, Kansas City, Missouri, U.S.A.

Christine J. Ren   New York University School of Medicine, New York, New York, U.S.A.

Tomasz Rogula   Department of Surgery, University of Pittsburgh Medical Center, Pittsburgh, Pennsylvania, U.S.A.

Crystal T. Schlösser   Center for Minimally Invasive Surgery, Department of Surgery, University of Minnesota, Minneapolis, Minnesota, U.S.A.

Benjamin E. Schneider   Harvard Medical School, Beth Israel Deaconess Medical Center, Boston, Massachusetts, U.S.A.

Scott A. Shikora   Obesity Consult Center, Center for Minimally Invasive Obesity Surgery, Tufts-New England Medical Center, Boston, Massachusetts, U.S.A.

Harvey J. Sugerman   Department of Surgery, Virginia Commonwealth University, Richmond, Virginia, U.S.A.

Jennifer E. Taylor   University of Missouri-Kansas City and Mid America Heart Institute, Kansas City, Missouri, U.S.A.

Michael Williams   Emory-Dunwoody Medical Center, Atlanta, Georgia, U.S.A.

Bruce Wolfe   Department of Surgery, University of California Davis School of Medicine, Sacramento, California, U.S.A.

1

Obesity: Pathogenetic Mechanisms

John G. Kral
Department of Surgery, SUNY Downstate Medical Center, Brooklyn, New York, U.S.A.

INTRODUCTION

The critical requirement for species' survival is securing nutrients. Surviving organisms either have primarily had characteristics enabling them to withstand all ambient environmental threats to their existence ("stressors") or have evolved through adaptability. Foremost among species in the latter group is *Homo sapiens*. Evolutionary pressure had quantitatively and qualitatively stimulated the development of mechanisms to detect, evaluate, ingest, digest, assimilate, store, and release nutrients to sustain life when humans appeared some 4 million years ago. It is only during the last 150 years that the efficiency of these mechanisms has become maladaptive, driving a life-threatening, civilization-related, global epidemic of a syndrome of metabolic obesity.

With this "ergocentric" (as in energy) view, it is reasonable to postulate that threats to nutrition, and thus to the integrity of an organism, are the ultimate stressors stimulating adaptation. The surgical treatment of obesity, as do all treatments of the disease, seeks to override the many protective mechanisms that have evolved through natural selection.

Tragically, in these affluent times, and largely ignored, social mechanisms have similarly evolved to "protect" the non-obese against the relative voracity of obese people, whose appetites threatened the previously limited food supplies of the group; bias, harassment, and frank ostracism of the obese became instinctive. With abundance of food, these "protective" mechanisms have remained and become social stressors for the obese. Perpetuation of these biases underlies the denial of obesity as a disease, limiting resources to treat or prevent it, thus maintaining a vicious cycle contributing to the disease.

The purpose of this chapter is to review publications relevant to ingestive behavior, the largest contributor to obesity, and thus the most logical target of surgical treatment. It is true that energy expenditure also contributes to the nutritional state and can be enhanced by some forms of surgery, but its contribution to energy balance is far smaller than caloric intake, except in the presence of complications or maladaptive behavior.

DETECTION AND EVALUATION OF FOOD

Plants and the most primitive unicellular organisms, with few exceptions, rely on chance encounters with nutrients in proximity to their stomata, although chemotactic mechanisms are involved in the tropism of plants and the protrusion of pseudopodia from amoebae. Plants are equipped with stomata and guard cells that regulate water flux and carbon gain (1), and have been demonstrated to rely on intracellular calcium-release channels for physiological processes (2). Similar channels are present in animals' enterocytes. In the brain, information processing, requiring increased blood flow for providing substrate, uses neurons that raise intracellular Ca^{2+} ions (3), demonstrating the fundamental role of calcium as a signal of the nutritive state of cells.

Early in phylogeny, the stoma was equipped with special cells for sensing nutrients. The brain has evolved from a collection of sensitive nerve cells surrounding the stoma (mouth) or the entry to the digestive system (4), enabling the identification, selection, and ingestion of nutrients and fluid. The anterior lobe of the pituitary is derived from pouching of the oral ectoderm, and is the source of the most important appetitive peptides. The primary function of the brain is to secure nutrition for the survival of the individual; the secondary function is to ensure reproduction for the survival of the species. Interestingly, there is evidence for reciprocity and cooperation between sexual behavior and ingestive behavior (5), and the related neural pathways associated with reward peptides colocalize in the brain.

The five classical senses vision, smell, touch, taste, and hearing contribute to the detection and evaluation of nutrients (solid or liquid) and water. It is teleologically attractive to hypothesize that the reliance of all senses on dopaminergic pathways mediating reward [e.g., (6)], implies a commonality of purpose, namely reinforcing nutritionally positive or rewarding stimuli. Only recently has it been determined that the process of estimating or evaluating rewards depends on dopamine neurons (7).

The evaluation of nutrients also requires the recognition of toxicity. The most important "tool" for this function is the tongue with its sense of taste. Recent research has identified the receptors necessary for detecting bitter taste, the most important characteristic of dangerous and inappropriate food (8).

PROCESSING OF NUTRIENTS

After detection and evaluation, followed by the "decision" (whether cognitive or reflexive) to reject or ingest a substance, processing begins. The expansion of the ectodermal stoma made possible by multicellularity, gave rise to the endodermal gut for food absorption via specialized cells (9). A different early function of the gut has been largely ignored, namely storage of excess nutrients. Interestingly, several species of snakes still exhibit an extraordinary storage capacity in the wall of the gut (10).

The mesoderm did not arise from the endoderm until after about 40 million years. Early in gut development, however, the pancreas, enhancing absorption, and the liver, synthesizing structural, transport, and functional proteins, developed from the foregut. A poorly recognized fact is that the liver took over the lipid-storing capacity of the gut and likely pre-dates the mesodermal formation of adipose tissue. Consequently it should not be surprising that the liver responds to diverse stressors by fatty metamorphosis (steatosis). Furthermore, lipodystrophy, adipose tissue knock-out models, and lipectomy all lead to fatty infiltration of the liver.

NUTRIENT SENSING

The most important aspect of energy balance and the central "problem" of obesity is determining the signal(s) driving ingestive behavior. Obviously the preceding elements of consummatory behavior do not require "consciousness" at any level; primitive organisms do not exhibit chronic overnutrition, as in obesity. Before addressing the topic of "hunger," operationally defined here as the cognitive correlate of undernutrition, it is important to consider the most basic signals of nutritive state. In this context, "set-point" theory has been a valuable construct.

Set-point theory evolved from the concept of sensors of body stores of macronutrients: lipostatic, glucostatic, or aminostatic or –privic signals regulating ingestive behavior. According to set-point theory there is a fixed level of body weight or some component of body composition toward which the organism will strive after deviations incurred by starvation or over-consumption (11). Since all three classes of macronutrients can function as signals, it is more logical to speak of a system based on energy: an ergostatic or nutristatic theory. In analogy with the carotid artery glomus cell, which is exquisitely sensitive to fluctuations in oxygen tension in the blood (12), considerable interest has been directed toward identifying nutritive sensors or "nutristats." Incidentally, the glomus cell itself responds to hypoxia by influx of calcium and release of dopamine, as described earlier for the regulation of substrate flux in plants and animals. Rather than engaging in the debate over whether glucostatic or lipostatic mechanisms take precedence, it is more enlightening to survey the most recent findings on nutrient signaling.

In a putative ranking of organs according to critical function, the brain comes to mind first, followed by the heart and the lungs, although it is questionable whether any ranking serves a practical purpose. Most "rankings" of nutrients begin with carbohydrate, owing to its role as the preferred substrate for the brain, and indeed, the tightly regulated blood glucose level is a key component in survival. Just recently the molecular mechanisms of glucose homeostasis were discovered, not surprisingly, in the liver (13). Thus, a "glucostat" has been detected.

Since most organs are made up of protein, the analyte best representing lean body mass, its importance is generally recognized, as evidenced in the interest in "protein-sparing" diets. The indispensable or "essential" amino acids are logical candidate signals serving a hypothetical "aminostat." Indeed, most species sense a diet deficient in indispensable amino acids within minutes (14). A basic mechanism functioning as an aminostat has also been discovered recently (15).

The last macronutrient, lipid, has as its basic and circulating components, fatty acids, some of which are essential. In the context of energy balance, especially its dysregulation in obesity, there has been a long-standing interest in "lipostatic" mechanisms. Lipid sensors were first discovered in a different context, however. Lipids are integral components of pathogenic microorganisms and have been identified as signals inducing septic shock. The toll-like receptor 2 (TLR2) is required for detecting various pathogens unrelated to any nutrient-sensing function. This aspect does not seem to have been investigated, although it is intriguing to speculate that TLR2 mediation of prostaglandin E2 release (16), with attendant vasodilation, might have a nutritive function.

Owing to the close relationships between lipids and glucose regulation, it is difficult to separate a specific lipostatic mechanism responsible for energy homeostasis. Nevertheless, long-chain fatty acids have been postulated to have an etiologic role in obesity and type 2 diabetes mellitus (T2DM), and they are metabolized in the brain (17). In a series of experiments manipulating fatty acid metabolism in the hypothalamus, the group led by L. Rossetti determined the presence of hypothalamic sensing of circulating fatty acids, thus providing evidence for a lipostat involved in glucose homeostasis (18). It remains to be shown whether these hypothalamic mechanisms directly influence ingestive behavior, although fatty acid synthetase inhibitors reduced food intake and body weight in mice (19).

Thus, it is obvious that humans are equipped with numerous overlapping mechanisms for detecting and signaling decreases in circulating nutrients. It is reasonable to postulate that they all contribute to "hunger," as was defined earlier. This narrow definition does not take into consideration the many manifestations of hunger explaining food-motivated behavior.

HUNGER AND MOTIVATION

It is not possible to perform a thorough review of this complicated topic here, although it is central to our understanding of ingestive behavior, obesity, and the effects of gastrointestinal operations. Hunger, as is the case with "beauty" and "quality of life," can only be interpreted subjectively, and the definitions may reflect situational, cultural, and socio-economic factors, making it much more esoteric than the "hunger" extrapolated from animal experimentation.

In keeping with our operational definition of hunger as the cognitive or conscious manifestation of dwindling cellular energy stores, it is appropriate to systematize the various symptoms of hunger (Table 1). "Satiety" is often proposed as the reciprocal of hunger; however, satiety implies satisfaction, with its hedonic connotation. "Nimiety," on the other hand, is an unpleasant sensation of fullness. Hunger could be interpreted as an absence of satiety, but such a simplification does not take into consideration the neutral, base-line, or "default" condition when neither hunger nor satiety is present. I make this distinction because there might be a wide variation in individual interpretations of "absence of satiety": some might accept its absence, while others, while under stress, for example, experience hunger (= desire) for "comfort food" providing "satiety."

This raises the issue of discriminating between hunger and appetite, both of which influence food-motivated behavior. The nutrition-related cues emanating from cellular deprivation drive hunger and appetite, which may be nutrient-specific (e.g., salt appetite), although the end result is the same, namely ingestive or consummatory behavior. This is a typical area where it is difficult, if not impossible, to translate animal experiments to the human condition. Although we have the benefit of language for subjective interpretation and communication of perceived inner states, the number of confounding factors is vastly greater than in animals. For a thorough

Table 1 Symptoms of Hunger

Physical	Psychological
Contractions of stomach	Craving
Gnawing, ache, pain	Desire, lust (to eat)
Light-headedness	Anxiety?
"Weakness"	Stress?
"Emptiness"	"Emptiness"

Table 2 Orexigenic Peptides

Central
    Agouti-related peptide (AGRP)
    α-Melanin-stimulating hormone (α-MSH)
    Corticotropin-releasing hormone (CRH)
    Growth hormone-releasing hormone (GHRH)
    Galanin
    Melanin-concentrating hormone (MCH)
    Neuropeptide Y (NPY)
    Orexin A, (B)/Hypocretin 1, (2)
Peripheral
    Ghrelin

---

exposition of hunger and appetite and their relation to ingestive behavior, the readers are referred to an excellent review by Blundell and Gillett in 2001 (20).

Motivation can be positive, as in rewarding and attractive, or negative, as in aversive or repulsive. Brain pathways or neural circuits of fear and aversion colocalize with those of reward and pleasure. Both rely on dopaminergic receptors and are associated with learning and memory, with reciprocal mechanisms for reinforcement. From this, it should be obvious that there cannot be any simple solutions to obesity, a condition that has evolved from the natural evolution of the human species. The discovery of appetitive peptides has been greeted with great expectations for developing pharmacological treatments of obesity. Unfortunately, the results are disappointing.

The preceding review of sensors and signals involved in detecting decreases in the substrate and the description of the multi-faceted aspects of interpreting hunger and appetite point to the difficulties in blocking ingestive behavior. For completeness, Table 2 provides a partial listing of orexigenic peptides and hormones. Three recent reviews provide in-depth analyses of relevant brain–gut peptides and mechanisms (21–23). The following section presents recent information on the place of operative treatment and its impact on these mechanisms.

SURGICAL TREATMENT OF OVEREATING

Recognizing the intractability and suffering of very obese patients, it is not surprising that a surgeon, with experience of unwanted weight loss after gastrointestinal resective operations, attempted small bowel resection. In 1952 Viktor Henriksson of Göteborg, Sweden published his experience with three patients, two sisters and an aunt, who had had small bowel resection two to three years earlier (24). This was reported by Philip Sandblom in *Annals of Surgery* in 1954 in his discussion of the landmark paper on intestinal bypass by Kremen et al. (25). Maintained weight loss after gastric resection and the clinical research on intestinal bypass stimulated Mason and Ito to perform animal experiments culminating in their first report of the clinical use of gastric bypass for obesity (26).

Table 3 groups anti-obesity operations according to mechanisms their inventors initially had in mind and mechanisms later discovered. The overarching principle is to achieve *controlled undernutrition* in patients unable to control overeating by

Table 3 Anti-Obesity Operations and Their Effects

Mechanical
  Decreased absorptive capacity
    Small bowel resection
    Intestinal bypass
      Jejuno-ileal
      Jejuno-colic
      Bilio-pancreatic diversion
  Foregut volume restriction/obstruction
    Gastroplasty
    Banding
    Esophageal banding
    Gastric bypass
    Bilio-pancreatic diversion
Appetitive
    Stereotactic hypothalamic lesions
    Jaw wiring
    Volume restriction
    Vagotomy
    Gastrointestinal bypass/diversion
      Intestinal bypass
      Gastric bypass
      Bilio-pancreatic diversion
      Intestinal interposition
    Electrostimulation
      Gastric wall
      Vagus

themselves. The table demonstrates that the operations originally conceived to decrease the absorptive capacity were earlier recognized to affect food intake. It is still unclear whether satiating or aversive consequences of the various operations dominate. It has often been suggested that obese patients have defects in achieving satiety, although there is no information on the prevalence of this phenomenon or its ability to predict outcome.

Since the early days of jejunoileal bypass there have been studies of the effects of bariatric operations on appetitive peptides, beginning with insulin in 1970 (27). Such studies focused exclusively on "satiating" peptides such as cholecystokinin and incretins [e.g., enteroglucagon, glucagon-like peptide 1 (GLP-1)] until ghrelin was recognized as a peripheral, gastrointestinal orexigenic peptide (28,29). There is ample evidence of the effects of generically different operations (diversionary versus obstructive) on gastrointestinal peptides, in step with the staggering pace of the discovery of new ones. The expectation is that new etiological factors for obesity will be discovered or that new methods for potentiating the release of appropriate peptides via intrinsic mechanisms in the surgically modified intestine can be developed from the information collected before and after various operations. Unfortunately there are so many counter-regulatory compensatory mechanisms activated by the reduction of in-continuity absorptive surface area that make it unlikely that such an approach in isolation will succeed over the long term.

The most important objective of current surgical investigation, while awaiting realistic measures to prevent obesity, should be to pursue the evolving sciences of functional neuro-imaging, genomics/proteomics, and metabolomics (30) in an effort to improve patient selection for generically different bariatric operations.

CONCLUSION

Threats to nutrition, the ultimate stressors, have exerted evolutionary pressure on the development of mechanisms to find, evaluate, ingest, assimilate, and store nutrients to sustain life. Although a "glomus cell" that specifically detects drops in energy has not yet been identified, considerable progress has been made in elucidating the many redundant mechanisms and pathways for maintaining "ergostasis." As this review has tried to demonstrate, the forces involved in the simple act of overeating are numerous and daunting, and are not easily overcome by individual "will-power" or available non-surgical methods. The technological advances of *Homo sapiens* have caused chronic dysregulation of energy balance leading to the worldwide epidemic of overnutrition. It is only recently that technological advances are being used to investigate obesity with a view to palliating exponentially increasing numbers of obese patients.

REFERENCES

1. Hetherington AM, Woodward FI. The role of stomata in sensing and driving environmental change. Nature 2003; 424(6951):901–908.
2. Peiter E, Maathuis FJM, Mills LN, Knight H, Pelloux J, Hetherington AM, Sanders D. The vacuolar Ca^{2+}-activated channel TPC1 regulates germination and stomatal movement. Nature 2005; 434(7031):404–408.
3. Faraci FM, Breese KR. Nitric oxide mediates vasodilatation in response to activation of N-methyl-D-aspartate receptors in brain. Circ Res 1993; 72(2):476–480.
4. Holland ND. Early central nervous system evolution: an era of skin brains? Nat Rev Neurosci 2003; 4(8):617–627.
5. Macias C, Ramirez G, Ramirez E. Evidence that sensory traps can evolve into honest signals. Nature 2005; 434(7032):501–505.
6. Dommett E, Coizet V, Blaha CD, Martindale J, Lefebvre V, Walton N, Mayhew JE, Overton PG, Redgrave P. How visual stimuli activate dopaminergic neurons at short latency. Science 2005; 307:1476–1479.
7. Tobler PN, Fiorillo CD, Schultz W. Adaptive coding of reward value by dopamine neurons. Science 2005; 307(5714):1642–1645.
8. Mueller KL, Hoon MA, Erlenbach I, Chandrashekar J, Zuker CS, Ryba NJ. The receptors and coding logic for bitter taste. Nature 2005; 434(7030):225–229.
9. Stainier DYR. No organ left behind: tales of gut development and evolution. Science 2005; 307(5717):1902–1909.
10. Starck JM, Beese K. Structural flexibility of the small intestine and liver of garter snakes in response to feeding and fasting. J Exp Biol 2002; 205(Pt 10):1377–1388.
11. Cohn C, Joseph D. Influence of body weight and body fat on appetite of "normal" lean and obese rats. Yale J Biol Med 1962; 34:598–607.
12. Hoshi T, Lahiri S. Cell biology. Oxygen sensing: it's a gas! Science 2004; 306(5704):2050.
13. Rodgers JT, Lerin C, Haas W, Gygi SP, Spiegelman BM, Puigserver P. Nutrient control of glucose homeostasis through a complex of PGC-1alpha and SIRT1. Nature 2005; 434(7029):113–118.

14. Koehnle TJ, Russell MC, Gietzen DW. Rats rapidly reject diets deficient in essential amino acids. J Nutr 2003; 133(7):2331–2335.

15. Hao S, Sharp JW, Ross-Inta CM, McDaniel BJ, Anthony TG, Wek RC, Cavener DR, McGrath BC, Rudell JB, Koehnle TJ, Gietzen DW. Uncharged tRNA and sensing of amino acid deficiency in mammalian piriform cortex. Science 2005; 307(5716):1176–1778.

16. Jimenez R, Belcher E, Sriskandan S, Lucas R, McMaster S, Vojnovic I, Warner TD, Mitchell JA. Role of toll-like receptors 2 and 4 in the induction of cyclooxygenase-2 in vascular smooth muscle. Proc Natl Acad Sci USA 2005; 102(12):4637–4642.

17. Miller JC, Gnaedinger JM, Rapoport SI. Utilization of plasma fatty acid in rat brain: distribution of (14C) palmitate between oxidative and synthetic pathways. J Neurochem 1987; 49(5):1507–1514.

18. Lam TKT, Pocai A, Gutierrez-Juarez R, Obici S, Bryan J, Aguilar-Bryan L, Schwartz GJ, Rossetti L. Hypothalamic sensing of circulating fatty acids is required for glucose homeostasis. Nat Med 2005; 11(3):320–327.

19. Loftus TM, Jaworsky DE, Frehywot GL, Townsend CA, Ronnett GV, Lane MD, Kuhajda FP. Reduced food intake and body weight in mice treated with fatty acid synthase inhibitors. Science 2000; 288(5475):2379–2381.

20. Blundell JE, Gillett A. Control of food intake in the obese. Obes Res 2001; 9(4): 263S–270S.

21. Näslund E, Hellström PM, Kral JG. The gut and food intake: an update for surgeons. J Gastrointest Surg 2001; 5(5):556–567.

22. Schwartz MW, Porte D, Jr. Diabetes, obesity, and the brain. Science 2005; 307(5708): 375–379.

23. Badman MK, Flier JS. The gut and energy balance: visceral allies in the obesity wars. Science 2005; 307(5717):1909–1914.

24. Henriksson V. Is small bowel resection justified as treatment for obesity? Nordisk Med 1952; 47:744.

25. Kremen AJ, Linner JH, Nelson CH. An experimental evaluation of the nutritional importance of proximal and distal small intestine. Ann Surg 1954; 140:439.

26. Mason EE, Ito C. Gastric bypass and obesity. Surg Clin North Am 1967; 47:1345–1352.

27. Rehfeld JF, Juhl E, Quaade F. Effect of jejunoileostomy on glucose and insulin metabolism in ten obese patients. Metabolism 1970; 19(7):529–538.

28. Tschop M, Smiley DL, Heiman ML. Ghrelin induces adiposity in rodents. Nature 2000; 407(6806):903–913.

29. Cummings DE, Weigle DS, Frayo RS, Breen PA, Ma MK, Dellinger EP, Purnell JQ. Plasma ghrelin levels after died-induced weight loss or gastric bypass surgery. N Engl J Med 2002; 346(21):1623–1630.

30. Lafaye A, Labarre J, Tabet JC, Ezan E, Junot C. Liquid chromatography-mass spectrometry and ^{15}N metabolic labeling for quantitative metabolic profiling. Anal Chem 2005; 77(7):2026–2033.

2

Epidemiology and Comorbidities of Morbid Obesity

Crystal T. Schlösser and Sayeed Ikramuddin
Center for Minimally Invasive Surgery, Department of Surgery, University of Minnesota, Minneapolis, Minnesota, U.S.A.

EPIDEMIOLOGY

Morbid obesity (MO) has been documented throughout history, even in times and cultures that had limited food supplies or excessive physical activity. Surprisingly, even in areas of the world where such limited food is available that growth stunting is found in the population, MO is seen in members of that cohort, and does not correlate with ingested calories (1). In the last 25 years, there has been an unprecedented growth in the proportion of the population above the ideal body weight. MO is the fastest-growing disease in the industrialized world with an estimated 1.7 billion affected worldwide (2,3). This disease is now surpassing undernourishment in prevalence (2). This rise is independent of age, education, ethnicity, sex, and smoking status. These changes, although most prominent in industrialized countries, are seen throughout most cultures and nations. With this rapid growth of obesity, sharp increases in the number of comorbid diseases have followed (4). The most serious are neoplasia of multiple organs, diabetes, hypertension, coronary artery disease (CAD) and its sequelae, pregnancy-related problems, arthritis, and extensive social consequences (4).

The U.S. National Heart, Lung, and Blood Institute published, in 1998, guidelines to stratify risk from increased body mass index (BMI) (4), calculated as: Weight (in kg)/Height (in m)^2.

Between 1986 and 2000, the incidence of mild to moderate obesity doubled to about 20% of the U.S. population; the prevalence of MO increased four times, but

Classification	Body mass index
Normal weight	20–24.9
Overweight	25–29.9
Mild obesity	30–34.9
Moderate obesity	35.0–39.9
Severe (morbid) obesity	≥ 40

the finding of a BMI ≥ 50 (superobesity) increased by a factor of 5 (5). Since 2000, the incidence of clinically severe obesity has continued to rise exponentially, and has outpaced the general rise in BMI. Currently, it is thought that one-third of the U.S. population is overweight, with another third having varying degrees of obesity, with no area of the country being spared (6).

This rise has been accompanied by disease of multiple organ systems (see separate sections later) and excess mortality from these illnesses. In the United States, an estimated 300,000 deaths yearly are attributable to obesity, a 33% increase from 1990. In addition, over $90 billion are incurred in annual direct costs for the treatment of obesity-related medical conditions (7).

In 2000, the most common underlying causes of death in the United States were related to tobacco (435,000 persons), poor diet and physical inactivity (400,000 persons), and alcohol consumption (85,000 persons) (8,9). It is estimated that within three years, obesity will become the number one underlying cause of death (10).

Fontaine et al. published recent estimates of the number of years of life lost due to the consequences of obesity, with significant differences seen when stratified by race and sex. The longest lifespan is seen in those persons with BMIs of 23 to 25 (whites) and 23–30 (blacks). In those who have elevated BMIs, there is a significant inverse correlation with age. The years of life lost for persons aged 20 to 30 with BMI > 45 were estimated as shown in the table below

Group	Years lost
Black males	20
White males	13
Black females	5
White females	8

Individuals older than 30 years have lesser years of life lost, even when controlling for average age-adjusted lifespan (11).

Trends in Oral Intake in the United States

The epidemiology of obesity is incomplete without examining the trends in oral intake. The National Health and Nutrition Examination Surveys of the US (NHANES) during four time periods (1971–1974, 1976–1980, 1988–1994, and 1999–2000) showed changes in several macronutrients. These included increased mean energy intake and percentage of calories from carbohydrates; decreases in the percentage of calories from total and saturated fat were observed (12). Decreased work and leisure physical activity, especially among children, have also been cited as etiologic (13). Even when combining these factors, the degree of rise in obesity cannot be completely explained.

Children

Obesity in varying degrees is being noted in ever-younger age groups, with even pre-school-age children showing alterations in body composition. In Japan a cross-sectional survey showed significant nationwide increases in the prevalence of obesity over a 13-year time period (1989–2002). Preschool boys showed the largest changes, although girls were also more obese (14,15). Mexican children tend to be highly overweight and obese, with geographic gradients related to closeness to the United States (16). Children were noted to have had increased BMIs over the last 20 years in all countries, with sex differences in many countries, and often with age-specific trends (17,18).

Socio-Economic Status

BMI is rising across all socio-economic lines, including in adverse social and economic conditions, with industrialized countries showing larger gains than agrarian societies. This is more common in women than in men, which is possibly related to gender roles in many parts of the world (19). Of the morbidly obese who present for surgical consideration in the United States, a disproportionate number are of African-American ancestry, poor, and with low levels of education. This sector makes up 38% of the population meeting criteria for bariatric surgery, but yet comprises only 13% of those that receive such treatment (20,21).

SOCIAL CONSEQUENCES OF OBESITY

The proliferation of obesity has grave consequences for health care systems and the economics of providing care due to the increasing numbers with obesity and more severe diseases. Health care spending on obesity-related conditions among people 50–69 years old is expected to increase by 50% by 2020 (22). There are obvious implications for public health policy and the need to educate the providers. The projections for gainful employment and contributions to society must also be considered in contemplating the economic effects of this disease. Most distressing is the prognosis for severely obese individuals. No effective long-term medical therapy currently exists. Effective surgical methods may be excluded or limited by health insurance providers, creating inequities (22). The thrust of research and public intervention must be toward identifying the cause and preventing the development of obesity (23).

COMORBID CONDITIONS

An interesting constellation of altered physiology and disease states accompanies the disease of MO. The number and severity of these comorbid conditions are related to age, duration and degree of MO, family history, and other less characterized risk factors, probably genetic in nature. The basic alterations that trigger MO have far-reaching effects on nearly every organ system; the mechanisms for most of these illnesses have been postulated, but not proven. A unifying theory has yet to be proposed and causation versus association not certain. Each system will be discussed separately, but not necessarily in the order of importance. Overall, men have more comorbidities than women when BMI is not considered, all of which are influenced by age and ethnicity. Of utmost concern is the association with neoplasia; given the long subclinical course of most cancers, the new epidemic of obesity has staggering implications on future cancer rates (24).

NEOPLASIA

In the United States in 2002, an estimated 41,383 (3.2%) incidences of cancers were thought to be potentially attributable to obesity, based on tumor registries and obesity prevalence trends (25). More recent data indicate that obesity in the United States could be responsible for 20% of cancer deaths in women and 14% in men. Death rates in MO (BMI ≥40) from all cancers combined were higher in both sexes. The increase observed was 62% in women [relative risk (RR) of death 1.62 (95% confidence interval (CI) 1.40, 1.87)] and 52% in men (RR 1.52, 95% CI 1.13, 2.05), when compared with non-obese persons (26).

Swedish researchers confirm an elevated risk with a 33% excess incidence of cancer, 37% in women and 25% in men (27). Multiple sites are involved, including the endometrium, breast, prostate, colon and rectum, gallbladder, esophagus, liver, pancreas, kidney, lymph nodes (non-Hodgkin's lymphoma), and bone marrow (multiple myeloma). Many of these sites have not previously been associated with obesity.

Carcinoma of endometrium. There has been a long association between obesity and the risk of endometrial cancer. Recently, attention has been directed to insulin resistance as a closer link between these two disease states. Lukanova et al. found that endometrial cancer risk increased with increasing levels of C-peptide, even when adjusted for BMI and insulin growth factor (28). Up to a 7-fold increase in the risk of endometrial cancer in obese women (BMI not reported) was noted by Brinton et al. (29).

Carcinoma of breast. Breast cancer, like other estrogen-sensitive cancers, is powerfully influenced by MO. In a report from Harvard, there was a 50% higher rate of breast cancer in women with MO (30). Second primary breast cancers are also higher in MO, with a hazard ratio of 1.58 (31). MO patients who carry BRCA1 or BRCA2 mutations also have an earlier onset of the disease, compared with those carriers with lower BMI (32).

Carcinoma of prostate. In a study of over 1000 men surgically treated for prostate cancer, MO (BMI ≥35) was associated with higher-grade tumors, a trend toward increased risk of positive surgical margins, and higher biochemical failure rates, especially in young men (33–35). A statistically significant correlation of prostate cancer with triglycerides and insulin resistance was noted by Zamboni et al. suggesting a mechanism outside the usual hormonal theories of prostate neoplasia (36).

Carcinoma of colon. A 40% higher rate of colon and rectal cancer has been seen in the MO population; other studies show a larger risk. In men, death rates from colon cancer have an odds ratio (OR) of 1.90 (95% CI 1.46, 2.47). Lesser associations for MO women were noted with an OR of 1.23 (95% CI 0.96, 1.59) (37). The adenoma–carcinoma sequence has been well established in colon cancer, and the increasing precursor lesions may influence cancer rates. Such an increase in the precursor adenomas is associated with abdominal obesity in middle age (38).

CARDIOVASCULAR

Hypertension. Elevated blood pressure (≥130/≥85) is present in 38% of the MO population, with 45% of these being undiagnosed. These numbers are slightly higher in blacks, and marginally less in Hispanics (39). Of hypertensive individuals, obesity *alone* accounts for 78% in males and 65% in females (40,41). The control of obesity can eliminate 48% of the hypertension in whites and 28% in blacks. Alterations in naturietic peptides, renal structural changes, multiple hormones, and genetic changes in beta-adrenergic receptors are the postulated mediators of obesity-related hypertension (42,43).

Left ventricular hypertrophy and heart failure. Independent of the arterial pressure, obesity increases the risk of left ventricular hypertrophy (LVH), especially the eccentric variant (44). Systolic function may remain intact in early obesity, but preload estimates suggest reduced contractility as measured by end-systolic wall stress and its relation to end–systolic volume index (45). Late systolic deterioration occurs through multiple mechanisms. Diastolic function also suffers, but these changes can be reversed by weight loss (46–48). In 74 MO patients, Alpert et al. found that 32% had clinical evidence of heart failure. After 20 and 25 years of MO, the probability of heart failure rose to 66% and 93%, respectively (47). The prognosis of obesity-related heart failure is not well established, but less severe disease is seen in many patients with higher BMI (49). This inverse correlation to BMI might suggest an alternate mechanism in the morbidly obese.

CAD. Multiple large studies [Framingham Heart Study (50), Nurses Health Study (51)] have clearly shown an association between the increasing levels of obesity and the risk of fatal and non-fatal myocardial infarction. A strong correlation between younger patients presenting with CAD and increased BMI has been noted. In Japan, those under 40 with CAD have an increasing prevalence of obesity, with 83% obese since childhood (52). Even with weight loss, previously obese individuals maintain a doubled risk for acute MI for at least 10 years, compared to never-obese controls (53). The prognosis for those requiring percutaneous or surgical revascularization is not clearly worsened by elevated BMI. Lean individuals show increased mortality, similar to the outcomes with heart failure (54,55), again suggesting a different pathophysiology.

Dyslipidemia (hypercholesterolemia hypertriglyceridemia, altered HDL/LDL ratios). Obesity is invariably associated with elevated triglycerides, and increased hepatic synthesis of VLDL drives this abnormality. Decreased HDL and abnormal LDL fractionation is also common. These alterations seem closely tied to insulin resistance, and together are a powerful initiator of atherosclerosis. Stepwise treatment is by weight loss, exercise, with the addition of pharmacologic lipid lowering agents as a last resort (56).

Metabolic syndrome. In 2001, the U.S. National Cholesterol Education Program Treatment Panel published the criteria to define a clinically recognized entity associated with excess cardiovascular morbidity and mortality, which was designated the *metabolic syndrome.* This was defined as the presence of at least three of these five abnormalities (57):

Measure	Criterion
Abdominal obesity (waist circumference)	>102 cm men, >88 cm women
Triglycerides	>150 mg/dL
HDL cholesterol	<40 mg/dL men, <50 women
Hypertension	≥130/≥85 mmHg
Insulin resistance (fasting glucose)	>110 mg/dL

In addition, hyperuricemia, microalbuminuria, and hypercoagulability are often noted in those who meet the criteria, but these are not part of the definition. The prevalence of metabolic syndrome in MO varies slightly with a specific regional group, but in general is approximately 50% and is independent of the BMI. This suggests that excess weight alone is not the root of metabolic syndrome, but rather a manifestation of the disease (58). The treatment is directed at the multiple clinical manifestations, and the most important modality may be insulin-sensitizing medications. These agents improve the endothelial function and reduce the vascular reactivity and inflammation. See section on "Diabetes" below.

Sudden death. To summarize the coronary risk of obesity, Hippocrates stated, "Sudden death is more common in those who are naturally fat than in the lean" (59). This highlights not only that MO was present even before fast food, cars, and video games, but that its coalescence of risk factors translates into true "mortal" obesity.

PULMONARY

Obstructive sleep apnea. Recurrent partial or total obstruction of airflow while sleeping leads to oxygen desaturation, increased effort, and partial to full arousal, causing sleep fragmentation and loss of REM sleep. Patients are often oblivious to their apnea or obstructed respirations, and diagnosis may be difficult in the absence of an observant bed partner. Obesity contributes to the redundancy of soft tissues of upper airways, including lateral pharyngeal walls and tongue, with the severity of symptoms often related to the degree of tissue enlargement. A cursory physical exam of the neck of an MO patient can often arouse suspicion for the presence of obstructive sleep apnea (OSA), by observing a concentration of fat and redundant tissue, especially laterally (60).

The major symptom of OSA is excessive daytime sleepiness, but other nonspecific acute and chronic neurocognitive and psychiatric symptoms occur, requiring a high index of suspicion by primary and consultative physicians. The prevalence of OSA in the general population is 25% to 58% of men and 10% to 37% of women aged 30 to 60 years. The *symptoms* were seen in only 4% of men and 2% of women, however (61,62). In the MO, 98% have mild apnea–hypopnea scores, and 33% have more severe forms of true sleep apnea. In obese individuals, anatomic and functional considerations of the pharyngeal airway, function of the central nervous system, mechanical effects of central obesity, and undefined actions of leptin all likely contribute to the manifestation of OSA. As a result, all MO patients should have polysomnography to diagnose sleep-disordered breathing and treatment of any identified abnormalities.

Independent of the effects of OSA and sleep-disordered breathing, associations of MO with insulin resistance and glucose intolerance have been noted. These may be directed by altered adrenergic function, direct effects of hypoxemia on glucose homeostasis, and increased levels of proinflammatory cytokines (63). The postulation of "syndrome Z," to include obesity, hypertension, diabetes, and OSA has been discussed (64). All these contribute to a vicious cycle of escalating disease, worsening comorbidity, and increased risk of cardiovascular and metabolic disorders. Treatment with continuous positive airway pressure may ameliorate this cycle by reducing the insulin resistance (65).

Obesity-hypoventilation syndrome. The obese have decreased lung volumes from increased intra-abdominal pressure. Subsequent elevation of the diaphragm impairs respiratory mechanics with incomplete excursion of this muscle. Increased pulmonary blood volume and right-sided cardiac output are associated. Decreased lung volumes cause chronic dyspnea, decreased expiratory reserve volume, increased oxygen consumption rates, and increased circulating carbon dioxide. Cumulative effects of these respiratory changes include pulmonary hypertension, right heart failure, and death. Significantly elevated levels of vascular endothelial growth factor are seen in these patients and those with severe sleep apnea; no similar association with interleukin 6 (IL-6) or tumor necrosis factor alpha (TNF-α) is present (66).

Pulmonary hypertension. Elevated pulmonary arterial pressures are common in OSA, up to 27%, with 18% having associated right ventricular changes (67). This may be related to the obesity-hypoventilation syndrome, with hypercapnia adding to the hypoxia of OSA, with resultant vasoconstriction (see above). Consideration should be given to preoperative cardiac echocardiography in patients with identified hypopnea or apnea.

ENDOCRINE

Diabetes mellitus. Type 2 diabetes mellitus (T2DM) and obesity are intimately connected. Of persons who are obese, the prevalence of T2DM is 30%, and of those, 33% are undiagnosed and 50% untreated (39). Conversely, patients with T2DM are obese or overweight 90% of the time. By the end of this decade, it has been estimated that between 200 million and 300 million people worldwide will meet World Health Organization's diagnostic criteria for T2DM (68). As an epidemic of T2DM has developed, there has been a concomitant rise in obesity (69). The previous demographics of T2DM was middle-aged to late-aged overweight people, but there has been a marked shift toward younger age groups, and now adolescents and children (70). The relationship is so strong that obesity is considered the number one risk factor for the onset of T2DM with a relative risk of 20.1 for a BMI 30 to 34.9, and 38 RR for BMI $\geq$ 35 (71). Central adiposity, regardless of the BMI, is also an independent risk factor for developing T2DM, and might suggest that waist–hip ratios are a better measure for predicting T2DM (72). The risk of dying from the development of cardiovascular disease (the number one cause of death in this population) is 2.5 to 3.3 times higher for mild to moderate obesity [20–30% over ideal body weight (IBW)] and 5.2 to 7.9 times higher for more severe obesity (> 40% over IBW) (68).

The basic mechanism of T2DM is obscure, but thought to be related to insulin resistance. This resistance creates increased glucose levels, triggering increased pancreatic beta-cell insulin production, with ever-increasing glucose resistance at peripheral sites. As the beta cells fail to satisfy the escalating demand for insulin, the complications of this disease occur. In addition, the coexistence of MO worsens insulin resistance, exacerbates hyperglycemia and dyslipidemia, and alters response to diabetic therapies such as oral hypoglycemic agents. These medications can also promote weight gain (73), again launching a downward spiral of metabolic disarray.

Modulators of insulin resistance have been theorized to include TNF-α and adiponectin via unidentified pathways. Further evidence suggests that after bariatric surgery, decreases in insulin resistance are independently and significantly correlated with the decrease in IL-6 concentrations, but decrease in BMI is related to decreases in C-reactive protein (CRP) (74). Gastric inhibitory polypeptide is reduced in another postoperative study (75), suggesting that multiple hormones are also involved in mediating surgical results. The thiazolidinediones, a class of oral hypoglycemic agents, act as insulin sensitizers and bind to nuclear receptor peroxisome proliferator-activated receptor gamma. Natural mutations in the gene that encodes this receptor is linked to abnormal glucose homeostasis, increased number of adipocytes, dyslipidemia, and abnormal blood pressure control. These mutations are seen in the offspring of patients with T2DM, and insulin resistance in the skeletal muscle of these children is associated with alterations of intramyocellular fatty acid metabolism (76). These findings may be a step closer to the basis of this illness, allowing greater understanding of this link to metabolic syndrome and more targeted therapies (77,78).

Hyperparathyroidism. Hyperparathyroidism (defined as parathyroid hormone levels >65 pg/mL) are common in the morbidly obese and are correlated with BMI. In a study of 165 patients undergoing duodenal switch, hyperparathyroidism was seen in 38.9% (BMI ≥50) and 14.9% (BMI <50). Postoperatively, these patients had only slight increases in PTH levels, with documented subnormal 25-hydroxy vitamin D levels in 10–17% (79). In another population of 213 patients, hyperparathyroidism was observed in 25.0% of all subjects at baseline. Despite elevated hormone levels, serum calcium levels were high in only 0.5%, and low in 3.5% (80). The cause of parathyroid elevations related to obesity is unclear.

GASTROINTESTINAL

Non-alcoholic steatohepatitis. Non-alcoholic steatohepatitis (NASH), also known as the fatty infiltration of the liver, is common in MO patients. Clinical diagnosis is made by typical ultrasonographic findings plus persistent elevation of alanine aminotransferase levels. Biopsy can show disease in the absence of these clinical findings, rendering such measurements insensitive. Beymer et al. showed in a prospective study of liver biopsies in MO patients that the prevalence of liver disease was high, with only 5% of biopsies being histologically normal. Some overlaps in groups were noted, but moderate to severe steatosis was seen in 65%, NASH in 33%, and severe fibrosis in 12%. When analyzing the findings, DM but not BMI is correlated with NASH and fibrosis (81). Others have suggested that insulin resistance and elevated ferritin levels are predictive of NASH (82).

Sakugawa et al. found that in 404 patients with cirrhosis, 40 (9.9%) had cryptogenic cirrhosis; NASH was considered the etiology in this group. These patients were more likely to be older, female, obese (53%), and have T2DM (40%) compared with the case-controls (83). Although fatty changes can regress with reduction in BMI, surveillance measurements of liver function tests, consideration of repeat biopsy, and hepatology consultation are suggested.

Gastroesophageal reflux. Gastroesophageal reflux disease (GERD) is common in the morbidly obese, with the increased intra-abdominal pressures thought to play an important role. The prevalence is high, with GERD seen in 40.3+/−18.9% and overt regurgitation in 29.9+/−19.0%, over twice that seen in age- and sex-matched controls. In addition, symptoms were felt more intensely in the MO population (84).

Cholelithiasis, microlithiasis, choledocholithiasis. The incidence of gallstones is very high in MO, anywhere from 35% to 70% depending on the ethnicity of the population. Microlithiasis, sludge, and cholesterolosis are also frequently seen, and some advocate routine removal of the gallbladder at the time of bariatric surgery, regardless of the ultrasonographic findings (85–90).

Acute pancreatitis. Due to hypertriglyceridemia and alterations in the bile composition, acute pancreatitis due to gallstones is common in this population. Estimates are difficult, but may be anywhere from 5% to 35% lifetime incidence, although most cases are mild. In a recent large meta-analysis, severe pancreatitis was significantly more frequent in BMI ≥ 30 (OR 2.6, 95% CI 1.5–4.6). More local complications (OR 4.3, 95% CI 2.4–7.9) and systemic illness (OR 2.0, 95% CI 1.1–4.6) is also seen. The risk of dying from the disease process, though, was 30% higher (OR 1.3, 95% CI 0.5–3.6) (91). This may suggest directions for management of asymptomatic gallbladder disease in this patient population.

GENITOURINARY

Menstrual irregularities/infertility. Due to the adipocyte steroid hormone uptake and conversion, infertility and menstrual aberrations are common. Irregular menses occur in 35% to 65% of premenopausal MO patients (92). Oligomenorrhea (18.3%) and amenorrhea (11.7%) were predominant in a recent Mexican study (93). After surgical therapy, the cycles were abnormal in only 4.6% (92). Primary or secondary infertility is frequent, ranging from 15% to 38% in MO women. Dietel et al. noted a 29.3% incidence in MO women, with 23% of patients regaining fertility after bariatric surgery (92). In those that undergo treatment for infertility, initial success is related to BMI, with higher loss after in vitro fertilization and intracytoplasmic sperm injection (94). Those that achieve conception, spontaneous abortion, ongoing pregnancy, or ectopic pregnancy in singleton gestations in the first trimester, are not affected by BMI (95).

In those that undergo treatment for infertility, initial implantation success is inversely related to BMI (94). Those that achieve singleton conception, spontaneous abortion, ongoing pregnancy, or ectopic pregnancy in the first trimester are not affected by BMI (95).

Pregnancy-related complications. Cedergren outlines the quantitative risk of obesity in pregnancy and delivery in a recent very large prospective study. Swedish women over a 10-year period (1/1/92–12/31/01) formed a cohort of 805,275 singleton pregnancies. This represented 88.2% of the total pregnant population during the time frame. Of these, 1.6% (12,698) were obese (BMI 35.1–39.9), and 0.4% (3480) met criteria for MO (BMI > 40). Women with MO showed the following adverse outcomes (expressed as adjusted OR with 95% CI) compared to normal weight women:

Complication (BMI > 40)	Odds ratio	95% CI
Pre-eclampsia	4.82	4.04–5.74
Large-for-gestational age	3.82	3.50–4.16
Early neonatal death	3.41	2.07–5.63
Shoulder dystocia	3.14	1.86–5.31
Meconium aspiration	2.85	1.60–5.07
Antepartum stillbirth	2.79	1.94–4.02
Cesarean (operative) delivery	2.69	2.49–2.90
Fetal distress	2.52	2.12–2.99
Instrumental delivery	1.34	1.16–1.56

The mothers with lesser obesity (BMI 35.1–39.9) showed a similar spectrum and distribution of complications but with slightly lower ORs. These risks were still elevated compared to women with normal BMI (96). This suggests that obesity places a higher pregnancy-related risk than previously thought. The higher rates of stillbirth and spontaneous abortion in MO are possibly mediated through other comorbidities. Alterations in cytokine levels, insulin resistance, and prothrombotic tendencies all may contribute to fetal loss. With the large number of children and adolescents with obesity, these pregnancy-related morbidities are expected to rise.

Birth defects. A Swedish prospective case-control study examined 6801 women who had infants with cardiovascular defects, excluding chromosomal aberrations and pre-existing maternal diabetes. The denominator was a delivered population of 812,457 women over a 10-year period. This showed a statistically significant correlation of MO (BMI ≥ 35) for ventricular and atrial septal defects (97). Another fetal risk is increased body fat in infants of women with gestational diabetes mellitus. Such increased fat is identified even when infants are of average weight for gestational age (98). The long-term effects of this excess fat on the health of the infant, and their future disposition toward obesity, requires further study.

Urinary incontinence. The reported prevalence rates for monthly incontinence vary depending on the population of women studied. The incidence ranges from 12% to 40% and is influenced by age and parity. Incontinence alters the quality of life and activities of daily living, often stigmatizing women to the point of unemployment and social isolation. Unfortunately, its role is often under-appreciated by health care providers, and patients may be reluctant to discuss these symptoms proactively.

The relative risk of stress incontinence in an obese population of women (BMI ≥ 30) was 1.74 (95% CI 1.22–2.48) compared with a risk of 1.25 (95% CI 0.94–1.67) for milder obesity. This statistically significant difference was also seen in overactive bladder (urgency) symptoms with a relative risk of 1.46 (95% CI 1.02–2.09) (99). The pathophysiology has traditionally been thought to relate to the increased intra-abdominal pressure, but neuromuscular function of the genito-urinary tract may also be altered, with the loss of protective compensation for such pressures (100).

Polycystic ovarian syndrome. Approximately 4% of women in the general population have chronic anovulation and androgen excess. Associated insulin resistance, hyperandrogenism, and altered gonadotropin homeostasis is seen, defining polycystic ovarian syndrome (PCOS). Obesity is not universal, and occurs in 50% of women (101). In most women with PCOS, the luteinizing hormone (LH) pulse frequency is increased. In obese patients, the *amplitude* and mean circulating LH values are lower than in lean patients. Higher levels of insulin, insulin resistance, leptin, catecholamines, and endorphin metabolism have all been implicated in these differences (102–104).

Diagnosis is made by history and physical examination treatment has historically included oral contraceptives with or without spironolactone, and ovulation induction. More recently, insulin-sensitizing agents such as metformin are being advocated, particularly in adolescents. Early treatment is thought to delay or prevent long-term complications of PCOS (105).

MUSCULOSKELETAL

Joint pain. Multiple joints are affected with varying degrees of pain in the MO population, regardless of the radiographically identified osteoarthritis. The most common joints affected include the lumbar spine, hips, knees, ankles, and feet, with relative sparing of hands. NHANES III data on U.S. adults ≥60 years showed a rising incidence of joint pain associated with increasing BMI. In the general population, the prevalence of knee, hip, and back pain is 21%, 14%, and 22%, respectively. In MO (BMI≥40), these figures rise to 55.7%, 23.3%, and 26.1%. When controlling for sex, race, and age, the prevalence of joint pain increased at increased levels of BMI (106).

Theories regarding the increased levels of cytokines and other inflammatory markers have shifted thinking about this comorbidity. The traditional weight-bearing or altered mechanics theory is being regarded as only part of the etiology of arthritis (107). Even before substantial amounts of weight are lost, rapid improvement is seen in joint pain after bariatric surgery. This might provide circumstantial evidence for such a mechanism.

Carpal tunnel syndrome. Increased pressure in the carpal tunnel of the wrist provokes median neuropathy with symptoms of pain, paresthesia, coolness, weakness, and exacerbation of symptoms with effort. An independent association with obesity has been known clinically, and was confirmed in a large case-control series with BMI $\geq$ 30 showing an OR of 2.90 (95% CI 2.25–3.73). A trend was noted for increasing OR with increasing BMI (108). Another study notes that although the risk of diagnosis of carpal tunnel syndrome increases with rising BMI, more *severe* symptoms do not correlate with those increases (109).

Plantar fasciitis. This common painful condition of the soft tissues of the foot is related to BMI, and patients with BMI >30 have an OR of 5.6 (95% CI 1.9–16.6) when compared with those of normal weight. Despite the association with BMI, the increased weight borne on the foot does not seem to be the cause, as BMI continues to be statistically significant when controlling for weight-bearing (110). This might suggest generalized soft tissue sensitivity, perhaps mediated through the chronic inflammatory state engendered by MO.

HEMATOLOGIC

Prothrombotic state. Deep venous thrombosis and pulmonary embolus incidences are higher in MO patients with multiple possible etiologies, including increased intra-abdominal pressure causing venous stasis (see below), decreased activity, and compression of veins by the surrounding tissues. More recently, especially in light of metabolic syndrome findings, a generalized prothrombotic state has been identified in MO individuals. The elements include endothelial activation, platelet hyperactivity, hypercoagulability, and decreased fibrinolysis due to elevated PAI-1 levels. Low grade inflammation with prolonged cytokine-mediated acute phase reaction is involved in these changes (111).

Varicose veins of the lower extremity and chronic venous insufficiency. Varicose veins are common in MO patients, and the degree of varices and severity of the associated chronic venous insufficiency (CVI) is statistically significantly correlated with BMI. Of interest is that in a recent evaluation by Padberg et al., two-thirds of the affected legs did not have anatomic evidence of venous disease. Their conclusion was that venous disease symptoms might be related to increased intra-abdominal pressure causing relative obstruction of both venous and lymphatic channels within the abdomen. Humoral factors and vascular inflammation may also contribute, but are not characterized as yet. The treatment of CVI is difficult in MO patients due to simple mechanistic problems of donning and doffing compressive hose, inability to see and assess wounds, and impaired sensation (112).

RENAL

Proteinuria/chronic renal disease. The relationship between MO and renal disease has been noted in the past, with glomerulopathy, focal-segmental glomerulosclerosis, hypertensive nephrosclerosis, and diabetic nephropathy (DN) as the most common pathology. Much attention is also being paid to chronic graft failure in previously transplanted individuals (113).

Klassen et al. (113) note that the incidence of obesity-associated glomerulopathy has markedly increased, again in tandem with obesity. This renal disease is manifested initially by asymptomatic microalbuminuria, but nephrotic syndrome levels of proteinuria are found in severe obesity (114). Adolescents may be particularly susceptible to the pathologic effects of proteinuria, and require careful monitoring if morbidly obese (115). A recent study by Chen et al. via NHANES III data examined whether metabolic syndrome criteria correlated with the risk of *chronic* renal disease (i.e., glomerular filtration rate <60 mL/min per 1.73 m^2):

Number of criteria met	Odds ratio	Confidence interval
2	2.21	1.16–4.24
3	3.38	1.48–7.69
4	4.23	2.06–8.63
5	5.85	3.11–11.0

In addition, they noted that microalbuminuria rates were also correlated with increasing metabolic syndrome criteria, although to a lesser extent than chronic renal disease (116).

The glomerulopathy of MO has its origins in alterations of hormones, metabolism, and hemodynamics, with hyperfiltration as a precursor to overt glomerulopathy. Hyperinsulinemia, the activated sympathetic nervous system, renin–angiotensin–aldosterone system, and hyperleptinemia have also been shown to have an etiologic role. In concert with the rise in T2DM, DN is rising, multiplied by the obesity-related renal derangements. As a result, diabetic nephropathy in the obese is the leading cause of end-stage renal disease (113). Weight loss reduces obesity-related glomerular hyperfiltration and this may prevent the progression to obesity-related glomerulopathy (117).

NEUROLOGIC

Intracranial hypertension (pseudotumor cerebri). This uncommon illness (0.1% incidence) is defined by an increased intracranial pressure without mass lesion or alteration in normal cerebrospinal fluid (CSF) composition. It is seen as a complication of MO rarely, predominantly in young women. Previously classified as "idiopathic," its origin seems to arise from the increased intra-abdominal pressure. Secondary effects on internal jugular venous, caval, and right atrial pressures result in symptoms (118). The symptoms are severe headache, pulsatile tinnitus, and temporary or permanent visual loss (119). Signs of papilledema, increased intrathecal pressure, and rarely spontaneous CSF rhinorrhea are seen. Any of the symptoms may be isolated, and therefore the diagnosis may be delayed. In a study by Rowe, 70.5% of patients with intracranial hypertension were obese, with increasing risk associated with the degree of obesity, as well as increasing age. MO (BMI > 40) was significantly associated with a poor visual outcome (120).

The postulated mechanism has been circumstantially validated by elegant experiments by Sugerman et al. using a mechanical external device to reduce intra-abdominal pressure. Decrease in the cross-sectional ultrasonographic area of the internal jugular vein but no alteration in flow was noted, supporting an elevated venous pressure theory. The device was able to relieve symptoms of tinnitus and headache; however the effects were limited temporally to the use of the device (121). Medical therapy, or surgical therapy with lumboperitoneal shunting, optic nerve sheath fenestration, or sinovenous stenting is not always successful. Surgical control of MO can induce remission in 81% to 93% (119,122,123).

Chronic daily headache. A significant association between obesity and chronic daily headache is noted, especially in the new-onset headache (124). Similarities to intracranial hypertension would suggest a common etiology, however this has not been proven.

Non-epileptic seizures. Psychogenic non-epileptic seizures (NES), physical manifestations of psychological distress, are associated with an increased risk of obesity. In a study by Marquez et al. of 46 NES patients and 46 age- and gender-matched epileptic controls, the NES patients had significantly higher BMIs (30.5 vs. 26.1, $P = 0.006$) than controls, even when accounting for the potential weight gain associated with some anti-epileptic drugs. Whether this is related to the underlying psychiatric comorbidities of obesity, or is a separate phenomenon, is unclear (125).

INFECTIOUS / IMMUNOLOGIC

Altered immunity. Neutrophils are altered in MO, with increased numbers/percentage of CD95+ T cells seen preoperatively, as well as increased expression of CD95 per T cell. Other immune alterations include lower numbers of naïve T cells [those lacking markers for CD62L (L-selectin)]. After surgical treatment of MO by gastric bypass, these changes resolve in three months. In addition, the number of natural killer T cells decline after surgery. These perturbations may allow "immune privilege" in sites, permitting or promoting neoplasia and infection (126).

Chronic inflammation. Whether the adipocyte, immune cells, or other tissues are the source, significant changes in multiple cytokines and other biologically active molecules are noted. These include adiponectin, resistin, leptin, ghrelin, plasminogen activator inhibitor-1, TNF-α, CRP, and IL-6 (74). Specifically, elevated levels of CRP and IL-6 are the primary mediators of chronic subclinical inflammation, and have been associated with features of the insulin-resistance syndrome and incident cardiovascular disease (74). Intensive research to delineate the source, message, and end result of these cytokines is ongoing, and is an area of great interest.

DERMATOLOGIC

Intertriginous dermatitis. Significant moistness, irritation, yeast overgrowth, and skin appendage infections are seen in the intertriginous areas under the breasts and pannus, and in the axillae, groins, gluteal cleft, and other skin folds. These skin manifestations contribute to chronic pain, odor, social embarrassment, sexual dysfunction, and increased medical costs.

PSYCHIATRIC

Mood disorders. Depression is a frequent concomitant illness in the morbidly obese. Women have a higher incidence than men, and adolescents show a lower percentage (127). In a Mexican population presenting for bariatric surgery, over 50% had at least one psychiatric disorder in axis 1 of DSM-IV, mostly anxiety and mood disorders (128). Daumit et al. report the correlation between NHANES data and a database for severe and persistent mental illness. They find a higher prevalence of obesity than in the general population and a fourfold association between atypical antipsychotics in men but not in women. It is unclear if obesity pre-dated mental illness in this study (129).

There is a continuing debate on whether obesity causes depression or vice versa. In a prospective cohort study of 9374 adolescents in 1995, 12.9% were overweight, 9.7% were obese, and 8.8% had depressed mood at initial evaluation. Baseline depression was not significantly correlated with baseline obesity. Having a depressed mood at baseline independently predicted obesity at follow-up with an OR of 2.05 (95% CI 1.18, 3.56) after controlling for multiple variables. Obesity did not predict follow-up depression in adolescents (127).

Self-esteem. In a study in Ohio, overweight children (>95th percentile) compared with normal weight children scored lower on Psychosocial Health Summary subscales measuring self-esteem (OR, 3.5; 95% CI, 1.9–6.3), physical functioning (OR 2.8, 95% CI 1.7–6.8), and effect on the parent's emotional well-being (OR 2.0, 95% CI, 1.1–3.6) (130).

Social isolation. Horchner et al. evaluated 104 patients with BMI 32–64 and mean age 36 years (90% female) for loneliness and coping skills. These patients had higher scores for loneliness than controls, and frequently used avoidance, "wait and see," and passive coping strategies. They express relationships as relatively unreliable and not very intimate. All of these may contribute to the ability of the MO patient to interact with health care providers, and ultimately to their success with interventions (131).

Stigmatization and stereotypes. Throughout U.S. society, stereotypes of MO patients are developed and displayed. Commercial television is a powerful influence, and of 1018 major television characters, only 14% of females and 24% of males were overweight or obese, less than half their true percentages. These characters were less likely to be considered attractive, to interact with romantic partners, and to display physical affection, and more likely to be viewed while eating (132).

Stigmatization of the obese by our society also contributes to the isolation of these patients, and appears to be increasing. Latner and Stunkard compared 4th to 6th grade children's perception of others in 1961 and again in 2001 via drawings. They were asked to arrange six drawings of the same-sex children with obesity, various disabilities, or no disability by how well they liked each person. Children in both the time periods liked the drawing of the obese child least, with a 40.8% greater response in terms of dislike from 1961 to 2001; girls showed more dislike than boys (133). The origins of this stigma are both individual and cultural, and new approaches are needed to correct this disparity (134).

SOCIAL / ECONOMIC

Unemployment, underemployment, barriers to promotion and advancement, discrimination against attaining public positions, lower wages, and barriers to public or private transportation, seating, clothing, and entertainment are all daily battles for the morbidly obese—and issues that persons of normal weight rarely consider. There is an open prejudice against the morbidly obese that contributes to an "anti-fat" bias that is pervasive and subversive. It influences attitudes about treatment of the morbidly obese, from the basic recognition of obesity as a disease, to health insurance payment for its treatment (135–137). Changing these biases is difficult, and educational interventions designed to alter such biases have not been effective (138,139).

Unfortunately, many physicians have little more factual information about the origins of obesity than the public, and may view obese patients with distaste and feel that they are responsible for their own medical problems. Patients with MO sense this, and fear the judgmental and discriminatory attitudes from their providers, leading to avoidance of health care (140,141). Due to preconceived attitudes about obesity and MO patients, physicians may not persist in dietary, behavioral, or medical treatment of obesity, and often consider obesity surgery as ideologically flawed and physically dangerous (142). Many insurers reject surgical treatment with similar arguments, presuming that MO is simply a character flaw or weakness. Many medical and health policy personnel do not accept obesity as a disease, which limits legal remedies that MO patients might seek to obtain bariatric surgery. Differing provider perceptions of what constitutes appropriate care also influence treatment (143). These multiple barriers and interacting patterns contribute to a lower standard of care for the obese (135,144).

These issues will become increasingly severe as a larger percentage of the population becomes morbidly obese. The strain on health care and economic resources, effects on productivity and restricted activity, and loss of years of life will have compounding effects on societies and communities. The estimated total cost of excess weight and obesity is $100 billion annually. In a given year in the United States, 40 million days of productive work are lost, 63 million health care visits are made, restricted activity occurs on 239 million days, and there are 90 million bed-bound days. Emotional suffering comes in the form of inability to meet societal visual expectations, as well as popular opinions that obese individuals are gluttonous, lazy, or both. The correlates to Christian beliefs that these traits are "sins," that one can and should avoid, also fuel negative attitudes toward the obese (141). Prejudice or discrimination in the job market, at school, and in social situations is common, accompanied by feelings of rejection, shame, and depression. The existing prejudices are not acceptable, and society needs to alter its perception of the etiology of obesity in order to effect improvement in public health (143,144).

SUMMARY

The trend toward increasing BMI worldwide is alarming, and the root causes not fully known. Drastic public health measures are needed to limit the extent of this epidemic, and to reduce the burden of comorbid diseases within the obese population. Research to delineate the basic mechanisms will enhance the ability to treat this illness efficaciously and compassionately.

REFERENCES

1. Florencio TT, Ferreira HS, Cavalcante JC, Luciano SM, Sawaya AL. Food consumed does not account for the higher prevalence of obesity among stunted adults in a very-low-income population in the Northeast of Brazil (Maceio, Alagoas). Eur J Clin Nutr 2003; 57(11):1437–1446.

2. Nishida C, Uauy R, Kumanyika S, Shetty P. The joint WHO/FAO expert consultation on diet, nutrition and the prevention of chronic diseases: process, product and policy implications. Public Health Nutr 2004; 7(1A):245–250.

3. Deitel M. Overweight and obesity worldwide now estimated to involve 1.7 billion people. Obes Surg 2003; 13(3):329–330.

4. National Heart, Lung, and Blood Institute. Clinical guidelines on the identification, evaluation, and treatment of overweight and obesity in adults. Bethesda, MD: US Department of Health and Human Services, National Institutes of Health, National Heart, Lung, and Blood Institute. Obes Res 1998; 6 (suppl 2):51S–209S.

5. Sturm R. Increases in clinically severe obesity in the United States, 1986–2000. Arch Intern Med 2003; 163(18):2146–2148.

6. Vastag B. Obesity is now on everyone's plate. JAMA 2004; 291(10):1186–1188.

7. Manson JE, Skerrett PJ, Greenland P, VanItallie TB. The escalating pandemics of obesity and sedentary lifestyle. A call to action for clinicians. Arch Intern Med 2004; 164(3):249–258.

8. Minino AM, Arias E, Kochanek KD, Murphy SL, Smith BL. Deaths: final data for 2000. Natl Vital Stat Rep 2002; 50(15):1–119.

9. Mokdad AH, Marks JS, Stroup DF, Gerberding JL. Actual causes of death in the United States, 2000. JAMA 2004; 291(10):1238–1246.

10. Allison DB, Fontaine KR, Manson JE, Stevens J, VanItallie TB. Annual deaths attributable to obesity in the United States. JAMA 1999; 282:1530–1538.

11. Fontaine KR, Redden DT, Wang C, Westfall AO, Allison DB. Years of life lost due to obesity. JAMA 2003; 289(2):187–193.

12. Centers for Disease Control and Prevention (CDC). Trends in intake of energy and macronutrients—United States, 1971–2000. MMWR Morb Mortal Wkly Rep. 2004; 53(4):80–82.

13. Giammattei J, Blix G, Marshak HH, Wollitzer AO, Pettitt DJ. Television watching and soft drink consumption: associations with obesity in 11-to 13-year-old schoolchildren. Arch Pediatr Adolesc Med 2003; 157(9):882–886.

14. Yoshinaga M, Shimago A, Koriyama C, Nomura Y, Miyata K, Hashiguchi J, Arima K. Rapid increase in the prevalence of obesity in elementary school children. Int J Obes Relat Metab Disord 2004; 28(4):494–499.

15. Matsushita Y, Yoshiike N, Kaneda F, Yoshita K, Takimoto H. Trends in childhood obesity in Japan over the last 25 years from the National Nutrition Survey. Obes Res 2004; 12(2):205–214.

16. Del Rio-Navarro BE, Velazquez-Monroy O, Sanchez-Castillo CP, et al. The high prevalence of overweight and obesity in Mexican children. Obes Res. 2004; 12(2):215–223.

17. Lissau I, Overpeck MD, Ruan WJ, Due P, Holstein BE, Hediger ML. Health Behaviour in school-aged children obesity working group. Body mass index and overweight in adolescents in 13 European countries, Israel, and the United States. Arch Pediatr Adolesc Med 2004; 158(1):27–33.

18. Rami B, Schober E, Kirchengast S, Waldhor T, Sefranek R. Prevalence of overweight and obesity in male adolescents in Austria between 1985 and 2000. A population based study. J Pediatr Endocrinol Metab 2004; 17(1):67–72.

19. Swinburn BA, Caterson I, Seidell JC, James WP. Diet, nutrition and the prevention of excess weight gain and obesity. Public Health Nutr 2004; 7(1A):123–146.

20. Livingston EH, Ko CY. Socioeconomic characteristics of the population eligible for obesity surgery. Surgery 2004; 135(3):288–296.

21. Choban P, Lu B, Flancbaum L. Insurance decisions about obesity surgery: a new type of randomization? Obes Surg 2000; 10(6):553–556.

22. Alt SJ. Bariatric surgery may become a self-pay service. Health Care Strateg Manage 2003; 21(12):1,12–19.

23. Ahluwalia IB, Mack KA, Murphy W, Mokdad AH, Bales VS. State-specific prevalence of selected chronic disease-related characteristics—behavioral risk factor surveillance system, 2001. MMWR 2003; 52(SS08):1–80.

24. Okasha M, McCarron P, McEwen J, Smith GD. Body mass index in young adulthood and cancer mortality: a retrospective cohort study. J Epidemiol Community Health 2002; 56(10):780–784.
25. Polednak AP. Trends in incidence rates for obesity-associated cancers in the US. Cancer Detect Prev 2003; 27(6):415–421.
26. Calle EE, Rodriguez C, Walker-Thurmond K, Thurn MJ. Overweight, obesity, and mortality from cancer in a prospectively studied cohort of U.S. adults. N Engl J Med 2003; 348(17):1625–1638.
27. Wolk A, Gridley G, Svensson M, Nyren O, McLaughlin JK, Fraumeni JF, Adam HO. A prospective study of obesity and cancer risk (Sweden). Cancer Causes Control 2001; 12(1):13–21.
28. Lukanova A, Zeleniuch-Jacquotte A, LundinE, Micheli A, Arslan AA, Rinaldi A, Muti P, Lenner P, Koenig KL, Biessy C, et al. Prediagnostic levels of C-peptide, IGFI, IGFBP -1, -2 and -3 and risk of endometrial cancer. Int J Cancer 2004; 108(2):262–268.
29. Brinton LA, Berman ML, Mortel R, Twiggs LB, Barrett RJ, Wilbanks GD, Lannom L, Hoover RN. Reproductive, menstrual, and medical risk factors for endometrial cancer: results from a case-control study. Am J Obstet Gynecol 1992; 167(5):1317–1325.
30. Harvard report on cancer prevention. Causes of human cancer. Obesity. Cancer Causes Control 1996; 7(suppl 1):S11–S13.
31. Dignam JJ, Wieand K, Johnson KA, Fisher B, Xu L, Mamounas EP. Obesity, tamoxifen use, and outcomes in women with estrogen receptor-positive early-stage breast cancer. J Natl Cancer Inst 2003; 95(19):1467–1476.
32. King MC, Marks JH, Mandell JB. New York Breast Cancer Study Group. Breast and ovarian cancer risks due to inherited mutations in BRCA1 and BRCA2. Science 2003; 302(5645):643–646.
33. Freedland SJ, Aronson WJ, Kane CJ, Presti JC Jr, Amling CL, Elashoff D, Terris MK. Impact of obesity on biochemical control after radical prostatectomy for clinically localized prostate cancer: a report by the Shared Equal Access Regional Cancer Hospital database study group. J Clin Oncol 2004; 22(3):446–453.
34. Amling CL, Riffenburgh RH, Sun L, Moul JW, Lance RS, Kusuda L, Sexton WJ, Soderdahl DW, Donahue TF, Foley JP, Chung AK, McLeod DG, Arroyo A, Laughlin GA. Pathologic variables and recurrence rates as related to obesity and race in men with prostate cancer undergoing radical prostatectomy. J Clin Oncol 2004; 22(3):439–445.
35. Rohrmann S, Roberts WW, Walsh PC, Platz EA. Family history of prostate cancer and obesity in relation to high-grade disease and extraprostatic extension in young men with prostate cancer. Prostate 2003; 55(2):140–146.
36. Zamboni PF, Simone M, Passaro A, Doh Dalla Nora E, Fellin R, Solini A. Metabolic profile in patients with benign prostate hyperplasia or prostate cancer and normal glucose tolerance. Horm Metab Res 2003; 35(5):296–300.
37. Murphy TK, Calle EE, Rodriguez C, Kahn HS, Thun MJ. Body mass index and colon cancer mortality in a large prospective study. Am J Epidemiol 2000; 152(9):847–854.
38. Kono S, Handa K, Hayabuchi H, Kiyohara C, Inoue H, Margugame T, Shinomiya S, Hamada H, Onuma K, Koga H. Obesity, weight gain and risk of colon adenomas in Japanese men. Jpn J Cancer Res 1999; 90(8):805–811.
39. Residori L, Garcia-Lorda P, Flancbaum L, Pi-Sunyer FX, Laferrere B. Prevalence of co-morbidities in obese patients before bariatric surgery: effect of race. Obes Surg 2003; 13(3):333–340.
40. Garrison RJ, Kannel WB, Stokes J III, Castelli WP. Incidence and precursors of hypertension in young adults: the Framingham Offspring Study. Prev Med. 1987; 16(2): 235–251.
41. Hall JE, Hildebrandt DA, Kuo J. Obesity hypertension: role of leptin and sympathetic nervous system. Am J Hypertens 2001; 14(6 Pt 2):103S–115S.
42. Hall JE, Crook ED, Jones DW, Wofford MR, Dubbert PM. Mechanisms of obesity-associated cardiovascular and renal disease. Am J Med Sci 2002; 324(3):127–137.

43. El-Atat F, Aneja A, Mcfarlane S, Sowers J. Obesity and hypertension. Endocrinol Metab Clin North Am 2003; 32(4):823–854.
44. Messerli FH. Cardiovascular effects of obesity and hypertension. Lancet 1982; 2: 1165–1168.
45. Garavaglia GE, Messerli FH, Nunez BD, Schmieder RE, Grossman E. Myocardial contractility and left ventricular function in obese patients with essential hypertension. Am J Cardiol 1988; 62:594–597.
46. Alpert MA, Lambert CR, Terry BE, Cohen MV, Mukerji V, Massey CV, Hashimi MW, Panayiotou H. Interrelationship of left ventricular mass, systolic function and diastolic filling in normotensive morbidly obese patients. Int J Obes Relat Metab Disord 1995; 19:550–557.
47. Alpert MA, Terry BE, Mulekar M, Cohen MV, Massey CV, Fan TM, Panayiotou H, Mukerji V. Cardiac morphology and left ventricular function in normotensive morbidly obese patients with and without congestive heart failure, and effect of weight loss. Am J Cardiol 1997; 80:736–740.
48. Alpert MA, Lambert CR, Terry BE, Kelly DL, Panayiotou H, Mukerji V, Massey CV, Cohen MV. Effect of weight loss on left ventricular mass in nonhypertensive morbidly obese patients. Am J Cardiol 1994; 73(12):918–921.
49. Horwich TB, Fonarow GC, Hamilton MA, MacLellan WR, Woo MA, Tillisch JH. The relationship between obesity and mortality in patients with heart failure. J Am Coll Cardiol 2001; 38:789–795.
50. Hubert HB, Feinleib M, McNamara PM, Castelli WP. Obesity as an independent risk factor for cardiovascular disease: a 26-year follow-up of participants in the Framingham Heart Study. Circulation 1983; 67:968–977.
51. Manson JE, Colditz GA, Stampfer MJ. A prospective study of obesity and risk of coronary heart disease in women. N Engl J Med 1990; 322:882–889.
52. Hiroshi I, Atsushi I, Ryuichi K, et al. Trends over the last 20 years in the clinical background of young Japanese patients with coronary artery disease. Circ J 2004; 68(3): 186–191.
53. Washio M, Hayashi R. Fukuoka Heart Study Group. Past history of obesity (overweight by WHO criteria) is associated with an increased risk of nonfatal acute myocardial infarction: a case-control study in Japan. Circ J 2004; 68(1):41–46.
54. Powell BD, Lennon RJ, Lerman A, Bell MR, Berger PB, Higano ST, Holmes DR Jr, Rihal CS. Association of body mass index with outcome after percutaneous coronary intervention. Am J Cardiol 2003; 91: 472–476.
55. Reeves BC, Ascione R, Chamberlain MH, Angelini GD. Effect of body mass index on early outcomes in patients undergoing coronary artery bypass surgery. J Am Coll Cardiol 2003; 42:668–676.
56. Howard BV, Ruotolo G, Robbins DC. Obesity and dyslipidemia. Endocrinol Metab Clin North Am 2003; 32(4):855–867.
57. Expert Panel on Detection, Evaluation, and Treatment of High Blood Cholesterol in Adults. Executive Summary of the Third Report of the National Cholesterol Education Program (NCEP) Expert Panel on Detection, Evaluation, and Treatment of High Blood Cholesterol in Adults (Adult Treatment Panel III). JAMA 2001; 285:2486–2497.
58. Lee WJ, Chen HH, Wang W, Wei PL, Lin CM, Huang MT. Metabolic syndrome in obese patients referred for weight reduction surgery in Taiwan. J Formos Med Assoc 2003; 102(7):459–464.
59. Chadwick J, Mann WN. In: Medical works of Hippocrates, Boston MA. Blackwell Scientific Publications, 1950:154.
60. Schwab RJ, Pasirstein M, Pierson R, Mackley A, Hachadoorian R, Arens R, Maislin G, Pack AI. Identification of upper airway anatomic risk factors for obstructive sleep apnea with volumetric magnetic resonance imaging. Am J Respir Crit Care Med 2003; 168(5):522–530.

61. Young T, Palta M, Dempsey J, Skatrud J, Weber S, Badr S. The occurrence of sleep-disordered breathing among middle-aged adults. N Engl J Med 1993; 328(17):1230–1235.
62. Young T, Shahar E, Nieto FJ, Redline S, Newman AB, Gottlieb DJ, Walsleben JA, Finn L, Enright P, Samet JM. Sleep Heart Health Study Research Group. Predictors of sleep-disordered breathing in community-dwelling adults: the Sleep Heart Health Study. Arch Intern Med 2002; 162(8):893–900.
63. Punjabi NM, Ahmed MM, Polotsky VY, Beamer BA, O'Donnell CP. Sleep-disordered breathing, glucose intolerance, and insulin resistance. Respir Physiol Neurobiol 2003; 136(2–3):167–178.
64. Wilcox I, McNamara SG, Collins FL, Grunstein RR, Sullivan CE. "Syndrome Z": the interaction of sleep apnoea, vascular risk factors and heart disease. Thorax 1998; 53(suppl 3):S25–S28.
65. Harsch IA, Schahin SP, Radespiel-Troger M, Weintz O, Jahreiss H, Fuchs FS, Wiest GH, Hahn EG, Lohmann T, Konturek PC, Ficker JH. Continuous positive airway pressure treatment rapidly improves insulin sensitivity in patients with obstructive sleep apnea syndrome. Am J Respir Crit Care Med 2004; 169(2):156–162.
66. Imagawa S, Yamaguchi Y, Ogawa K, Obara N, Suzuki N, Yamamoto M, Nagasawa T. Interleukin-6 and tumor necrosis factor-alpha in patients with obstructive sleep apnea-hypopnea syndrome. Respiration 2004; 71(1):24–29.
67. Bady E, Achkar A, Pascal S, Orvoen-Frija E, Laaban JP. Pulmonary arterial hypertension in patients with sleep apnoea syndrome. Thorax 2000; 55(11):934–939.
68. Maggio CA, Pi-Sunyer FX. Obesity and type 2 diabetes. Endocrinol Metab Clin N Am 2003; 32:805–822.
69. Mokdad AH, Ford ES, Bowman BA, Dietz WH, Vinicor F, Bales VS, et al. Prevalence of obesity, diabetes, and obesity-related health risk factors, 2001. JAMA 2003; 289(1):76–79.
70. Kaufman FR. Type 2 diabetes mellitus in children and youth: a new epidemic. J Pediatr Endocrinol Metab 2002; 15(suppl 2):737–744.
71. Hu FB, Manson JE, Stampfer MJ, Colditz G, Liu S, Solomon CG, et al. Diet, lifestyle, and the risk of type 2 diabetes mellitus in women. N Engl J Med 2001; 345(11):790–797.
72. Rosenthal AD, Jin F, Shu XO, Yang G, Elasy TA, Chow WH, Ji BT, Xu HX, Li Q, Gao YT, Zheng W. Body fat distribution and risk of diabetes among Chinese women. Int J Obes Relat Metab Disord 2004; 28(4):594–599.
73. Fonseca V. Effect of thiazolidinediones on body weight in patients with diabetes mellitus. Am J Med 2003; 115(suppl 8a):42S–48S.
74. Kopp HP, Kopp CW, Festa A, Krzyzanowska K, Kriwanek S, Minar E, Roka R, Schernthaner G. Impact of weight loss on inflammatory proteins and their association with the insulin resistance syndrome in morbidly obese patients. Arterioscler Thromb Vasc Biol 2003; 23(6):1042–1047.
75. Clements RH, Gonzalez QH, Long CI, Wittert G, Laws HL. Hormonal changes after Roux-en Y gastric bypass for morbid obesity and the control of type-II diabetes mellitus. Am Surg 2004; 70(1):1–4; discussion 4–5.
76. Petersen KF, Dufour S, Befroy D, Garcia R, Shulman GI. Impaired mitochondrial activity in the insulin-resistant offspring of patients with type 2 diabetes. N Engl J Med 2004; 350(7):664–671.
77. Gurnell M, Savage DB, Chatterjee VK, O'Rahilly S. The metabolic syndrome: peroxisome proliferator-activated receptor gamma and its therapeutic modulation. J Clin Endocrinol Metab 2003; 88(6):2412–2421.
78. Pickup JC. Inflammation and activated innate immunity in the pathogenesis of type 2 diabetes. Diabetes Care 2004; 27(3):813–823.
79. Hamoui N, Kim K, Anthone G, Crookes PF. The significance of elevated levels of parathyroid hormone in patients with morbid obesity before and after bariatric surgery. Arch Surg 2003; 138(8):891–897.

80. Hamoui N, Anthone G, Crookes PF. Calcium metabolism in the morbidly obese. Obes Surg 2004; 14(1):9–12.
81. Beymer C, Kowdley KV, Larson A, Edmonson P, Dellinger EP, Flum DR. Prevalence and predictors of asymptomatic liver disease in patients undergoing gastric bypass surgery. Arch Surg 2003; 138(11):1240–1244.
82. Hsiao TJ, Chen JC, Wang JD. Insulin resistance and ferritin as major determinants of nonalcoholic fatty liver disease in apparently healthy obese patients. Int J Obes Relat Metab Disord 2004; 28(1):167–172.
83. Sakugawa H, Nakasone H, Nakayoshi T, Kawakami Y, Yamashiro T, Maeshiro T, Swinburn BA, Caterson I, Seidell JC, James WP. Diet, nutrition and the prevention of excess weight gain and obesity. Public Health Nutr 2004; 7(1A):123–146.
84. Foster A, Richards WO, McDowell J, Laws HL, Clements RH. Gastrointestinal symptoms are more intense in morbidly obese patients. Surg Endosc 2003; 17(11):1766–1768.
85. Csendes A, Burdiles P, Smok G, Csendes P, Burgos A, Recio M. Histologic findings of gallbladder mucosa in 87 patients with morbid obesity without gallstones compared to 87 control subjects. J Gastrointest Surg 2003; 7(4):547–551.
86. Freeman JB, Meyer PD, KJ, Mason BE, Denbesten L. Cholelithiasis in morbid obesity. Analysis of gallbladder bile in morbid obesity. Am J Surg 1975;129:163–166.
87. Oria HE. Pitfalls in the diagnosis of gallbladder in clinically severe obesity. Obes Surg 1998; 8:444–451.
88. Shiffman ML, Sugerman HJ, Kelhum JH, Brewer WH, Moore EW. Gallstones in patients with morbid obesity. Relationship to body weight, weight loss and gallbladder bile cholesterol solubility. Int J Obes Relat Metab Disord 1993; 17:153–158.
89. Thilt MD, Mittelstaedt CA, Herbst CA, Buckwalter JA. Gallbladder disease in morbid obesity. South Med J 1984; 77:415–417.
90. Worobetz IS, Inglis FG, Shaffer EA. The effect of ursodeoxycolic acid therapy on gallstone formation in the morbidly obese during rapid weight loss. Am J Gastroenterol 1993; 88:1705–1710.
91. Martinez J, Sanchez-Paya J, Palazon JM, Suazo-Barahona J, Robles-Diaz G, Perez Mateo M. Is obesity a risk factor in acute pancreatitis? A meta-analysis. Pancreatology 2004; 4(1):42–48.
92. Deitel M, Stone E, Kassam HA, Wilk EJ, Sutherland DJ. Gynecologic-obstetric changes after loss of massive excess weight following bariatric surgery. Am Coll Nutr 1988; 7(2):147–153.
93. Castillo-Martinez L, Lopez-Alvarenga JC, Villa AR, Gonzalez-Barranco J. Menstrual cycle length disorders in 18- to 40-y-old obese women. Nutrition 2003; 19(4):317–320.
94. Wang JX, Davies MJ, Norman RJ. Obesity increases the risk of spontaneous abortion during infertility treatment. Obes Res 2002; 10(6):551–554.
95. Roth D, Grazi RV, Lobel SM. Extremes of body mass index do not affect first-trimester pregnancy outcome in patients with infertility. Am J Obstet Gynecol 2003; 188(5):1169–1170.
96. Cedergren MI. Maternal morbid obesity and the risk of adverse pregnancy outcome. Obstet Gynecol 2004; 103(2):219–224.
97. Cedergren MI, Kallen BA. Maternal obesity and infant heart defects. Obes Res 2003; 11(9):1065–1071.
98. Catalano PM, Thomas A, Huston-Presley L, Amini SB. Increased fetal adiposity: a very sensitive marker of abnormal in utero development. Am J Obstet Gynecol 2003; 189(6):1698–1704.
99. Dallosso HM, McGrother CW, Matthews RJ, Donaldson MM. Leicestershire MRC Incontinence Study Group. The association of diet and other lifestyle factors with overactive bladder and stress incontinence: a longitudinal study in women. BJU Int 2003; 92(1):69–77.
100. Cummings JM, Rodning CB. Urinary stress incontinence among obese women: review of pathophysiology therapy. Int Urogynecol J Pelvic Floor Dysfunct 2000; 11(1):41–44.

101. Salehi M, Bravo-Vera R, Sheikh A, Gouller A, Poretsky L. Pathogenesis of polycystic ovary syndrome: what is the role of obesity? Metabolism 2004; 53(3):358–376.
102. Arroyo A, Laughlin GA, Morales AJ, Yen SS. Inappropriate gonadotropin secretion in polycystic ovary syndrome: influence of adiposity. J Clin Endocrinol Metab 1997; 82(11):3728–3733.
103. Morales AJ. Inappropriate gonadotropin secretion in polycystic ovary syndrome: influence of adiposity. J Clin Endocrinol Metab 1997; 82:3728–3733.
104. Morales AJ, Laughlin GA, Butzow T. Insulin, somatotropic, and luteinizing hormone axes in lean and obese women with polycystic ovary syndrome: common and distinct features. J Clin Endocrinol Metab 1996; 81:2854–2864.
105. Homburg R, Lambalk CB. Polycystic ovary syndrome in adolescence—a therapeutic conundrum. Hum Reprod 2004.
106. Andersen RE, Crespo CJ, Bartlett SJ, Bathon JM, Fontaine KR. Relationship between body weight gain and significant knee, hip, and back pain in older Americans. Obes Res 2003; 11(10):1159–1162.
107. Manek NJ, Hart D, Spector TD, MacGregor AJ. The association of body mass index and osteoarthritis of the knee joint: an examination of genetic and environmental influences. Arthritis Rheum 2003; 48(4):1024–1029.
108. Becker J, Nora DB, Gomes I, Stringari FF, Seitensus R, Panosso JS, Ehlers JC. An evaluation of gender, obesity, age and diabetes mellitus as risk factors for carpal tunnel syndrome. Clin Neurophysiol 2002; 113(9):1429–1434.
109. Kouyoumdjian JA, Morita MD, Rocha PR, Miranda RC, Gouveia GM. Body mass index and carpal tunnel syndrome. Arq Neuropsiquiatr 2000; 58(2A):252–256.
110. Riddle DL, Pulisic M, Pidcoe P, Johnson RE. Risk factors for plantar fasciitis: a matched case-control study. J Bone Joint Surg Am 2003; 85-A(5):872–877.
111. Juhan-Vague I, Morange PE, Alessi MC. The insulin resistance syndrome: implications for thrombosis and cardiovascular disease. Pathophysiol Haemost Thromb 2002; 32(5–6): 269–273.
112. Padberg F Jr, Cerveira JJ, Lal BK, Pappas PJ, Varma S, Hobson RW II. Does severe venous insufficiency have a different etiology in the morbidly obese? Is it venous? J Vasc Surg 2003; 37(1):79–85.
113. Klassen A, Bahner U, Sebekova K, Heidland A. The importance of overweight and obesity for the development and progression of renal diseases. Dtsch Med Wochenschr 2004; 129(11):579–582.
114. Cohen AH. Pathology of renal complications in obesity. Curr Hypertens Rep 1999; 1(2):137–139.
115. Adelman RD, Restaino IG, Alon US, Blowey DL. Proteinuria and focal segmental glomerulosclerosis in severely obese adolescents. J Pediatr 2001; 138(4):481–485.
116. Chen J, Muntner P, Hamm LL, Jones DW, Batuman V, Fonseca V, Whelton PK, He J. The metabolic syndrome and chronic kidney disease in U.S. adults. Ann Intern Med 2004; 140(3):167–174.
117. Chagnac A, Weinstein T, Herman M, Hirsh J, Gafter U, Ori Y. The effects of weight loss on renal function in patients with severe obesity. J Am Soc Nephrol 2003; 14(6):1480–1486.
118. Brazis PW. Pseudotumor cerebri. Curr Neurol Neurosci Rep 2004; 4(2):111–116.
119. Michaelides EM, Sismanis A, Sugerman HJ, Felton WL III. Pulsatile tinnitus in patients with morbid obesity: the effectiveness of weight reduction surgery. Am J Otol 2000; 21(5):682–685.
120. Rowe FJ, Sarkies NJ. The relationship between obesity and idiopathic intracranial hypertension. Int J Obes Relat Metab Disord 1999; 23(1):54–59.
121. Sugerman HJ, Felton WL III, Sismanis A, Saggi BH, Doty JM, Blocher C, Marmarou A, Makhoul RG. Continuous negative abdominal pressure device to treat pseudotumor cerebri. Int J Obes Relat Metab Disord 2001; 25(4):486–490.

122. Sugerman HJ, Felton WL III, Salvant JB Jr, Sismanis A, Kellum JM. Effects of surgically induced weight loss on idiopathic intracranial hypertension in morbid obesity. Neurology 1995; 45(9):1655–1659.

123. Sugerman HJ, Felton WL III, Sismanis A, Kellum JM, DeMaria EJ, Sugerman EL. Gastric surgery for pseudotumor cerebri associated with severe obesity. Ann Surg 1999; 229(5):634–640; discussion 640–642.

124. Scher AI, Stewart WF, Ricci JA, Lipton RB. Factors associated with the onset and remission of chronic daily headache in a population-based study. Pain 2003; 106 (1–2):81–89.

125. Marquez AV, Farias ST, Apperson M, Koopmans S, Jorgensen J, Shatzel A, Alsaadi TM. Psychogenic nonepileptic seizures are associated with an increased risk of obesity. Epilepsy Behav 2004; 5(1):88–93.

126. Cottam DR, Schaefer PA, Shatfan GW, Angus LD. Dysfunctional immune-privilege in morbid obesity: implications and effect of gastric bypass surgery. Obes Surg 2003; 13(1): 49–57.

127. Goodman E, Whitaker RC. A prospective study of the role of depression in the development and persistence of adolescent obesity. Pediatrics 2002; 110(3):497–504.

128. Sanchez-Roman S, Lopez-Alvarenga JC, Vargas-Martinez A, Tellez-Zenteno JF, Vazquez-Velazquez V, Arcila-Martinez D, Gonzalez-Barranco J, Herrera-Hernandez MF, Salin-Pascual RJ. Prevalence of psychiatric disorders in patients with severe obesity waiting for bariatric surgery [Article in Spanish]. Rev Invest Clin 2003; 55(4): 400–406.

129. Daumit GL, Clark JM, Steinwachs DM, Graham CM, Lehman A, Ford DE. Prevalence and correlates of obesity in a community sample of individuals with severe and persistent mental illness. J Nerv Ment Dis 2003; 191(12):799–805.

130. Friedlander SL, Larkin EK, Rosen CL, Palermo TM, Redline S. Decreased quality of life associated with obesity in school-aged children. Arch Pediatr Adolesc Med 2003; 157(12):1206–1211.

131. Horchner R, Tuinebreijer WE, Kelder H, van Urk E. Coping behavior and loneliness among obese patients. Obes Surg 2002; 12(6):864–868.

132. Greenberg BS, Eastin M, Hofschire L, Lachlan K, Brownell KD. Portrayals of overweight and obese individuals on commercial television. Am J Public Health 2003; 93(8):1342–1348.

133. Latner JD, Stunkard AJ. Getting worse: the stigmatization of obese children. Obes Res 2003; 11(3):452–456.

134. Puhl RM, Brownell KD. Psychosocial origins of obesity stigma: toward changing a powerful and pervasive bias. Obes Rev 2003; 4(4):213–227.

135. Pryor W. The health care disadvantages of being obese. NSW Public Health Bull 2002; 13(7):163–165.

136. Rand C, Macgregor A. Morbidly obese patients' perceptions of social discrimination before and after surgery for obesity. South Med J 1990; 83(12):1390–1395.

137. Wadden T, Stunkard A. Social and psychological consequences of obesity. Ann Intern Med 1985; 103(6):1062–1067.

138. Teachman BA, Brownell KD. Implicit anti-fat bias among health professionals: is anyone immune? Int J Obes Relat Metab Disord 2001; 25(10):1525–1531.

139. Teachman BA, Gapinski KD, Brownell KD, Rawlins M, Jeyaram S. Demonstrations of implicit anti-fat bias: the impact of providing causal information and evoking empathy. Health Psychol 2003; 22(1):68–78.

140. Culbertson MJ, Smolen DM. Attitudes of RN students toward obese adult patients. J Nurs Educ 1999; 38(2):84–87.

141. Kaminsky J, Gadaleta D. A study of discrimination within the medical community as viewed by obese patients. Obes Surg 2002; 12(1):14–18.

142. Schwartz MB, Chambliss HO, Brownell KD, Blair SN, Billington C. Weight bias among health professionals specializing in obesity. Obes Res 2003; 11(9):1033–1039.

143. Zhang Q, Wang Y. Socioeconomic inequality of obesity in the United States: do gender, age, and ethnicity matter? Soc Sci Med 2004; 58(6):1171–1180.

144. Wellman NS, Friedberg B. Causes and consequences of adult obesity: health, social and economic impacts in the United States. Asia Pac J Clin Nutr 2002; 11(suppl 8): S705–S709.

3

Treating the Morbidly Obese Patient: A Lifestyle Approach to a Chronic Condition

Jennifer E. Taylor, Sara A. Pyle, and Walker S. Carlos Poston
University of Missouri-Kansas City and Mid America Heart Institute,
Kansas City, Missouri, U.S.A.

John P. Foreyt
Baylor College of Medicine, Houston, Texas, U.S.A.

INTRODUCTION

The prevalence of obesity has grown to epidemic proportions in the United States and many other industrialized and developing nations (1–4). Currently, 65% of the adult population in the United States is either overweight [defined as a Body Mass Index (BMI; kg/m^2) between 25 and <30] (2) or obese (a BMI of ≥ 30 or more) (1,2,5–7). Thirty percent of the entire adult population can be classified as obese (1,2,7). There are three classifications of obesity: Class I (BMI 30–34.9), Class II (BMI 35–39.9) and Class III (BMI 40 or more). Morbid or severe obesity is considered to include classes II and III (4,8).

The pervasiveness of the problem in industrialized cultures has led to a great deal of treatment research. Medically, morbidly obese individuals face more health complications and are more likely to suffer from a variety of comorbid conditions (9). For instance, the likelihood of developing type 2 diabetes is 42 times greater for morbidly obese men when compared to nonobese men (10). Women who are classified as morbidly obese also have a higher likelihood of contracting endometrial and cervical cancers than their non-obese peers (11). Individuals who are morbidly obese have a higher incidence of a broad range of other medical problems including hypertension, heart disease, musculoskeletal pain, hypercholesterolemia, coronary heart disease (CHD), gall bladder disease, sleep apnea, and osteoarthritis (8,9,12–17).

The findings on the psychological adjustment of morbidly obese individuals are somewhat mixed. Some studies have found significantly higher rates of eating, mood, anxiety, substance abuse, and personality disorders in the morbidly obese (18,19) while others have not (20–23). Kolotkin et al. (24) suggest that as the weight or BMI increases, the quality of life decreases. Thus, the potentially greater prevalence of psychological disorders is believed to be the result, in part, of negative attitudes and prejudices that are acceptable in our culture (25). As a result, morbidly obese individuals report a higher prevalence of depression, i.e., 22% for those with a BMI $\geq$ 35 vs. 12% for individuals in the normal BMI range (9).

Similarly, Higgs et al. (26) found that morbidly obese individuals were significantly more depressed than the non-obese individuals. In addition, morbidly obese participants who sought medical treatment for their obesity were significantly more depressed than their peers who sought lifestyle modification treatment. De Zwaan et al. (27) found a positive relationship between binge eating and feelings of ineffectiveness, lower self-esteem, stronger perfectionistic attitudes, increased impulsivity, and less introceptive awareness.

LIFESTYLE MODIFICATION

Although the treatment of obesity may seem like a daunting task, many of these comorbid conditions are significantly decreased with modest weight losses of 5% to 10% of the initial body weight (2,28). Current guidelines suggest that the most effective way to medically manage obese patients involves an interdisciplinary lifestyle modification program that combines behavioral modification of diet and physical activity alone or with pharmacotherapy (2,29). Some of the more effective components of lifestyle modification, which is a systematic method for modifying eating, exercise, and other behaviors that may contribute to or maintain morbid obesity (30), include self-monitoring, stimulus control, cognitive restructuring, goal setting, social support, problem solving, relapse prevention, and stress management. These techniques are applied to make changes in a patient's dietary and activity patterns, which are thought to contribute most to obesity. These techniques, diet and exercise recommendations, current Food and Drug Association (FDA)-approved medications for long-term obesity management, and surgery are discussed below.

Self-monitoring is the observation and recording of one's behaviors. The primary purpose of this technique is to help patients become aware of behaviors that influence their weight-loss attempts in order to modify those behaviors. In the treatment of obesity, self-monitoring can include the use of food diaries, physical activity logs, and body weight scales. Food diaries can be used to record the type and amount of food that one consumes during the day, the amount of calories in those foods, the total grams of fat consumed, the food groups eaten, and the situations and emotions occurring when one ate the food. For example, someone who ate a bowl of cereal with 2% milk, orange juice, a bagel with cream cheese, and five pieces of bacon for breakfast would record 300, 120, 220, 100, and 180 calories, respectively (values are approximate); 5, 0, 8, and 10 g of fat, respectively (values are approximate); food groups eaten include dairy, fruit, carbohydrates/grains, and meat; and finally, the situation, i.e., breakfast on Tuesday morning and the patient was anxious about an upcoming presentation at work.

Physical activity logs record the amount of exercise engaged in by the patient. Typically, the frequency, duration, and intensity of the exercise are recorded. For example, if someone starts walking regularly, the monthly log would indicate that person normally walks four days a week for 40 minutes at a moderate pace. Weight scales are used to record the progress of an individual who is attempting to lose weight by regularly measuring actual body weight.

Patients consistently report that self-monitoring is one of the most helpful tools for weight loss and maintenance, and research confirms that self-monitoring is associated with improved treatment outcomes (31–33).

Stimulus control is based on the old adage "out of sight, out of mind." Stimulus control attempts to limit the cues associated with eating by modifying the patients' immediate environment. Patients are taught how to modify their environments and cues so that they will increase the amount of physical activity and appropriate eating behavior, while decreasing the inappropriate behaviors that contribute to weight gain. Examples of stimulus-control activities include keeping their house free of snack foods, packing a gym bag the night before, and eating only at the kitchen table without television or other distractors. Patients should work with their health care providers to help create a stimulus-control strategy that works best for them. Foreyt and Goodrick (34) found that patients who utilize stimulus-control strategies are more successful in sustaining their weight-loss attempts and in long-term maintenance. This is possibly due to the assumption that exposure to obesity-promoting cues (e.g., high-fat snack foods) can trigger a relapse. Therefore, limiting these cues or exposures helps avoid returning to old behaviors.

Cognitive restructuring involves helping patients reframe their thoughts and perceptions associated with food and their weight. This technique involves teaching patients to change their internal dialogue with regard to weight management. For example, there are many types of self-defeating thoughts that can lead to rationalizations or excuses for inappropriate eating behavior or inactivity.

A particular challenge that obesity professionals often address is the topic of an "ideal weight." Our culture imposes an unrealistic image of what is ideal, and this perception of "normal" can lead to unattainable expectations for many morbidly obese patients. For example, Foster et al. (28) found that almost half of the patients enrolled in an obesity-treatment program had substantially greater weight loss expectations than the 10% weight reduction suggested by experts. This discrepancy could lead to substantial dissatisfaction with reasonable weight loss goals promoted by obesity experts (2), and lead to greater attrition, unrealistic weight loss goals, etc. (28). Thus, the goal of cognitive restructuring is to teach patients to feel better about themselves and be realistic about weight loss and how it will affect their lives.

Goal setting is a valuable tool for weight loss and maintenance. The emphasis when selecting goals should be on small, but achievable goals (35). Therefore, once one goal is accomplished, attention can be shifted to the next small goal with a greater sense of confidence and motivation. In most lifestyle modification weight reduction programs, the goal is to lose between 1 and 2 pounds a week, starting with an overall goal to lose 10% of one's current weight. For example, if someone weighs 250 pounds, the initial goal should be to lose 25 pounds, which should take approximately 13 weeks (at a minimum) if they are reasonably committed to the weight loss program and there are no circumstances that would interfere with weight loss (e.g., being placed on a medication that tends to cause weight gain).

The setting of appropriate goals helps patients realize that modest changes in weight, i.e., a 5–10% reduction in weight maintained for a year (15), are realistic and considered successful, as opposed to more dramatic goals imposed by cultural standards. For example, as noted earlier, Foster et al. (28) found a dramatic disparity between patient expectations for weight loss goals and current professional recommendations. In this study, the average goal weight desired by the study participants was a 32% reduction in body weight, which was three times lower than their reported previous weight loss (average of 4.4 attempts). A 17% (42.5 lbs) loss of initial body weight was defined by participants as disappointing, while a 25% loss (55 lbs) was viewed as acceptable. Although both of these goals are unrealistic for most behavioral weight loss programs and are much larger than those recommended by the experts, almost 50% of patients still set these as their goals. These unrealistic expectations can lead to greater patient dissatisfaction (28) and possibly to greater attrition and feelings of personal failure. Thus, helping patients set more realistic goals that are consistent with expert expectations and improvements in health can help to lessen this problem.

Social support can play an important role in patient participation, adherence, and the ultimate success of a patient's weight management program (33,36). Social support can involve everything from letting family and friends know that the patient is trying to lose weight to getting family and friends involved in the treatment program. Social support also can involve having the patient become involved in other outside activities or community-based programs that are not necessarily oriented toward weight reduction. For example, having the patient become active in a church group is a form of gaining social support that can help the patient develop stronger interpersonal skills and become more self-accepting (33,34). Additionally, it has been demonstrated that people who have more social support tend to have greater success in achieving a weight loss goal and maintaining weight loss in the future (33).

Problem solving involves learning how to identify situations and circumstances that pose a problem to eating healthy and exercising and developing solutions to these problems. Problem solving also involves trying out solutions that one has generated and evaluating their effectiveness. If the solution is ineffective, then another solution is attempted. This strategy can be used to tailor group lifestyle modification approaches to individual patients. Recently, Perri et al. (37) compared extended problem solving therapy to a standardized behavior therapy program without additional contacts. Participants who completed the additional problem-solving therapy intervention achieved clinically significant weight losses (10% or more of initial body weight) more frequently than those in the behavior therapy alone (i.e., 35% vs. 6%). In addition, participants who were randomly assigned to and completed the problem-solving intervention had significantly greater long-term weight reductions than those in the behavior therapy alone intervention without additional contacts (37).

Relapse prevention is utilized in a variety of treatments to help patients anticipate and prevent a lapse, or a minor slip, from becoming a relapse into an earlier behavior pattern (38). Developing coping strategies for these lapses is the major goal of relapse prevention. Thus, relapse-prevention training should instruct patients to interpret slips as learning opportunities and signals to work at a program rather than as failures that lead to a complete relapse to old behaviors.

A study by Baum et al. (39) compared the relative effectiveness of a therapist-supported maintenance condition, which provided relapse prevention skills, to a minimal contact condition, with presumably no relapse-prevention skill development, following a 12-week obesity treatment program. At the three- and six-month follow-ups, participants in the therapist-supported maintenance condition continued to lose weight or maintain their weight loss significantly more often that those in the no-contact condition. These results persisted for 1 year as well (39).

Stress management involves teaching patients a variety of techniques to control their stress. This is an extremely important component of any lifestyle modification weight management program, because stress and its accompanying mood states (e.g., depression and anxiety) often have been found to be predictors of relapse to overeating (33,40). Specifically, Schlundt et al. (41) found three high-risk situations that can lead to unplanned meals and impulsive overeating: positive social interaction, negative emotions, and physiological cravings. Techniques to help manage stress include tension and relaxation exercises, progressive muscle relaxation, meditation, and diaphragmatic breathing. These techniques, and a few others, have been shown highly effective for reducing stress, and presumably reducing relapse, in morbidly obese patients (42).

Outcomes associated with behavior modification. Incorporation of these techniques generally has been found to be effective for producing gradual and moderate weight loss, i.e., one to two pounds a week. Behavior modification interventions typically last 18 weeks and can include any of the previously discussed techniques. The average weight loss across numerous studies over the last two decades is one pound per week with an average of 8 kg (17.6 lbs) over the total treatment time. Attrition rates are generally low (<18%), and the use of multiple behavioral strategies appears to be associated with greater weight loss (2,43). Patients are able to maintain, on average, about two-thirds of their initial weight loss 9 to 10 months after treatment termination, but without continued treatment, patients gradually regain all of their lost weight over a 3- to 5-year period (2,43). Behavior modification techniques, in conjunction with extended treatment and physical activity, have been found consistently to predict weight loss during treatment (33,36,40).

DIETARY CHANGES

Nutritional counseling is one of the main components of a good weight reduction program (44). Nutritional counseling involves teaching patients how to choose and prepare foods that will promote their health goals. These lessons focus on topics such as learning the nutritional values in items, increasing the intake of complex carbohydrates and fiber, and decreasing the intake of dietary fat. For example, learning the food pyramid and the amounts of each food group one should consume daily would be the topic of one session. Specific skills also are focused on teaching patients to read nutrition labels, modify recipes, prepare healthy foods, and how to eat nutritionally in a restaurant.

In a study with obese children, Johnson et al. (45) found that providing nutrition counseling that resulted in a change in eating habits within the context of a cognitive-behavioral program that was paired with an exercise component produced modest, but significant, reduction in weight and blood lipids in morbidly obese children. These weight reductions and lipid profiles were maintained at a five-year follow-up whereas children in the information only condition remained morbidly obese (45).

Balanced deficit diets, which are sometimes referred to as low-calorie diets (LCD), call for a moderate reduction in caloric intake. The NHLBI (2) guidelines suggest that people who want to lose weight should reduce their caloric intake by 500 to 1000 kcal per day. This reduction in kilocalories produces weight loss in the range of one to two pounds (0.5–1.0 kg) per week (46). In addition, according to these guidelines, women who are attempting to lose weight should choose a diet of 1000 to 1200 kcal per day and men who want to lose weight should choose a diet of 1200 to 1500 kcal per day.

A popular variation of the LCD is a low-fat diet, which involves reducing the intake of dietary fat. This diet has been used alone or in conjunction with diets that attempt to reduce one's overall caloric intake. The premise of low-fat diets is that fat is the primary contributor to total caloric intake. Thus, if fat intake is reduced, total caloric intake also should drop, even though intake of other macronutrients may not change. This approach has been demonstrated to be effective in the short term, but it does not produce greater weight loss than traditional LCDs in the long term. For example, Viegener et al. (47) compared the efficacy of a continuous 1200 kcal/day LCD + behavior therapy with an intermittent low-fat 800 kcal/day (used four days per week) + behavior therapy. At the early evaluation points (e.g., months 1–4), women randomized to the intermittent low-fat diet demonstrated greater weight loss; however, by one year, there were no differences between the groups with respect to weight loss.

Schlundt et al. (48) conducted a randomized trial comparing a low-fat diet with ad libitum carbohydrate intake with a low-fat, low-calorie diet. Both groups received instructions in behavior modification. The low-fat, low-calorie group lost significantly more weight (males 11.8 ± 6.4 kg, females 8.2 ± 4.2 kg) than the low-fat group only (males 8.0 ± 1.3 kg; females 3.9 ± 3.7 kg) at the end of 20 weeks. In addition, while both groups experienced similar losses of lean body mass, participants in the low-fat, low-calorie group lost significantly more body fat. However, follow-up at 12 months after treatment demonstrated no significant difference between the two groups in weight loss from baseline (low-fat group 2.6 kg; low-calorie group 5.5 kg).

Jeffery et al. (49) evaluated the effectiveness of dietary counseling focusing on fat reduction (20 g/day) compared to calorie reduction (1000–1200 kcal/day) in promoting long-term weight loss in a randomized 18-month study with 122 obese women. Among the completers, women assigned to the fat-reduction group averaged larger weight loss than those in the low-calorie group (4.6 kg vs. 3.7 kg) at 6 months. However, by the end of the trial (18 months), women in both groups returned to baseline weight, despite continued intervention. Finally, a recent meta-analysis of the literature evaluating the efficacy of these diets found that they produced an average weight loss of 3.2 kg, a 10.2% reduction in fat intake, and a substantial reduction in energy intake (113 kJ/day) (50).

Very low calorie diets consist of consuming less than 800 kcal per day. Normally, very low calorie diets (VLCDs) involve consuming a prepared liquid formula or lean meat, fish, or fowl (51). These diets, while stringent, have been demonstrated to be safe if conducted under medical supervision. Results from studies on this type of diet have shown initial weight loss in the range of 9 kg (19.84 lbs) in 12 weeks (47,52–54). VLCDs are a promising approach for the treatment of obesity, producing weight loss two or three times greater than conventional LCD (2).

While VLCDs produce greater initial weight loss in patients, long-term weight-loss maintenance is not optimal and VLCDs need to be medically supervised (2). For example, Torgerson et al. (55) compared patients randomized to a 12-week VLCD combined with a two-year behavioral maintenance program versus patients only given the behavioral program. At the end of the study, both groups of patients achieved significant weight loss (-9.2 ± 14.2 kg vs. -6.3 ± 9.4 kg), a difference that was not statistically significant. Thus, there was no overall advantage for the VLCD group in the long term. However, when the data were examined by gender, men in the VLCD group lost significantly more weight than men in the behavioral support group only (-15.5 ± 17.2 kg vs. -5.3 ± 9.8 kg, respectively). In addition, intermittent administration of VLCDs appears to produce results similar to continuous administration, at least in the short term (56). Intermittent administration may be more palatable to patients who experience significant side effects to continuous administration.

Studies combining VLCD and behavioral intervention have been more successful than VLCDs alone; however, some weight is regained. When VLCDs are combined with behavior therapy, the one- and two-year results are significantly better than a VLCD alone. For example, patients using a combination of a VLCD plus behavior modification regained significantly less weight than patients using only a VLCD (i.e., -22.9 kg vs. -8.9 kg, respectively; $p < 0.001$) (26). These same results held up at the five-year follow-up as well (-16.9 kg vs. -4.9 kg, respectively; $p = 0.03$) (57).

PHYSICAL ACTIVITY

As part of any comprehensive weight loss and maintenance program, physical activity should be included. However, this may initially be a difficult task. A short-term goal in physical activity for obese patients includes moderate levels, such as brisk walking, for 30 to 45 minutes per session for three to five days a week (2). This will allow for an expenditure of about 150 to 225 kcal per session.

The types of physical activity with which morbidly obese patients should start include the ones that are non-weight-bearing and lifestyle activity modifications (29). Non-weight-bearing exercise options include activities such as water aerobics, swimming, and the use of an elliptical trainer. Lifestyle activities involve adapting one's daily routine to include more physical activity. Examples include parking one's car further away from the door in order to increase the time spent walking, using a motorized push mower instead of a riding mower, and using stairs rather than elevators when possible and safe.

These short-term goals should be followed by the intermediate goal of engaging in moderate exercise sessions on most or all days of the week (29). Gradually, patients can pursue the long-term goal of increasing the intensity of the physical activity to reach the guidelines set by the American College of Sports Medicine. These guidelines recommend that adults who are attempting to lose weight should exercise a minimum of 150 minutes per week and, when possible, progress to greater than 200 minutes per week (58).

Engaging in regular physical activity has been found to be associated with reductions in most of the comorbidities associated with severe obesity (2,59). However, some studies suggest that there is a "healthy" obese patient, one in which the person is obese but is physically fit. A study by Barlow et al. (60) found that moderately and highly fit men experienced significantly lower age-adjusted risk for all-cause mortality compared to sedentary or low-fit men. This finding was irrespective of their weight or BMI.

More recently, Wei et al. (61) conducted a prospective observational cohort study to evaluate the impact of low cardiorespiratory fitness as an objective marker of physical inactivity, on cardiovascular disease (CVD)- and all-cause mortality in normal-weight, overweight, and obese men. Low fitness level was defined as age-dependent. MET values, i.e., 20 to 39 years, 10.5 METs; 40 to 49 years, 9.9 METs; 50 to 59 years, 8.8 METs; and ≥ 60 years, 7.5 METs. Using high-fit, normal weight men as the reference group, risk of all-cause mortality was two to three times greater among low-fit overweight (Risk ratio (RR) 2.5, 95% CI 2.1–3.0) and low-fit obese men (RR 3.1, 95% CI 2.5–3.8). There was no significant increase in risk for all-cause mortality for overweight (RR 1.1, 95% CI 1.0–1.3) or obese men (RR 1.1, 95% CI 0.8–1.5) who were fit. The results were even more striking when risk for CVD-related mortality was examined. Figure 1 illustrates the relationship between fitness level and CVD-mortality across weight status groups.

As can be seen, low fitness is a strong, independent risk factor for both CVD- and all-cause mortality, regardless of the weight status.

Finally, Blair and Brodney (62) conducted a meta-analysis of studies examining the impact of activity level or fitness on mortality. In particular, they were interested in

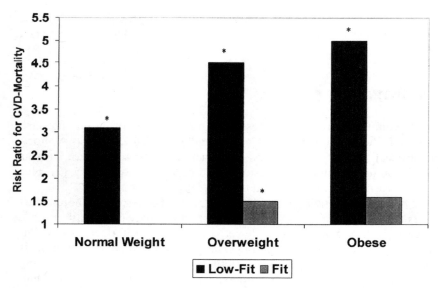

Figure 1 CVD-mortality risk by fitness level and weight status. *Statistically significant differences from reference group (high-fit, normal weight men). *Source*: Adapted from Ref. 61.

whether physical activity may attenuate health risks associated with overweight and obesity, and whether sedentary lifestyle is a more important predictor of morbidity and mortality than weight status.

They evaluated 24 studies that met all inclusion criteria and included outcomes such as all-cause mortality, cardiovascular disease mortality, CHD, hypertension, and type 2 diabetes. In general, they found that active or fit women and men appeared to be protected against the hazards of overweight or obesity, and the protective effect of fitness or activity often was stronger in obese individuals than in those of normal weight or who were overweight. They concluded that there is significant evidence that regular physical activity can attenuate health risks associated with overweight and obesity and inactivity, or low fitness, are strong, independent risk factors, and as important as overweight and obesity as mortality predictors.

COMBINING BEHAVIOR MODIFICATION AND PHARMACOTHERAPY

Pharmacotherapy is an adjunctive intervention that can be added to a behavior modification program. According to the current guidelines, appropriate patients may include those who have a $BMI \geq 30$ or a $BMI \geq 27$ in the presence of obesity-related comorbidities (2). However, many obesity clinical trials include only minimal lifestyle modification programs. For example, Poston et al. (63,64) conducted a meta-analysis of 108 randomized, controlled obesity pharmacotherapy trials over the last 40 years. They found that lifestyle interventions such as behavioral techniques and exercise were included in less than 30% of the published trials. Only dietary changes were included in the majority of drug studies, usually in the form of a balanced deficit diet (BDD). However, most studies in the meta-analysis provided little or no documentation on how they implemented lifestyle changes (64).

A few studies have specifically examined the additive benefit of obesity medications to lifestyle modification programs. For example, Craighead et al. (65) conducted a study using both pharmacotherapy and behavior modification. Patients were assigned to receive: (1) drug but no behavioral counseling, (2) behavior modification only, and (3) both the drug plus 26 weekly group behavior modification sessions. The drug-only group lost an average 6.0 kg in 6 months, while those in the behavior modification only group lost 10.9 kg. The combined medication and behavior modification group lost 15.3 kg, which was significantly more than the drug- and behavior modification only groups. Thus, in the short term, the combination of medication plus behavior modification was superior to either approach used separately. However, at one year, behavior therapy alone produced the greatest net weight loss (9.0 kg), while pharmacotherapy alone only produced a net weight loss of 6.3 kg and the combined group's net weight loss was 4.6 kg, suggesting that lifestyle interventions are an important part of weight loss maintenance. These data suggest that while the combined approach may be most helpful in the beginning of the treatment, lifestyle modification alone is important for weight loss maintenance.

Another study provided similar results (66). Two groups of patients received the same amount of fenfluramine and phentermine each day[a] (29). All patients were given a lifestyle modification workbook in which the program assigned tasks and homework. The first group received 10 monthly brief behavioral counseling sessions from a physician during office visits throughout the year. The second group attended a total of 32 group behavior modification classes during the year, each one lasting about 75 minutes. Patients in both groups lost approximately 15% of their initial body weight. These findings suggest that physicians trained in behavior modification can provide effective lifestyle modification using brief office visits by following a structured behavioral approach such as the to lifestyle exercise attitudes relationships nutrition (LEARN) program.

Wadden et al. (67) also demonstrated similar results in a randomized trial comparing drug-only, drug combined with group behavior modification, and a combination of drug, group behavior modification, and a portion-controlled diet for the first 16 weeks of the study. The first two groups were instructed to consume a BDD (1200–1500 kcal/day) consisting of 55% carbohydrates, 30% fat, and 15% protein. All three groups also were encouraged to increase their exercise four to five sessions per week lasting 30 to 40 minutes each session. At the end of the 12-month study, patients treated with the drug-only lost an average of 4.1% of their initial body weight. Patients in the drug plus behavior modification group lost an average of 10.8% of their initial body weight, significantly more than the drug-only group. The combined group lost an average of 16.5% of their initial body weight, which also was significantly more than the drug-only group. Thus, patients in the two behavior modification groups lost significantly more weight than patients in the drug-only group, suggesting that drug therapy is more effective when combined with a behavior modification program.

There are two broad categories of medications approved for weight loss in the United States: appetite suppressants, which decrease food intake by reducing one's appetite or increasing satiety, and nutrient absorption blockage, which decreases the amount of nutrients that are absorbed (68). Currently, there are two anti-obesity

[a] Fenfluramine was removed from the market after safety concerns were reported to the FDA.

medications that are effective and approved for long-term use: sibutramine (Meridia®) and orlistat (Xenical®).

Sibutramine is an appetite suppressant medication that inhibits the reuptake of the neurotransmitters, norepinephrine and serotonin, and to a lesser extent dopamine. Normally, sibutramine is taken once a day in a dose of 10 to 15 mg; however, a 5-mg dose can be substituted for those patients who do not tolerate the 10-mg dose well. The results of the clinical trials have shown sibutramine to be effective. In a six-month period, patients receiving the active drug lose 5% to 8% of their pre-intervention weight as compared to a 1% to 4% weight loss for those patients receiving a placebo (69–72). Generally, published studies have shown that this weight loss is maintained for up to one year (73).

Orlistat is the only FDA-approved weight loss drug that inhibits the absorption of nutrients by binding to gastrointestinal lipases in the lumen of the stomach. This prevents the hydrolysis of triglycerides (dietary fat) into absorbable fatty acids. Generally, patients are instructed to take a 120-mg dose of orlistat up to one hour before each meal. This dose has been shown to produce approximately a third less absorption of dietary fat, thereby reducing calorie and fat intake. Studies have also reported that orlistat produces an average of a 9% decrease in weight from the patients' pre-intervention weight, compared to a 5.8% weight loss for those patients taking an inactive substance (74). Orlistat, like sibutramine, has been shown to slow the rate of weight regain (75).

SURGERY

Surgical treatment can achieve substantial sustained weight loss in the majority of eligible obese patients. Eligible patients generally are those with a BMI ≥ 40 (2,8). There are three main types of surgical anti-obesity interventions: physical or mechanical, regulatory (influencing appetite regulation), and a combination of both physical and regulatory (76). The main surgical principles involved are bypass of the intestinal tract (resulting in malabsorption), restriction or obstruction of transit, and neuroregulation that does not disrupt gastrointestinal continuity.

Weight loss due to surgical intervention alone has been found to range from 50 kg (110 lbs) to 100 kg (222 lbs) over a period of six months to one year with gastric bypass (2,8,77). The Swedish Obesity Study, which is following 1879 matched patients for 10 years, found that surgically treated patients lost 28 ± 15 kg vs. 0.5 ± 9 kg among the obese controls at two year post-treatment (78). After eight years, surgically treated patients' weight loss was 20 ± 16 kg while the controls gained 0.7 ± 12 kg (78). Surgically treated patients also experienced significant reductions in the incidence of obesity-related comorbidities. For example, surgically treated patients had a 32- and 5-fold decrease in the incidence of type 2 diabetes at two and eight years post-surgery, respectively, when compared to obese controls (78). In addition, they had a three- to four-fold decrease in the development of hypertension and other cardiovascular risk factors (2,8). Surgically treated patients also experience significant improvements in mood- and health-related quality of life when compared to obese controls (79). A greater proportion of surgically treated patients also discontinue the use of cardiovascular (35% vs. 14%; RR 0.77, 95% CI 0.67–0.88) and diabetes (31% vs. 0%; RR 0.71, 95% CI 0.56–0.89) medications at six years post-treatment relative to controls (80).

There are several important risks associated with anti-obesity surgery. Depending on the type of surgery, these risks can include: micronutrient deficiencies, neuropathy, post-operative complications, "dumping syndrome," and post-operative depression (76). However, it has been suggested that, unlike other surgical complications, these risks can be modified with behavior modification techniques. For example, vomiting can occur in approximately 10% of patients post-surgically which is most often due to non-adherence to eating small portion sizes (4).

In conclusion, surgery is an extremely effective weight management treatment for the morbidly obese (81). However, there are risks involved in all of the currently available surgical procedures. Fortunately, if a multidisciplinary approach to treatment is taken that considers surgery as part of a comprehensive arsenal of treatments, patients who receive this treatment can experience significant long-term weight control, resulting in improvement in a variety of other comorbid conditions (82). As part of this comprehensive approach, lifestyle modification can play an important role in the success of surgical interventions by helping patients to manage problematic eating behaviors (e.g., binge eating), non-adherence to other dietary restrictions, and mood disorders (76).

SUMMARY AND CONCLUSIONS

Lifestyle modification is the cornerstone of obesity management because patients have to make long-term changes in their eating and physical activity habits in order to lose weight and maintain those changes. The strategies discussed have been shown to assist patients in making the necessary changes in diet and physical activity for both weight loss and improved health status. In addition, as noted in the chapter, increasing physical activity can be particularly important, not only for its benefit in weight loss maintenance, but because it appears to attenuate health risks associated with obesity. Finally, the addition of pharmacotherapy also can be helpful, particularly medications that are approved for long-term use, as obesity is now recognized as a chronic disorder that requires lifetime management (68).

REFERENCES

1. Flegal KM, Carroll MD, Ogden CL, Johnson CL. Prevalence and trends in obesity among US adults, 1999–2000. JAMA 2002; 288:1723–1727.
2. National Heart, Lung, and Blood Institute, National Institute of Diabetes and Digestive and Kidney Diseases. Clinical guidelines on the identification, evaluation, and treatment of overweight and obesity in adults: the evidence report. Washington, D.C.: U.S. Government Press, 1998. Guidelines available at http://www.nhlbi.nih.gov/guidelines/obesity/ob_gdlns.htm.
3. Pinhas-Hamiel O, Zeitler P. "Who is the wise man?—the one who forsees consequences": childhood obesity new associated comorbidity prevention. Prev Med 2000; 31:702–705.
4. World Health Organization. Obesity: preventing and managing the global epidemic. Report of the WHO Consultation on Obesity, Geneva, 3–5 June, 1997. Geneva: World Health Organization, 1998.
5. Koplan JP, Dietz WH. Caloric imbalance and public health policy. JAMA 1999; 282:1579–1581.
6. Sokol RJ. The chronic disease of childhood obesity: the sleeping giant has awakened. J Pediatr 2000; 136:711–713.
7. Centers for Disease Control and Prevention (CDC) (2000). Prevalence of overweight and obesity among adults: United States, 1999. www.cdc.gov/nchs/products/pubs/pubd/hestats/obese/obse99.htm.

8. U.S. Department of Health and Human Services. The Surgeon General's call to action to prevent and decrease overweight and obesity. Rockville, MD: U.S. Department of Health and Human Services, Public Health Service, Office of the Surgeon General, 2001. Available from U.S. GPO, Washington.

9. Quesenberry CP, Caan B, Jacobson A. Obesity, health service use and health care costs among members of a health maintenance organization. Arch Intern Med 1998; 158: 466–472.

10. Chan JM, Rimm EB, Colditz GA, Stampfer MJ, Willett WC. Obesity, fat distribution and weight gain as risk factors for clinical diabetes in men. Diabetes Care 1994; 17: 961–969.

11. Garfinkel L. Overweight and cancer. Ann Intern Med 1995; 103:1034–1036.

12. Barakat HA, Mooney N, O'Brien K, Long S, Khazani PG, Pories W, Caro JF. Coronary heart disease risk factors in morbidly obese women with normal glucose tolerance. Diabetes Care 1993; 16:144–149.

13. Bray GA. Pathophysiology of obesity. Am J Clin Nutr 1992; 55:488S–494S.

14. Colditz GA, Willett WC, Stampfer MJ, Manson JE, Hennekens CH, Arky RA, Speizer FE. Weight as a risk factor for clinical diabetes in women. Am J Epid 1990; 132:501–513.

15. Institute of Medicine (IOM). Weighing the options: criteria for evaluating weight-management programs. Washington, D.C.: National Academy Press, 1995.

16. Soloman CG, Manson JE. Obesity and mortality: a review of the epidemiological data. Am J Clin Nutr 1997; 66:1044S–1050S.

17. Troiano RP, Frongillo EA, Sobal J, Levitsky DA. The relationship between body weight and mortality: a quantitative analysis of combined information from existing studies. Int J Obes Relat Metab Disord 1996; 20:63–75.

18. Black DW, Goldsten RB, Mason EE. Prevalence of mental disorder in 88 morbidly obese bariatric clinic patients. Am J Psychiatry l992; 149:224–227.

19. Goldsmith SJ, Anger-Friedfield K, Beren S, Rudolph D, Boeck M, Aronne L. Psychiatric illness in patients presenting for obesity treatment. Int J Eat Disord 1992; 12:62–71.

20. Moore ME, Stunkard AJ, Srole L. Obesity, social class, and mental illness. JAMA 1962; 181:962–966.

21. Stewart AL, Brook RH. Effects of being overweight. Am J Pub Health 1983; 73:171–178.

22. Fitzgibbon ML, Kirschenbaum DS. Heterogeneity of clinical presentation among obese individuals seeking treatment. Add Behav 1990; 15:291–295.

23. Kayloe JC. Food addiction. Psychother 1993; 30:268–275.

24. Kolotkin RL, Head S, Hamilton M, Tse CJ. Assessing impact of weight on quality of life. Obes Res 1995; 3:49–56.

25. Stunkard AJ, Sorenson TI. Obesity and socioeconomic status: a complex relation. N Engl J Med 1993; 329:1036–1037.

26. Higgs ML, Wade T, Cescato M, Atchinson M, Slavotinek A, Higgins B. Differences between treatment seekers in obese populations: medical interventions vs. dietary restrictions. J Behav Med 1997; 20:391–405.

27. De Zwaan M, Mitchell JE, Seim HC, Specker SM, Pyle RL, Raymond NC, Crosby RB. Eating related and general psychopathology in obese females with binge eating disorder. Int J Eat Disord 1994; 15:43–52.

28. Foster GD, Wadden TA, Vogt RA, Brewer G. What is a reasonable weight loss? Patients expectations and evaluations of obesity treatment outcomes. J Consult Clin Psychol 1997; 65:79–85.

29. Poston WSC, Suminski RR, Foreyt JP. Physical activity level and the treatment of severe obesity. In: Bouchard C, ed. Physical Activity and Obesity. Champaign, IL: Human Kinetics, 2000:295–310.

30. Stunkard AJ, Stinnett JL, Smoller JW. Psychological and social aspects of the surgical treatment of obesity. Am J Psychiatry 1986; 143:417–429.

31. Baker RC, Kirschenbaum DS. Self monitoring may be necessary for successful weight control. Behav Ther 1993; 24:377–394.

32. Boutelle KN, Kirschenbaum DS. Further support for consistent self-monitoring as a vital component of successful weight control. Obes Res 1998; 6:219–224.

33. Kayman S, Bruvold W, Stern JS. Maintenance and relapse after weight loss in women: behavioral aspects. Am J Clin Nutr 1990; 52:800–807.

34. Foreyt JP, Goodrick GK. Evidence for success of behavior modification in weight loss control. Ann Intern Med 1993; 119:698–701.

35. Bandura A, Simon KM. The role of proximal intentions in self-regulation of refractory behavior. Cogn Ther Res 1977; 1:177–193.

36. McGuire MT, Wing RR, Klem ML, Hill JO. Behavioral strategies of individuals who have maintained long-term weight loss. Obes Res 1999; 7:334–341.

37. Perri MG, Nezu AM, McKelvey WF, Shermer RL, Renjilian DA, Viegener BJ. Relapse prevention training and problem-solving therapy in the long-term management of obesity. J Consult Clin Psychol 2001; 69:722–7266.

38. Marlatt GA, Gordon JR. Determinants of relapse: implications for the maintenance of behavior change. In: Davidson PO, Davidson SM, eds. Behavioral Medicine: Changing Health Lifestyles. New York: Brunner/Mazel, 1979:410–452.

39. Baum JG, Clark HB, Sandler J. Preventing relapse in obesity through posttreatment maintenance systems: comparing the relative efficacy of two levels of therapist support. J Behav Med 1991; 14:287–302.

40. McGuire MT, Wing RR, Klem ML, Hill JO. What predicts weight regain in a group of successful weight losers? J Consult Clin Psychol 1999; 67:177–185.

41. Schlundt DG, Sbrocco T, Bell C. Identification of high-risk situations in a behavioral weight loss program: application of the relapse prevention model. Int J Obes Relat Metab Disord 1989; 13:223–234.

42. Everly GS. A Clinical Guide to the Treatment of the Human Stress Response. New York: Plenum Press, 1989.

43. Wing RR. Behavioral approaches for the treatment for obesity. In: Bray GA, Bouchard C, James WPT, eds. Handbook of Obesity. New York: Marcel Dekker Inc., 1998:855–874.

44. Brownell KD. The LEARN Program for Weight Control. Dallas, TX: American Health Publishing Company, 1991.

45. Johnson WG, Hinkle LK, Carr RE, Andreson DA, Lemmon CR, Engler LB, Bergeron KC. Dietary and exercise interventions for juvenile obesity: long-term effect of behavioral and public health models. Obes Res 1997; 5:257–261.

46. VanGaal LF. Dietary treatment of obesity. In: Bray GA, Bouchard C, James WPT, eds. Handbook of Obesity. New York: Marcel Dekker Inc., 1998:875–890.

47. Viegener BJ, Perri MG, Nezu AM, Renjilian DA, McKelvey WF, Schein RL. Effects of an intermittent, low-fat, low-calorie diet in the behavioral treatment of obesity. Behav Ther 1990; 21:499–509.

48. Schlundt DG, Hill JO, Pope-Cordle J, et al. Randomized evaluation of a low fat "ad libitum" carbohydrate diet for weight reduction. Int J Obes 1993; 17:623–629.

49. Jeffery RW, Hellerstedt WL, French SA, Baxter JE. A randomized trial of counseling for fat restriction versus calorie restriction in the treatment of obesity. Int J Obes Relat Metab Disord 1995; 19:132–137.

50. Astrup A, Grunwald GK, Melanson EL, Saris WHM, Hill JO. The role of low-fat diets in body weight control: a meta-analysis of ad libitum dietary intervention studies. Int J Obes Rel Metab Disord 2000; 24:1545–1552.

51. Jeffery RW, Hellerstedt WL, French SA. A randomized trial of counseling for fat restrictions versus calorie restriction in the treatment of obesity. Int J Obes Rel Metab Disord 1995; 19:132–137.

52. Wing RR, Marcus MD, Salata R. Effects of a very-low-calorie diet on long-term glycemic control in obese type II diabetics. Arch Intern Med 1991; 151:1334–1340.

53. Wadden TA, Stunkard AJ. Controlled trial of very low calorie diet, behavior therapy, and their combination in the treatment of obesity. J Consult Clin Psychol 1986; 54:482–488.

54. Wadden TA, Foster GD, Letizia KA. One-year behavioral treatment of obesity: comparison of moderate and severe caloric restriction and the effect of weight maintenance therapy. J Consult Clin Psychol 1994; 62:165–171.
55. Torgerson JS, Lissner L, Lindroos AK, Kruijer H, Sjostrom L. VLCD plus dietary and behavioural support versus support alone in the treatment of severe obesity: a randomised two-year clinical trial. Int J Obes Rel Metab Disord 1997; 21:987–994.
56. Rossner S. Intermittent vs continuous VLCD therapy in obesity treatment. Int J Obes Rel Metab Disord 1998; 22:190–192.
57. Pekkarinen T, Mustajoki P. Comparison of behavior therapy with and without very-low-energy diet in the treatment of morbid obesity. Arch Intern Med 1997; 157:1581–1585.
58. Jakicic JM, Clark K, Coleman E, Donnelly JE, Foreyt J, Melanson E, Volek J, Volpe SL. American College of Sports Medicine. American College of Sports Medicine position stand. Appropriate intervention strategies for weight loss and prevention of weight regain for adults. Med Sci Sports Exerc 2001; 33:2145–2156.
59. U.S. Department of Health and Human Services, Office of the Surgeon General. Physical Activity and Health: A Report of the Surgeon General. Atlanta, GA: U.S. Department of Health and Human Services, Centers for Disease Control and Prevention, National Center for Chronic Disease Prevention and Health Promotion, 1996.
60. Barlow CE, Kohl HW III, Gibbons LW, Blair SN. Physical fitness, mortality, and obesity. Int J Obes Relat Metab Disord 1995; 19:S41–S44.
61. Wei M, Kampert JB, Barlow CE, Nichaman MZ, Gibbons LW, Paffenbarger RS Jr, Blair SN. Relationship between low cardiorespiratory fitness and mortality in normal-weight, overweight, and obese men. JAMA 1999; 282:1547–1553.
62. Blair SN, Brodney S. Effects of physical inactivity and obesity on morbidity and mortality: current evidence and research issues. Med Sci Sports Excer 1999; 31:S646–S662.
63. Haddock CK, Poston WSC, Dill PL, Foreyt JP, Ericsson M. Pharmacotherapy for obesity: a quantitative analysis of four decades of published randomized clinical trials. Int J Obes Relat Metab Disord 2002; 226:262–273.
64. Poston WSC, Haddock CK, Dill PL, Thayer B, Foreyt JP. Lifestyle treatments in randomized clinical trials of pharmacotherapies for obesity: data from 40 years of research. Obes Res 2001; 9:552–563.
65. Craighead LW, Stunkard AJ, O'Brien RM. Behavior therapy and pharmacotherapy for obesity. Arch Gen Psychiatry 1981; 38:763–768.
66. Wadden TA, Berkowitz RI, Vogt RA, et al. Lifestyle modification in the pharmacologic treatment of obesity: a pilot investigation of a potential primary care approach. Obes Res 1997; 5:218–226.
67. Wadden TA, Berkowitz RI, Sarwer DB. Benefits of lifestyle modification in the pharmacologic treatment of obesity: a randomized trial. Arch Intern Med 2001; 161:218–227.
68. Yanovski SZ, Yanovski JA. Drug therapy: obesity. New Engl J Med 2002; 346:591–602.
69. Fanghanel G, Cortinas L, Sanchez-Reyes L, Berber A. A clinical trial of the use of sibutramine for the treatment of patients suffering essential obesity. Int J Obes Relat Metab Disord 2002; 24:144–150.
70. Ryan DH. Use of sibutramine and other noraderenergic and serotonergic drugs in the management of obesity. Endocrine 2002; 13:193–199.
71. Fujioka K, Seaton TB, Rowe E, et al. Weight loss with sibutramine improves glycaemic control and other metabolic parameters in obese patients with type 2 diabetes mellitus. Diabetes Obes Metab 2000; 2:175–187.
72. Bray GA, Blackburn GL, Ferguson JM, et al. Sibutramine produces dose-related weight loss. Obes Res 1999; 7:189–198.
73. McMahon FG, Fujioka K, Singh BN, et al. Efficacy and safety of sibutramine in obese white and African American patients with hypertension: a 1-year, double-blind, placebo-controlled, multicenter trial. Arch Intern Med 2000; 160:185–191.
74. Heck AM, Yanovski JA, Calis KA. Orlistat, a new lipase inhibitor for the management of obesity. Pharmacotherapy 2000; 20:270–290.

75. Davidson MH, Hauptman J, DiGirolamo M, et al. Weight control and risk factor reduction in obese subjects treated for 2 years with orlistat: a randomized controlled trial. JAMA 1999; 281:235–242.

76. Kral JG. Surgical treatment of obesity. In: Bray GA, Bouchard C, James WPT, eds. Handbook of Obesity. New York: Marcel Dekker, Inc., 1998:977–993.

77. Mun EC, Blackburn GL, Matthews JB. Current status of medical and surgical therapy for obesity. Gastroenterology 2001; 120:669–681.

78. Torgerson JS, Sjostrom L. The Swedish obesity subjects (SOS) study: rationale and results. Int J Obes Relat Metab Disord 2001; 25:S2–S4.

79. Karlsson J, Sjostrom L, Sullivan M. Swedish obese subjects (SOS)—an intervention study of obesity: two-year follow-up of health-related quality of life (HRQL) and eating behavior after gastric surgery for severe obesity. Int J Obes Relat Metab Disord 1998; 22:113–126.

80. Sugerman HJ, DeMaria EJ, Kellum JM. Surgery for morbid obesity. In: Foreyt JP, McGinnis KJ, Poston WSC, Rippe JM, eds. Lifestyle Obesity Management. New York: Blackwell Publishing, 2003:147–166.

81. Agren G, Narbro K, Naslund I, Sjostrom L, Peltonen M. Long-term effects of weight loss on pharmaceutical costs in obese subjects: a report from the SOS intervention study. Int J Obes Relat Metab Disord 2002; 26:184–192.

82. Benotti PN, Forse RA. The role of gastric surgery in the multidisciplinary management of severe obesity. Am J Surg 1995; 169:361–367.

4

Preoperative Evaluation and Intraoperative Care of the Obese

Rodrigo Gonzalez, Scott F. Gallagher, Lisa Saff Koche, and Michel M. Murr
Interdisciplinary Obesity Treatment Group, Department of Surgery, University of South Florida Health Sciences Center, Tampa, Florida, U.S.A.

INTRODUCTION

Obesity is an independent risk factor for postoperative morbidity and mortality. Obese patients are at a greater risk of developing postoperative pulmonary complications as well as wound infections, deep venous thrombosis (DVT), and cardiac events compared to non-obese patients (1). Additionally, obesity is associated with several chronic diseases that are also independent risk factors for postoperative complications such as diabetes, atherosclerosis, hypertension, and obstructive sleep apnea (OSA).

Obese patients develop acute, critical, and unanticipated cardiopulmonary events and are more likely than non-obese patients to have cardiac problems requiring admission to the intensive care unit (2). Patient-specific factors, which are predictive of a complicated postoperative course in patients undergoing Roux-en-Y gastric bypass (RYGB), include male gender, age greater than 55 years, body mass index (BMI) greater than $50 \, \text{kg/m}^2$, hypertension, and a preoperative abnormal electrocardiogram (3,4). Identification of patients at highest risk for developing complications is essential to ensure favorable outcomes, especially if modifiable risk factors can be controlled or resolved. Nevertheless, the criteria for risk stratification have not been established, and the impact of preoperative intervention for comorbidities on operative outcomes has not been clearly documented either.

This chapter will review an interdisciplinary approach to patients with clinically significant obesity, and will outline evidence-based preoperative evaluations to improve immediate and long-term outcomes in patients who are considered candidates for bariatric surgery.

PREOPERATIVE EVALUATION

The Role of the Bariatric Surgeon

There is consensus that weight-loss surgery should be undertaken by surgeons with a strong interest in bariatric surgery. As bariatric practices evolve from a single practitioner to an interdisciplinary team, the role of the surgeon becomes that of the leader who coordinates the bariatric team and supervises preoperative evaluation. Once the patient is considered a candidate for surgery, the evaluation process begins under the supervision of both the bariatrician and the bariatric surgeon. Nevertheless, the surgeon should independently assess the adequacy of preoperative work-up, and determine whether or not to proceed with the operative treatment. Integral to this preoperative preparation is partnering with patients through the process of informed consent and setting realistic expectations.

We have adopted a fully interdisciplinary approach similar to the model of cardiologist–cardiac surgeons as well as transplant nephrologists/hepatologist–transplant surgeons. The interdisciplinary team approach not only taps into a vast array of resources and expertise, but it also maximizes utilization of a surgeon's time and technical experience, providing the foundation for a cooperative effort in the long-term follow-up care for the escalating number of bariatric patients.

The Role of the Bariatrician

As bariatric surgery evolves into a distinct area of specialization within surgery, bariatrics is evolving as a specialty for the treatment and prevention of obesity and its related comorbidities. The role of a bariatrician, who may be an internist or a family practitioner with a strong interest in bariatrics, is to ensure proper evaluation and treatment of comorbidities before and after weight-loss surgery. The task of caring for patients with clinically significant obesity can be overwhelming in light of the fact that many physicians lack the proper training or desire to treat obese patients (5).

We screen and treat comorbidities to minimize the adverse outcomes of bariatric surgery, because many obesity-related comorbidities are often neglected or untreated by primary providers. Although extensive diagnostic work-up is being undertaken in many centers, its utility is not fully proven (6). The bariatrician, as necessary, consults with cardiologists, pulmonologists, gynecologists, and other specialists to address these comorbidities while coordinating the evaluation of the psychologists and nutritionists prior to issuing the final medical clearance and referring on to the bariatric surgeon.

The Role of the Bariatric Nutritionist

As contrary as it may seem, many obese patients suffer from nutritional deficiencies. Nearly every obese patient has undergone energy-restrictive dietary regimens, most of which include reducing daily caloric intake. The implementation of low-fat, low-energy diets typically results in an increased intake of vegetables, counterbalanced by a decreased consumption of milk and dairy products, cereals, fruit, meat products, and added fats, which may result in a significant decreased daily intake of phosphorus, zinc, magnesium, iron, as well as vitamins B_1, B_2, and B_6 (7). These nutritional deficiencies, in particular that of iron and vitamin B_1, should be replenished prior to any planned bariatric procedure, especially in patients with previously failed bariatric operations.

The role of the nutritionist is to assess eating habits and preferences, to screen for nutritional deficiencies, and to educate patients on dietary ramifications after bariatric surgery. Patients are instructed to keep a seven-day food record, which becomes the basis to evaluate food preferences, food patterns, and possible areas of change. Specifically, food diaries unmask unrecognized high consumption of junk food, simple sugar and fat, binge eating, and night eating. In addition, the nutritionist educates patients about the importance of chewing food thoroughly (because of the restrictive nature of most bariatric procedures) and the value of nutritional supplements (to avoid protein deficiency), as well as teaching exercises to relearn hunger and satiety. The utility of preoperative weight-reducing diets to facilitate laparoscopic surgery is unfounded and cannot be recommended at this time.

The Role of the Bariatric Psychologist/Psychiatrist

Obesity has a considerable negative impact on psychological and social dynamics, and patients with clinically significant obesity have a higher prevalence of psychological comorbidities including depression, anxiety, binge eating, and body dysmorphic disorders. Patients who do not meet the Diagnostic and Statistical Manual of Mental Disorders symptom criteria for depression, have an increased risk of developing a major depressive episode within one year following surgery (8). It is generally agreed, although inconsistently documented, that patients with active psychosis, active substance abuse, suicidal ideation, mental retardation, delirium, dementia, and amnestic disorders should not be considered for bariatric surgery, because these disorders interfere with the process of informed consent as well as compliance with postoperative care and instructions.

Intuitively, patients who undergo psychological evaluation and counseling, both pre- and postoperatively, have better outcomes in terms of weight loss (9). Nevertheless, psychological instruments designed to predict postoperative outcomes have been inconsistent and inconclusive; therefore, clear guidelines for psychological screening to predict outcomes are lacking.

We recommend a thorough evaluation by a psychologist/psychiatrist to screen for severe psychopathology and eating disorders, to assess patient motivation and social support system, and to develop a treatment plan. Our psychologist conducts a semi-structured interview and utilizes a battery of psychological instruments (PDS, MCSDI, BDI-II, STAI-Y, and EDI-2) in addition to counseling on postoperative psychological changes. Currently, the impact of interventions designed to address and ameliorate major psychopathology while eliminating disordered eating for at least three months prior to surgery via behavior modification, cognitive therapy, or pharmacotherapy is under investigation.

Cardiovascular Evaluation

Not uncommonly, full evaluation may not be technically feasible because of body habitus and the weight limitations of diagnostic equipment. Obesity increases PR interval and QRS complex duration and significantly prolongs the QT interval; however, the clinical significance of these abnormalities is uncertain (10).

In general, cardiac risk assessment for bariatric procedures should be similar to that for other abdominal operations. Tools such as the Modified Cardiac Risk Index by Detsky et al. (11) and the additional low-risk variable calculations should be utilized in order to determine which patients should undergo further evaluation by exercise stress testing, dobutamine stress echocardiogram (DSE), or nuclear myocardial scintigraphy (performed when DSE is unsuccessful). However, most studies have shown that nuclear imaging or DSE do not accurately predict the occurrence of perioperative cardiac events, and their low, positive predictive value in patients undergoing major non-cardiac vascular procedures limits their usefulness. Patients with a history of recent myocardial infarction ($<$6 months), significant dysrhythmia, congestive heart failure, angina, and diabetes are at a higher risk for postoperative myocardial events and therefore, we often recommend stress testing with a high dose thallium two-day protocol (in a sitting position if the patient's weight exceeds the weight limit of the equipment) as part of the preoperative evaluation. Our experience has been that there is no real diagnostic benefit to attempt stress testing in patients over 450 pounds. In addition, we recommend that patients with more than two risk factors as outlined above are considered for perioperative beta-blockade, unless otherwise contraindicated. We commonly use atenolol 50 mg/day prior to surgery, which is continued daily until discharged from the hospital.

Management of hypertension in obese patients is frequently challenging, as many patients require a combination of two or more antihypertensive medications to achieve satisfactory results. We aggressively pursue control of hypertension to help patients tolerate the normal catecholamine surge that accompanies surgery. We recommend that patients take their antihypertensive medications the morning of surgery with a sip of water. Postoperatively, patients usually require about one-half the amount and dosage of antihypertensive medications they needed prior to surgery. The medications can be administered intravenously until the patients resume oral intake on the first or second postoperative day. In case of patients who are taking diuretics for lower extremity edema, these medications should be stopped several days before surgery to avoid volume contraction and hypotension during general anesthesia. However, diuretics for other indications (i.e., hypertension, congestive heart failure) should not be discontinued.

Based on this protocol, extensive testing has detected significant cardiovascular diseases that resulted in deferring bariatric surgery in less than 1% of our patients (unpublished data). However, preoperative testing was very important in detecting and treating modifiable risk factors such as hypertension. Consequently, the incidence of postoperative cardiac events in our practice has been less than 1%. We currently do not recommend bariatric surgery for patients with uncompensated cardiomyopathy and poor ejection fraction or for patients with refractory, moderate-to-severe pulmonary hypertension.

Obstructive Sleep Apnea (OSA)

Obesity is the single most important physical characteristic associated with obstructive sleep apnea (OSA) in adults (60–90% incidence). Table 1 summarizes the prevalence of OSA in patients undergoing RYGB at our institution (12,13). Both OSA and obstructive sleep hypopnea repeatedly disrupt sleep due to increased ventilatory

Table 1 Prevalence of Obstructive Sleep Apnea in Patients Undergoing Roux-en-Y Gastric Bypass as Determined by the Respiratory Disturbance Index (RDI) During Polysomnography

Obstructive sleep apnea	RDI	Patients (%)
None	$<$5	13
Mild	6–20	29
Moderate	21–40	16
Severe	$\geq$41	42

Source: From Refs. 12, 13.

effort-induced arousal, which in turn causes daytime sleepiness and altered cardio-pulmonary function. Repetitive sleep-time oxygen desaturation may cause bradycardia and dysrhythmias. Long-standing OSA causes alveolar hypoventilation and pulmonary hypertension as the reduction in arterial oxygen tension (PaO_2) induces pulmonary vasoconstriction. Pulmonary hypertension worsens with the severity and duration of OSA as intrathoracic pressure progressively becomes more negative with increasing ventilatory effort to overcome airway obstruction (14).

A presumptive clinical diagnosis of OSA can be made in patients with classical signs and symptoms including large neck circumference, snoring, apnea during sleep as witnessed by a bed partner, periodic snorting, arousal, and daytime sleepiness. The Epworth Sleepiness Scale (ESS) can be implemented as a non-invasive bedside tool to screen for the presence of OSA. Since neither the ESS nor the BMI predicts the severity of OSA (13), we refer all patients who score 6 points or more for consultation with a pulmonologist and to undergo polysomnography. Using this approach we documented that 60% of all bariatric patients had moderate-to-severe OSA, which otherwise was undiagnosed and untreated (13). These patients were treated with CPAP/BiPAP for at least two weeks prior to surgery to recruit all alveoli and reverse alveolar hyperventilation. The use of CPAP/BiPAP should continue postoperatively starting in the recovery room as many adverse events of hypoventilation and atelectasis can be prevented. We have used this approach on all patients with OSA with no untoward events such as pouch blow out or Roux limb dilatation. More importantly, the incidence of respiratory failure requiring artificial ventilation has been less than 1% in our cohort and we have not undertaken any elective tracheostomy to manage OSA in the perioperative period.

Diabetes

Obesity has long been recognized as a significant risk factor for the development of type 2 diabetes and is quite prevalent in bariatric patients (more than 30%). In preparation for bariatric surgery, we require all diabetic patients to strictly adhere to medications and dietary guidelines to maintain serum glucose below 150 mg/dL or HbA_{1c} below 7%. We also recommend these patients undergo additional dietary education regarding nutritional changes after the operation. All extended-release diabetic medications are changed to immediate-release forms to afford close and accurate monitoring of glucose, especially in the postoperative period where food intake is limited.

Weight loss has beneficial effects on virtually every aspect of type 2 diabetes. This early reduction in fasting glucose induced by the postoperative restriction of caloric intake is paralleled by reductions in hepatic glucose production and urinary glucose excretion. We use non-glucose containing intravenous solutions in diabetic patients during and after the operation and determine blood glucose levels (finger stick) every six hours postoperatively, employing a sliding scale insulin treatment for close control of glucose levels. Tight control of serum glucose levels is of paramount importance in the subset of patients who have severe glucosuria despite serum glucose of ≤ 300 mg/dL, because of the propensity of these patients to develop non-ketotic hyperosmolar acidosis and subsequent volume contraction. We treat these patients with a continuous insulin drip intravenously and postoperatively for 24 to 48 hours to keep serum glucose ≤ 150 mg/dL.

Gastrointestinal Evaluation

Gastroesophageal Reflux Disease

Routine preoperative endoscopic evaluation has revealed a prevalence of reflux esophagitis in >30% and peptic gastroduodenal lesions in 37% to 59% of morbidly obese patients (15). Moreover, preoperative 24-hour pH testing documented abnormal esophageal acid exposure in 35% to 50% of patients undergoing bariatric surgery (16). Neither weight nor BMI is correlated with the percentage of time with pH < 4. We recommend endoscopic evaluation of the stomach for patients with acute symptoms of peptic ulcer disease (<1% of patients) to ensure complete healing prior to the proposed bariatric procedure. Routine surveillance endoscopy, upper gastrointestinal study, and screening for *Helicobacter pylori* are not supported by vigorously tested data.

Although the incidence of hiatal hernias has been reported to be high (15), these hernias are small and usually asymptomatic defects that rarely require further intervention when performing a bariatric procedure. In our experience, only one large crural defect required closure in more than 600 patients who underwent gastric bypass. On the other hand, it may be important to screen for hiatal hernias in patients undergoing gastric banding, since a defect larger than 3 cm in diameter is considered a contraindication.

Gallstone Disease

Controversy still surrounds whether to undertake prophylactic cholecystectomy in patients at the time of a bariatric operation. The incidence of developing symptomatic gallstones within the first year following RYGB is in the range of 36% to 53% (17). Proponents of selective cholecystectomy cite the lack of significant morbidity of the procedure in patients developing gallstones following bariatric surgery, and recommend it only in patients with evidence of gallstones. Others advocate postoperative replacement of the cholecystectomy with bile salt therapy for the treatment of gallstones. However, concerns of this modality are the potential side effects (which can occur in approximately 25% of patients), increased costs, and its inherent high rate of patient non-compliance (reported in up to 60% of patients) (18). On the other hand, the lack of morbidity justifies concomitant cholecystectomy, as it adds little time to the bariatric procedure (19) and reduces costs compared to both selective and deferred management of the gall bladder (20).

Non-Alcoholic Steatohepatitis

Non-alcoholic steatohepatitis (NASH) represents a spectrum of disorders defined by the presence of hepatic steatosis and inflammatory infiltrates in the absence of alcohol use or other chronic liver disease (i.e., viral hepatitis, autoimmune hepatitis, hereditary hemochromatosis) and is the most common cause of cryptogenic cirrhosis. Currently, all non-invasive modalities such as serum liver tests and imaging studies do not accurately predict the stage of NASH. Imaging studies, including abdominal ultrasound, computed tomography (CT) scan, and magnetic resonance imaging, cannot distinguish simple fatty liver from NASH. Therefore, liver biopsy remains the most sensitive diagnostic test, but its use is heavily curtailed because of its invasive nature as well as the absence of a definitive treatment for NASH (23).

Since preoperative liver biopsy is not practical in the majority of bariatric patients, we routinely undertake an intraoperative liver biopsy to screen for NASH.

Table 2 Prevalence of Non-Alcoholic Steatohepatitis in Patients Undergoing Roux-en-Y Gastric Bypass as Determined by Intraoperative Liver Biopsy

Non-alcoholic steatohepatitis	Patients (%)
None	49
Mild	34
Moderate	9
Severe	2
Cirrhosis	6

Source: From Refs. 12, 22.

More than 8% of bariatric patients have cirrhosis or severe fibrosis and an additional 9% have moderate NASH (Table 2). Patients with moderate to severe NASH are referred for further work-up of viral etiologies and may benefit from future clinical trials. These data will provide valuable information on the natural history of NASH after bariatric surgery, and can be used to determine the effect of rapid weight loss on the natural history of NASH, fibrosis, cirrhosis, and liver insufficiency (23).

Deep Venous Thrombosis (DVT)

Obesity is also a risk factor for deep venous thrombosis (DVT). The adjusted risk ratio of pulmonary embolism (PE) according to weight increases from 1.0 in patients with $BMI < 25 \, kg/m^2$ to 2.7 in patients with $BMI > 40 \, kg/m^2$ (24, 25). The reported incidence of PE in patients undergoing bariatric surgery is between 1.4% and 2.6% (24). However, widespread screening of asymptomatic patients undergoing bariatric surgery for thrombophilic risk factors is not practical, akin to prophylactic and routine use of inferior vena cava (IVC) filters.

Preoperatively, we require patients who are ambulatory to start a vigorous daily walking program. Patients who have a previous history of PE are treated with an IVC filter. We do not place an IVC filter in all patients with a history of DVT, but will strongly consider it in patients who are non-ambulatory or currently on anticoagulation therapy. Because optimal dosing of heparin and fractionated heparin for prophylaxis in patients with $BMI > 40 \, kg/m^2$ is not known, it is suspected that adequate prophylaxis may not be attainable in many bariatric patients. We have consequently instituted a regimen of high-dose, fractioned, low–molecular weight heparin albeit data to support this approach are lacking. The use of sequential compression devices adds another layer of prophylaxis. These devices should be employed prior to transfer to the operating room and until the patient is fully ambulatory.

Patients may present with venous stasis ulcers in the lower extremities or chronically infected wounds in the abdominal panus. In addition to aggressive wound care to promote epithelization and formation of granulation tissue, we recommend a long-term use of oral antibiotics in the perioperative period to minimize the chance of uncontrolled skin infections postoperatively.

REVISIONAL BARIATRIC SURGERY

Patients with failed previous bariatric procedure deserve special consideration. The indications for revisional surgery are multiple, although the most common is inadequate weight loss. However, depending on the type of the original bariatric operation, revisional surgery is undertaken for strictures, stomal ulcers, gastro-gastric fistulas, gastroesophageal reflux disease, and metabolic complications. There-fore, it is imperative that the surgeon fully understands the anatomic reasons for failure in each patient. In addition to undergoing the same type of preoperative evaluation as for a primary bariatric procedure, including counseling with a nutri-tionist and a psychologist, patients should undergo evaluation of the causes and con-sequences of the failed operation. Endoscopy, barium swallow, and CT scan should be used liberally, not only as diagnostic tools, but also to fully elucidate the anatomy of the previous procedure and to plan the revisional procedure beforehand. Docu-mentation of the failed procedure may be sought by a review of the operative report.

The majority of these patients will develop nutritional and/or electrolyte abnormalities due to malabsorption or inability to maintain adequate intake, and some patients will develop complications (i.e., diarrhea, vomiting, food intolerance, etc.) resulting in anemia and protein-calorie malnutrition. Although infrequent, micronutrient deficiencies, particularly of iron, folate, vitamin B_{12}, potassium, and magnesium have been reported (26). Optimization of the nutritional status and elec-trolyte abnormalities may necessitate the use of total parenteral nutrition for some patients in preparation for revisional surgery.

INTRAOPERATIVE CARE

Airway Management

Airway management is a major source of morbidity and mortality in critically ill and anesthesized obese patients. A BMI greater than 26 kg/m^2 results in a three-fold increased incidence of difficult ventilation via a mask and a 10-fold difficulty of endotracheal intubation (27). Commonly used anesthetic agents such as propofol, thiopental, narcotics, benzodiazepines, neuromuscular blockers, and nitrous oxide have been demonstrated to cause pharyngeal collapse (28). Obese patients should therefore be carefully evaluated for airway difficulty. History of sleep apnea, limited neck movement, limited mouth opening, large tongue, and short thyromental dis-tance all increase the risk for difficulty in airway management and, hence, fiber-optic-guided intubation is frequently recommended in these patients.

An emergency tracheostomy is challenging in obese patients and may not be practical or safe. In case of airway loss or accidental extubation during surgery, several alternatives have been proposed. The intubating laryngeal mask airway (ILMA) has been reported to be a safe alternative to endotracheal intubation, with a successful rate of tracheal intubation of 96% with no adverse effects related to the technique (29). In patients whose airway is characterized as difficult and who have severe OSA, an elective tracheostomy before bariatric surgery has been advocated, but we have not used this approach because of the universal success of the current approach to endotracheal intubation with or without fiber-optic guidance.

Respiratory Mechanics

General anesthesia profoundly affects respiratory function in morbidly obese patients, and may reduce functional residual capacity (FRC), expiratory reserve volume (ERV), and total lung volume (TLV). Pulmonary atelectasis occurs in 85% to 90% of healthy adults within minutes after induction of general anesthesia, and up to 15% of the lungs may be atelectatic particularly in the basal regions (30), resulting in a right-to-left intrapulmonary shunting of approximately 10% of cardiac output (31). Because awake obese patients (BMI > 35 kg/m^2) exhibit severe alterations in their respiratory mechanics, including decreased chest wall and lung compliance and decreased FRC, they are particularly vulnerable to intra- and postoperative atelectasis, which is associated with postoperative pulmonary morbidity (particularly pneumonia) and increased length of hospital stay (32,33).

To counteract this, patients are frequently ventilated with high tidal volumes (which can result in barotrauma and reduced venous return), PEEP (which can result in hemodynamic compromise), or receive intermittent vital capacity "recruitment maneuvers" in an attempt to reinflate alveoli that have collapsed. Newer modes of ventilation have been adopted in an attempt to prevent alveolar collapse, and the initial results of trials with airway pressure release ventilation (APRV) have been promising in obese patients and those undergoing RYGB in our institution, with decreased work of breathing, improved ventilation, and reduced requirement for supplemental oxygen delivery (34).

End tidal CO_2 monitoring provides additional useful information such as correct position of the tracheal tube, a ventilator disconnection, and analysis of the waveform. Furthermore, pCO_2 can frequently rise due to the pneumoperitoneum delivered for prolonged periods of time and at higher pressures than that needed for non-obese patients.

Intraoperative Physiologic Pulmonary and Hemodynamic Changes

Some of the changes in pulmonary and cardiac physiology that occur in obese patients may impede normal adaptation to respiratory and hemodynamic changes that take place during anesthesia. In most instances, patients are placed in reverse Trendelenburg position, which is an independent factor for the development of venous stasis. Combining this position and pneumoperitoneum further reduces femoral peak systolic velocity and, consequently, increases venous stasis as well as femoral vein cross-sectional area (35). Increasing experience of the surgical and anesthetic teams has resulted in reduced utilization of invasive monitoring, as we no longer require routine central venous access or arterial line placement.

CONCLUSION

The safety of bariatric surgery hinges not only on the intra- and postoperative care but also on the adequacy of preoperative evaluation and screening. Efforts should be aimed at identifying modifiable risk factors and treating them prior to the planned bariatric procedure. Greater efforts to identify predictors of outcomes are lacking, and will be crucial to the progress of bariatric surgery.

ACKNOWLEDGMENT

The authors are grateful to Dr. Roy G. Soto, from the Department of Anesthesiology, University of South Florida College of Medicine for his critical review of the manuscript.

REFERENCES

1. Choban PS, Flanchaum L. The impact of obesity on surgical outcomes: a review. J Am Coll Surg 1997; 185:593–603.
2. Rose DK, Cohen MM, Wigglesworth DF, DeBoer DP. Critical respiratory events in the post anesthesia care unit. Patient, surgical, and anesthetic factors. Anesthesiology 1994; 81:410–418.
3. Livingston EH, Huerta S, Arthur D, Lee S, De Shields S, Heber D. Male gender is a predictor of morbidity and age a predictor of mortality for patients undergoing gastric bypass surgery. Ann Surg 2002; 236:576–582.
4. Gonzalez R, Bowers SP, Venkatesh KR, Lin E, Smith CD. Preoperative factors predictive of complicated postoperative management after Roux-en-Y gastric bypass for morbid obesity. Surg Endosc 2003; 17:1900–1904.
5. Banasiak M, Murr MM. Medical school curricula do not address obesity as a disease. Obes Surg 2001; 11:677–679.
6. Ramaswamy A, Gonzalez R, Smith CD. Extensive preoperative testing is not necessary in morbidly obese patients undergoing gastric bypass. J Gastrointest Surg 2004; 8: 159–165.
7. Grzybek A, Klosiewicz-Latoszek L, Targosz U. Changes in the intake of vitamins and minerals by men and women with hyperlipidemina an overweight during dietetic treatment. Eur J Clin Nutr 2002; 56:1162–1168.
8. Dixon JB, Dixon ME, O'Brien PE. Depression in association with severe obesity. Changes with weight loss. Arch Intern Med 2003; 163:2058–2065.
9. Clark MM, Balsiger BM, Sletten CD, Dahlman KL, Ames G, Williams DE, Abu-Lebdeh HS, Sarr MG. Psychosocial factors and 2-year outcome following bariatric surgery for weight loss. Obes Surg 2003; 13:739–745.
10. El-Gamal A, Gallagher D, Nawras A, Gandhi P, Gomez J, Allison DB, Steinberg JS, Shumacher D, Blank R, Heymsfield SB. Effects of obesity on QT, RR, and QTc intervals. Am J Cardiol 1995; 75:956–959.
11. Detsky AS, Abrams HB, Forbath N, Scott JG, Hilliard JR. Cardiac assessment for patients undergoing noncardiac surgery. A multifactorial clinical risk index. Arch Intern Med 1986; 146:2131–2134.
12. Serafini FM, MacDowell Anderson W, Rosemurgy AS, Strait T, Murr MM. Clinical predictors of sleep apnea in patients undergoing bariatric surgery. Obes Surg 2001; 11:28–31.
13. Rasheid V, Banasiak M, Gallagher SF, Lipska A, Kaba S, Ventimiglia D, Anderson WM, Murr MM. Gastric bypass is an effective treatment for obstructive sleep apnea in patients with clinically significant obesity. Obes Surg 2003; 13:58–61.
14. Benumof JL. Obstructive sleep apnea in the adult obese patient: implications for airway management. Anesthesiol Clin North Am 2002; 20:789–811.
15. Frigg A, Peterli R, Zynamon A, Lang C, Tondelli P. Radiologic and endoscopic evaluation for laparoscopic adjustable gastric banding: preoperative and follow-up. Obes Surg 2001; 11:594–599.
16. Iovino P, Angrisani L, Tremolaterra F, Nirchio E, Ciannella M, Borrelli V, Sabbatini F, Mazzacca G, Ciacci C. Abnormal esophageal acid exposure is common in morbidly obese patients and improves after successful Lap-band system implantation. Surg Endosc 2002; 16:1631–1635.
17. De Oliveira CIB, Chaim EA, da Silva BB. Impact of rapid weight reduction on risk of cholelithiasis after bariatric surgery. Obes Surg 2003; 13:625–628.
18. Scott DJ, Villegas L, Sims TL, Hamilton EC, Provost DA, Jones DB. Intraoperative ultrasound and prophylactic ursodiol for gallstone prevention following laparoscopic gastric bypass. Surg Endosc 2003; 17:1796–1802.
19. Fobi M, Lee H, Igwe D, Felahy B, James E, Stanczyk M, Fobi N. Prophylactic cholecystectomy with gastric bypass operation: incidence of gallbladder disease. Obes Surg 2002; 12:350–353.

20. Matter SG, Bowers SP, Lin E, Gonzalez LR, Venkatosh KR, Smith CD. Should chole-cystectomy be a routine part of laparoscopic gastric bypass for obesity: a cost analysis? [abstr]. Surg Endosc 2002; 16:S243.

21. Clark JM, Diehl AM. Nonalcoholic fatty liver disease. An unrecognized cause of crypto-genic cirrhosis. JAMA 2003; 289:3000–3004.

22. Shalhub S, Parsee A, Gallagher SF, Haines KL, Willkomm C, Brantley SG, Pinkas H, Saff-Koche L, Murr MM. The importance of routine liver biopsy in diagnosing nonalco-holic steatohepatitis in bariatric patients. Obes Surg 2004; 14:54–59.

23. Kral JG, Thung SN, Biron S, Hould FS, Lebel S, Marceau S, Simard S, Marceau P. Effects of surgical treatment of the metabolic syndrome on liver fibrosis and cirrhosis. Surgery 2004; 135:48–58.

24. Eriksson S, Backman L, Ljungstrom KG. The incidence of clinical postoperative throm-bosis after gastric surgery for obesity during 16 years. Obes Surg 1997; 7:332–336.

25. Schauer PR, Ikramuddin S, Gourash W, Ramanathan R, Luketich J. Outcomes after laparoscopic Roux-en-Y gastric bypass for morbid obesity. Ann Surg 2000; 232:515–529.

26. Brolin RE. Gastric bypass. Surg Clin North Am 2001; 81:1077–1095.

27. El-Ganzouri AR, McCarthy RJ, Tuman KJ, Tanck EN, Ivankovich AD. Preoperative airway assessment: predictive value of a multivariate risk index. Anesth Analg 1996; 82:1197–1204.

28. Benumof JL. Obstructive sleep apnea in the adult obese patient: implications for airway management. Anesthesiol Clin North Am 2002; 20:789–811.

29. Frappier J, Guenoun T, Journois D, Philippe H, Aka E, Cadi P, Silleran-Chassany J, Safran D. Airway management using the intubating laryngeal mask airway for the mor-bidly obese patient. Anesth Analg 2003; 96:1510–1515.

30. Lundquist H, Hedenstierna G, Strandberg A, Tokics L, Brismar B. CT-assessment of dependent lung densities in man during general anesthesia. Acta Radiol 1995; 36:626–632.

31. Rothen HU, Sporre B, Engberg G, Wegenius G, Hedenstierna G. Re-expansion of atelectasis during general anesthesia: a computed tomography study. Br J Anaesth 1993; 71:788–795.

32. Pelosi P, Croci M, Ravagnan I, Cerisara M, Vicardi P, Lissoni A, Gattinoni L. Respira-tory mechanics in sedated, paralyzed, morbidly obese patients. J Appl Physiol 1997; 82:811–818.

33. Eichenberger A, Proietti S, Wicky S, Frascarolo P, Suter M, Spahn DR, Magnusson L. Morbid obesity and postoperative pulmonary atelectasis: an underestimated problem. Anesth Analg 2002; 95:1788–1792.

34. Soto RG, Murr MM, Smith RA, Downs JB. Apneustic anesthesia ventilation (AAV) during laparoscopy. American Society of Anesthesiologists Meeting, New Orleans, LA, Oct 14, 2002.

35. Perilli V, Sollazzi L, Modesti C, Annetta MG, Sacco T, Bocci MG, Tacchino RM, Proietti R. Comparison of positive end-expiratory pressure with reverse Trendelenburg position in morbidly obese patients undergoing bariatric surgery: effects on hemody-namics on pulmonary gas exchange. Obes Surg 2003; 13:605–609.

5
Essentials of a Bariatric Surgery Program

Samer G. Mattar and Tomasz Rogula
*Department of Surgery, University of Pittsburgh Medical Center,
Pittsburgh, Pennsylvania, U.S.A.*

INTRODUCTION

The incidence of morbid obesity is increasing in epidemic proportions (1). This alarming trend is being accentuated by daily media-driven highlights and periodic calls for action from government officials (2). General surgeons are coming under increasing market pressures to provide surgical solutions for these patients who seek significant and durable weight loss. Morbidly obese patients often carry multiple diagnoses, and many surgeons who had embarked on this speciality rapidly realized that the safest and most effective approach to managing these patients successfully is through a comprehensive management program.

In this chapter, we will present a brief outline of the scope of the obesity problem that we face as health care providers and the criteria that are required for patient eligibility for weight loss surgery. We will describe the components of a successful, comprehensive bariatric program including essential staff, ancillary personnel, material infrastructure, and educational and patient support strategies.

OVERVIEW OF ETIOLOGY AND EPIDEMIOLOGY
OF MORBID OBESITY

Obesity is increasing in epidemic proportions worldwide. Even mild degrees of obesity have adverse health effects and are associated with diminished longevity. For this reason aggressive dietary intervention is recommended. Patients with body mass indices exceeding 40 have medically significant obesity in which the risk of serious health consequences is substantial, with concomitant significant reductions in life expectancy. For these patients, sustained weight loss rarely occurs with dietary intervention. For the appropriately selected patients, surgery is beneficial. Surgical treatment is associated with sustained weight loss for obese patients who uniformly fail non-surgical treatment. Following weight loss there is a high resolution rate for diabetes and sleep apnea, with significant decreases in other comorbidities of obesity such as hypertension and osteoarthritis (3).

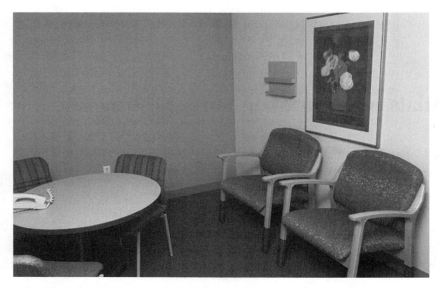

Figure 1 Bariatric clinic office furniture. Chairs are oversized.

Morbid obesity is reaching epidemic proportions in the United States. Since 1960, surveys of the prevalence of obesity have been conducted every decade by the National Center for Health Statistics. Twenty-five percent of adult Americans were overweight in 1980 compared to 34% as of 1990. Presently over 58 million adult Americans (one-third of the adult population) are overweight. Approximately four million Americans have a body mass index between 35 and $40 \, \text{kg/m}^2$. An additional four million have a body mass index exceeding $40 \, \text{kg/m}^2$. Despite the expenditure of over 30 billion dollars annually on weight-loss products, the prevalence of obesity is increasing. Obesity is most common in minorities, low-income groups, and women. Nearly half of African-American, Mexican-American, and Native-American women are overweight (4).

CRITERIA FOR SELECTION OF PATIENTS FOR BARIATRIC SURGERY

Not all individuals who are obese or who consider themselves overweight are candidates for bariatric surgery. Patients with body mass index of $40 \, \text{kg/m}^2$ or more, or those with a body mass index of $35 \, \text{kg/m}^2$ or more and co-morbidity are generally eligible for bariatric surgery. They must have attempted weight loss in the past by medically supervised diet regimens, exercise, or medications. Furthermore, they must be motivated to comply with postoperative dietary and exercise regimens and follow-up. Traditionally, surgeons offered obesity surgery to patients aged 18 to 60 years. However, bariatric surgery is now offered to older adults at some institutions, with no increase in morbidity or mortality. Adolescent patients with morbid obesity may be considered for bariatric surgery under select circumstances. The patient must be committed to the appropriate work-up for the procedure and for continuing long-term postoperative medical management. He or she must be cognizant of the potential perioperative complications, and every effort is made to eliminate the occurrence of any undesired

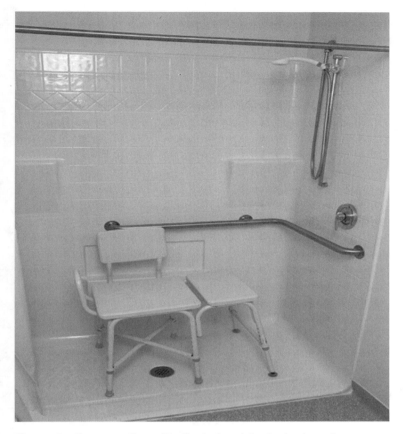

Figure 2 Shower stall specifically designed for bariatric patients.

outcomes. Screening of the patients to ensure appropriate selection is a critical responsibility of the surgeon and the supporting health care team.

Patients who are unable to undergo general anesthesia because of cardiac, pulmonary, or hepatic disease, or those who are unwilling or unable to comply with postoperative lifestyle changes, diet, supplementation, or follow-up, are considered unsuitable candidates.

COMPONENTS OF A BARIATRIC SURGERY PROGRAM

Personnel

Dietary Evaluation

There is a growing movement among bariatric surgeons to consider themselves metabolic surgeons, in recognition of the preponderantly beneficial metabolic effects that result from either restrictive or malabsorptive operations. Malnutrition, however, is an undesirable outcome that is associated with all bariatric operations, particularly of the malabsorptive type. It is largely preventable if proper patient selection, thorough preoperative nutritional education, and postoperative nutritional follow-up are incorporated in the program. A well-known characteristic of all surgical options is

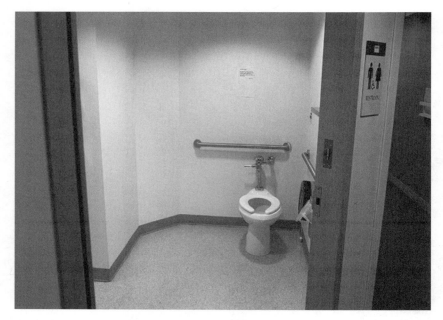

Figure 3 Bathroom with floor mounted commode and wide entrance.

the complete elimination of appetite, at least for the first six months after surgery. Although this is a facilitating feature of the operations, patients will often forget to eat and will require reminders to take in sustenance. Patients and family members should be made aware of this side effect. The dumping syndrome is an additional,

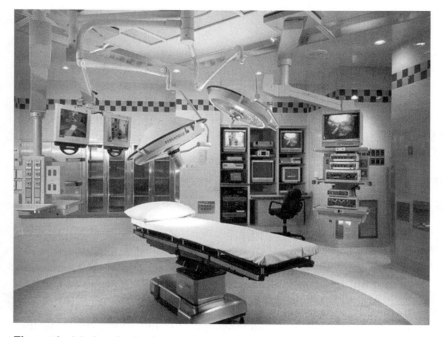

Figure 4 Modern bariatric operating room.

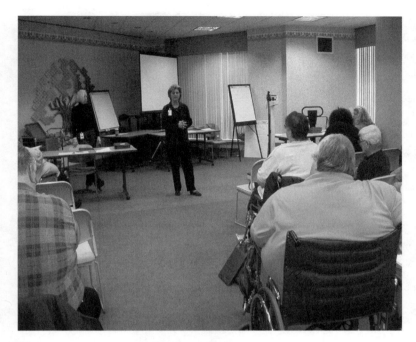

Figure 5 Preoperative educational workshop.

often considered beneficial, effect of operations that are designed to bypass the duodenum. Patients must be made aware of this phenomenon and understand its causes and, more importantly, how to avoid precipitating its occurrence.

Of all the food elements, proteins are the most valuable and essential. Patients' dietary regimens must meet their daily requirements for these nutrients. Nutritional counselors are trained to deliver advice on the proper identification of protein sources and the preparation of foodstuffs to render them more palatable. They will also advise patients on proper chewing and swallowing techniques, and give tips on how to avoid consuming liquids concomitantly with solids. Patients are required to know the hazards of insufficient fluid intake and are counseled to imbibe through the day, pausing before meals. The daily administration of vitamins and supplements is a critical requisite for postoperative patients and it is incumbent on surgeons to ensure that patients are meeting their nutritional needs. Surgeons have been held liable for complications of vitamin deficiencies, particularly neurological manifestations that may result from inadequate intake. The provision of appropriate access to nutritional counselors and opportunities for periodic laboratory assessment of nutritional parameters may reduce the occurrence of these indefensible and undesirable outcomes.

An additional important role for nutritional counselors is the assessment of a candidate's ability to comply with the required dietary modifications imposed by bariatric surgery. Patients should have an appreciable degree of motivation to accept and reliably follow dietary guidelines, and should have a minimum level of understanding of the potential repercussions of non-adherence. Nutritionists are in an ideal position to gauge patients' eligibility and compliance from a cognitive and motivational perspective.

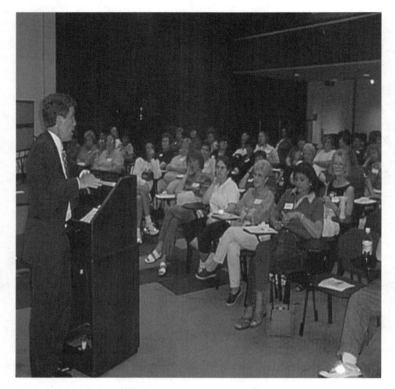

Figure 6 Support groups.

Psychological Evaluation

Unlike the nutritional component of any comprehensive bariatric program, an integral psychological support is less critical. Many successful programs do not count psychologists as basic members of their staff, and patients are often referred to "outside" mental health specialists for evaluation. Nevertheless, psychological support for the morbidly obese patient is essential. Morbidly obese patients often carry a diagnosis of depression, anxiety, and other stress-related conditions. There are often problems with body image and with low and demoralized self-esteem. Psychologists offer invaluable support in assessing patients' mental conditions and counsel the patient to withstand the lifelong changes imposed by bariatric surgery. Several instruments for psychological assessment of morbidly obese patients in the preoperative and postoperative periods have been developed and validated, and are in wide use. The Moorehead-Ardelt questionnaire is an example of such a tool that is in wide use (5).

Pre- and postoperative education of patients presenting for weight-loss surgery is more critical as compared to that of patients preparing for non-bariatric surgery. For example, knowledge of the "rules of eating" and the "rules of vomiting" is essential for the positive outcome of gastric restrictive surgery (6). However, although outcome predictors are not quite understood, it is recognized that patient knowledge, psychosocial adaptation, and motivational factors including secondary gain and other benefits of not remaining obese are important. Discrepancies between patients' weight goals, "ideal" or healthy weight for post-obese individuals and realistic weight loss based on body composition and energy balance, contribute to subjective assessment of quality of life after bariatric surgery. Well-designed observational studies that are both ethically and scientifically valid are needed to improve patient selection (6).

It is common for bariatric patients to experience postoperative nausea, depression, and possibly remorse for several months following surgery. Many patients who successfully lose weight experience jealousy from close friends and relatives. Difficulty exists for the surgeon in delineating the physical from the psychological etiologies of many postoperative symptoms that afflict patients. Preoperative education, evaluation, and preparation, although essential, will not identify nor eliminate all the potential problems. Psychological intervention is sometimes useful in achieving overall patient stability and emotional well-being, thereby underscoring its important role throughout the entire course of a patient's treatment experience (7).

Expert Consultants

Morbidly obese patients often have associated comorbid factors that negatively affect quality of life, and often pose a significant risk on a day-to-day basis. Additionally, if unrecognized or inappropriately managed, these factors may be a cause of perioperative complications. Serious medical conditions associated with morbid obesity include cardiovascular, pulmonary, endocrine, metabolic, hematological, and many other diseases (Table 1). The availability of consultants and experts in these fields is critical. These individuals should be familiar with the particular pathophysiologic consequences of morbid obesity, and should be able to ascertain with a certain degree of confidence the eligibility of candidates to withstand the rigors of major surgery and the required physical demands on patients in the postoperative period. Such consultants should be proficient in adequately preparing patients for general anesthesia, particularly regarding cardiac and pulmonary reserve, and the implementation of special preoperative patient training for those afflicted with sleep apnea. Patients with life-threatening myocardial ischemia should be revascularized prior to weight-loss surgery. These experts need to be readily available both in the immediate postoperative period and in the long term, should circumstances demand their presence.

All patients should undergo extensive evaluation prior to weight-loss surgery. Careful initial history taking and clinical examinations will guide clinicians to diagnose hitherto unrecognized diseases. By following appropriate algorithms and considering particular risk factors, many known and undiagnosed conditions can be evaluated, not in an attempt to discourage or prevent operations, but with the goal of fully optimizing surgical outcomes by taking special perioperative precautions and additional supportive measures.

Anesthesiology for Bariatric Surgery

Just as pediatric patients are not merely "little people," morbidly obese patients are not typical patients who happen to be very large. Failure to fully appreciate the sequelae of morbid obesity will result in unacceptable morbidity and mortality.

Anesthesiologists who are charged with managing bariatric patients undergoing major surgery should be experienced in diagnosing and treating immediate or imminent life-threatening conditions, such as a difficult airway, hypoventilation syndrome, sleep apnea, congestive heart failure, renal insufficiency, venous thrombo-embolism,

Table 1 Diseases Coexisting with Morbid Obesity and Requiring Preoperative
Multidisciplinary Evaluation

System/organ/discipline	Disease related to obesity
Cardiovascular	Arterial hypertension
	Chronic venous insufficiency
	Leg ulcers difficult to treat
	Deep venous thrombosis
	Pulmonary thrombo-embolism
	Peripheral edema
	Cardiac dysrhythmia
	Arteriosclerosis
	Ischemic heart disease
	Ventricular volume overload
	High cardiac output
	Increased oxygen consumption
	Pulmonary hypertension
	Peripheral vascular disease
Respiratory	Asthma
	Sleep apnea
	Chronic obstructive pulmonary disease
	Asthmatic bronchitis
	Dyspnea and fatigue
	Picwickian syndrome
	Pulmonary embolism
	Reduced vital capacity, total lung capacity, and expiratory reserve volume
Metabolic and endocrine	Non-insulin-dependent diabetes mellitus
	Dyslipidemia
	Hypertriglicerydemia
	Hypercholesterolemia
	Glucose intolerance
	Decreased serum testosterone
	Increased serum estradiol and estrone
	Plasma cortisol reduced or increased
	Diminished growth hormone secretion in response to hypoglycemia
	Hirsutism
Musculoskeletal	Osteoarthritis and arthralgias
	Degenerative joint disease
	Scoliosis, kyphosis, hyperlordosis
	Hyperuricemia
	Gout
	Abdominal wall hernias
Gastrointestinal	Gallstones
	Cirrhosis of the liver
	Gastroesophageal reflux disease (GERD)
	Hepatic steatosis
	Colon carcinoma
	Hepatic fibrosis
	Accelerated transit of nutrients and rapid intestinal absorption

(*Continued*)

Table 1 Diseases Coexisting with Morbid Obesity and Requiring Preoperative Multidisciplinary Evaluation (*Continued*)

System/organ/discipline	Disease related to obesity
Dermatology	Intertriginous dermatitis
	Acanthosis nigricans
	Fungal skin infections
Neurology	Pseudotumor cerebri
	Migraine headache
	Wernicke-Korsakoff syndrome (very uncommon)
	Peripheral neuropathy (very uncommon)
Psychiatry	Depression
	Anxiety
	Somnolence
Genitourinary and reproductive	Urinary stress incontinence
	Infertility problems
	Endometrial hyperplasia and endometrial carcinoma
	Breast carcinoma
	Prostate carcinoma
	Hypogonadic hypogonadism
	Obstetric complications
	Polycystic ovary syndrome
	Focal glomerulosclerosis
	Diabetic nephropathy
	Menstrual abnormalities
	Anovulatory cycles
	Dysfunctional uterine bleeding
	Early menopause
	Eclampsia and pre-eclampsia
	Gestational diabetes
	Average length of labor
	Need for cesarean section
Socio-economic and other medical	Educative, labor, and social discrimination
	Social isolation
	Loss of self-esteem
	Stressful mobilization and immobility
	Accident propensity

to name a few. Those anesthesiologists who will manage bariatric patients undergoing laparoscopic operations must be cognizant of the pulmonary and hemodynamic changes that occur upon establishing and maintaining prolonged pneumoperitoneum. These are cases that are not to be taken lightly and certainly not to be delegated to inexperienced staff. Special consideration of these facts should be taken when selecting anesthesiology staff. There should, at all times, be more than one experienced anesthesiology staff member available, or he or she should be assisted by qualified, similarly experienced, anesthesia nursing personnel.

The collaboration of experienced bariatric surgeons and anesthesiologists represents a powerful intellectual combination that greatly benefits patients. Perioperative recommendations by "bariatric" anesthesiologists are invaluable in promoting favorable outcomes in patient safety and comfort.

Preoperative Workshops and Support Groups

Although bariatric surgery has been practiced for several decades, it remains an evolving discipline. Many biological features of the metabolic, endocrine, nutritional, and psychological manifestations of morbid obesity are just now being revealed. Patients undergo dramatic changes in almost every aspect, often by unclear mechanisms. There is, however, a constant accrual of voluminous information as more research is expended on this growing field. Understandably, morbidly obese patients considering weight-loss surgery, or who are recovering from these operations, often possess insatiable appetites for information. Although all members of a bariatric surgery program should be reasonably abreast of established and emerging knowledge, it is incumbent on the physicians to assume the role of experts in the scientific aspects of bariatric medicine. Physicians, and their physician assistants and nurses, represent an invaluable reference source to patients. Their information is best delivered in a group setting where discussion can flow freely between inquisitive patients (and their family members) and bariatric program personnel. Informal group settings provide the most efficient method of disseminating information. Two examples of effective group activities are the preoperative educational workshops and the support groups.

The Preoperative Educational Workshop

The primary purpose of the preoperative educational workshop is to gain information. This is a mutually beneficial exercise between prospective patients and bariatric program health providers. Patients gain acquaintance, in a broad sense, with the scheme of the program, the pathway they will follow in their preoperative evaluation, the inherent features that pertain to different laparoscopic and open operations, the risks and benefits of each procedure, and the importance of adhering to feeding and exercise guidelines. Particular emphasis is placed on the need for lifelong follow-up and periodic assessment of nutritional parameters. Program health providers, on the other hand, perform initial evaluations of the patients, review their nutritional and medical backgrounds, and consider patients' eligibility for surgery. Patients who are deemed to require specialist work-ups are appropriately referred. The duration of these workshops is usually a half-day and preferably includes informative presentations by the program staff with audio-visual aids and printed material for future review. Family members should be encouraged to attend. Patients and their family members should be given ample opportunity to participate in a dedicated free-flowing discussion.

Support Groups

Support groups are designed for patients who are in the recovery phase of their operations. Although prospective patients are encouraged to attend, these sessions should be primarily targeted to addressing medical, nutritional, psychological, and social issues experienced by postoperative patients. Patients undergo dramatic changes that affect every sphere of life, some of which may be difficult to accept. Patients greatly benefit from the tips and advice delivered by more experienced patients and from the program staff. Additional gain may be achieved by holding informal educational lectures, in lay terms, by a variety of invited speakers. It is important that these support group sessions be consistently attended by members

Table 2 Goals of Preoperative Patient Education and Teaching

Encouragement for compliance and praise for success
Education about life after surgery, including nutrition, exercise and dieting techniques
Identification of problems
Identification and development of new kinds of self-nurturing
Participation in a forum where others really "understand" the challenges and difficulties
    associated with "change," even when the change is for the better
Creation of a friendly, safe atmosphere where patients can bring spouses, parents, and
    significant others so that they may also understand, encourage continuing success, and
    recognize their own personal issues related to the major changes that they are also
    experiencing with their loved one
Opportunity for curious potential patients in the community to come and learn from the
    "experts" in an atmosphere of true caring and concern

of the bariatric program staff to act as moderators, and to monitor the discussion so as to ensure that false information or misconceptions are not disseminated.

Following bariatric surgery, the inclusion of a support group as part of the treatment plan makes after-care easier and more efficient for the patients, as well as for the physicians. Table 2 outlines the elements required for the education of patients for achieving effective after-care.

HOSPITAL REQUIREMENTS

It is inconceivable that any bariatric surgery program can be established without the full support and commitment of the health care institution within which it resides. The decision to initiate and nurture a bariatric program represents a major shift in paradigm of standard hospitals. Commitment towards achieving a safe and successful bariatric program includes the adoption of a holistic, institution-wide acceptance of the responsibilities required for a project of this magnitude. There must be a generalized intellectual acceptance of morbid obesity as a disease. All staff, including administrative and non-medical personnel, must recognize obese patients as special individuals with specific needs. Only in an atmosphere of total institutional commitment can bariatric programs flourish. Once this fundamental attitude is achieved, efforts are then placed on creating the material infrastructure necessary for a bariatric program.

Morbidly obese patients must feel welcome upon entering an institution. These patients must be accommodated with appropriate furniture in the waiting areas and examination rooms. Weight scales, sphygmomanometer cuffs, and other paraphernalia used to manage patients should be appropriately sized. The same applies for hospital clothing, hospital beds, wheelchairs, doorways, and toilet facilities. This principle should extend to all areas that patients attend, such as laboratories and radiology suites.

The operating-room environment should be designed with the supreme concern for the safety of the morbidly obese patient. Investing in stretchers and operating tables that can accommodate these patients exemplify this. Operating on morbidly obese patients requires the possession of adequate instruments and lighting equipment. Clearly, the safety of operating-room staff is equally important, and the recent availability of powered air mattresses (Hovermat) for patient transfer practically eliminates the occurrence of lower back injuries.

As mentioned above, there needs to be a generalized commitment toward achieving a successful bariatric program, and this must include provisions for managing the complicated morbidly obese patient. Intensive care units should be prepared to accept these patients and should be in possession of the appropriate staff and equipment to treat challenging obese patients. Radiology suites must have modalities that are able to accommodate heavy and wide patients. This pertains to all imaging equipment including CT scanners and image intensifiers. These are essential minimal requirements, and the prudent bariatric program director will not initiate a program in their absence.

BARIATRIC SURGERY DATABASE

An important requirement for any bariatric program is the ability to maintain a repository of information that includes patient demographics, co-morbid factors, operative characteristics, and follow-up. Such a database will prove to be an invaluable resource for both clinical and research purposes. Ideally, patients will be followed for life and there will occasionally be the need for rapid access to patient information. By collating and sorting data, a well-maintained database will demonstrate past program performance and help predict future trends. The periodic interrogation of the database allows an intelligent analysis of patient outcomes, thereby indicating program components that may require special attention. There are several commercial databases that have been specifically created for bariatric programs, and any of these represent a worthy investment.

BARIATRIC SURGERY PROGRAM WEB SITE

The ability to instantly obtain information on any topic is the result of the tremendous advancements made in the field of cyber technology. This achievement, however, is a double-edged sword. Internet content is not regulated or controlled. For the most part, web sites that are obesity-related are beneficial and informative, but there are sites that do disseminate erroneous and false information.

For this reason, it is highly advisable to invest in creating an electronic onsite resource that accurately reflects the mission and purpose of the bariatric surgery program. Such a web site should, in lay terms, contain an explanation of the problems of obesity and the available medical and surgical solutions. It should describe the physical and personnel set-up of the program, and the preoperative and postoperative pathways patients will follow. Additionally, it would be of great benefit for the web site to possess the ability to accept initial patient application forms electronically, to be used as a basic screening tool prior to inviting the patient for the educational workshop. A chat room for patients and/or an area where patients could directly contact the surgery program personnel may result in a modality that is more efficient and practical than relying on conventional telephonic arrangements.

CONCLUSION

As the worldwide epidemic of obesity continues its exponential growth, the demand on surgeons to safely and effectively treat patients with this disease will strengthen accordingly. Because morbid obesity is a disease that globally affects patients, it can only be managed by a diverse group of skilled individuals, all of whom are united in the common purpose of its eradication. The aim of surgical solutions should be permanent weight loss, and this will require the prolonged services of bariatricians, nutritionists, physical therapists, perhaps even spiritual healers and marriage counselors. The fact is, there has to be a comprehensive program in place to be able to fully evaluate prospective patients, and to prepare them mentally and physically for the rigors of surgery and permanent lifestyle changes they will need to adopt. Such a comprehensive program requires dedicated personnel, a strong fundamental infrastructure, and total institutional commitment. Most important of all, there needs to be a pervasive philosophy that stretches across all institutional departments, and that accepts morbid obesity as a disease process, the management of which is a noble and dramatically rewarding mission.

REFERENCES

1. Mokdad AH, Ford ES, Bowman BA, Dietz WH, Vinicor F, Bales VS, Marks JS. Prevalence of obesity, diabetes, and obesity-related health risk factors, 2001. JAMA 2003; 289(1):76–79.
2. International Food Information Council Foundation. Trends in obesity-related media coverage, 2003 (http://www.ific.org/research/obesitytrends.cfm).
3. Livingston EH. Obesity and its surgical management. Am J Surg 2002; 184(2):103–113.
4. Kuczmarski RJ, Flegal KM, Campbell SM, Johnson CL. Increasing prevelance of overweight among US adults. The National Health and Nutrition Examination Surveys, 1960 to 1991. JAMA 1994; 272(3):205–211.
5. DiGregoria JM, Moorehead MK. The psychology of bariatric surgery. Obes Surg 1994; 4(4):361–369.
6. Kral JG. Selection of patients for anti-obesity surgery. Int J Obes Relat Metab Disord 2001; 25(suppl 1):S107–S112.
7. Higa KD, Ho T, Boone KB, Roubicek MC. Narcotic withdrawal syndrome following gastric bypass—a difficult diagnosis. Obes Surg 2001; 11(5):631–634.

6

Nutrition and Roux-en-Y Gastric Bypass Surgery

Jeanne Blankenship and Bruce Wolfe
Department of Surgery, University of California Davis School of Medicine, Sacramento, California, U.S.A.

INTRODUCTION

Nutrition assessment and dietary management in surgical weight loss is thought to be an important correlate of success. In the simplest explanation, obesity is the result of an imbalance in energy intake versus expenditure. While obese individuals are over-nourished from an energy standpoint, sufficient evidence exists that certain micronutrient deficiencies are more common in the overweight. The incongruity in nutrition status despite adequate intake must be explored preoperatively with a comprehensive nutrition assessment conducted by a dietitian, physician, or a well-informed nurse practitioner or physician assistant. In addition to assessing the nutrition status of the surgical candidate, the psychosocial aspects of nutrition along with general nutrition knowledge should be evaluated. This chapter will describe a comprehensive approach to the nutrition management of both surgical candidates and postoperative patients, focusing on Roux-en-Y gastric bypass (RYGB).

PRE-SURGICAL NUTRITION ASSESSMENT AND MANAGEMENT

Pre-surgical assessment of nutrition status includes the evaluation of anthropometric, biochemical, clinical, and dietary intake data (1). The accurate heights of all patients should be measured rather than relying on self-reported data. In addition to weight, excess body weight (EBW) should be calculated. EBW is defined as the difference between ideal body weight (IBW) and current body weight. Different methods for determining IBW are listed in Table 1. The percent change in EBW is thought to be more reflective of surgical impact post-operative than weight loss expressed in pounds alone (2). Informing patients that historically surgical weight loss patients lose approximately 60% to 70% EBW (3) is important in helping establish realistic long-term weight loss goals and expectations prior to surgery. Studies suggest that with appropriate patient selection, education, and long-term follow-up,

Table 1 Methods Used for Determining Ideal Body Weight (IBW)

1. Hamwai equation		
a. Women	1st 5 feet	Allow 100 lbs and add 5 lbs/inch
Small frame subtract 10%		
Large frame add 10%		
b. Men	1st 5 feet	Allow 106 lbs and add 5 lbs/inch
Small frame subtract 10%		
Large frame add 10%		
2. BMI equal to 24		
3. Metropolitan Life tables		

up to 80% of patients will have successful weight loss of >50% of EBW at two years (4).

In addition to height and weight measurements used to calculate body mass index (BMI), many centers collect a waist circumference measurement, though its application with BMIs $\geq 35\,kg/m^2$ may not be any more predictive of a disease risk than BMI alone in the morbidly obese (5). Skinfold measurements to assess visceral protein stores are not routinely used in clinical practice due to time constraints in conjunction with the technical challenges of accurately collecting reliable data from obese subjects. Body composition analysis using bioelectrical impedance or alternate methods can be useful in determining lean mass and fat mass before and after surgery (6).

Biochemical analysis should include nutrition markers to assess pre-surgical status as described in Table 2. Laboratory studies should also include markers that are specific to the individual. For example, if the individual has followed a low-calorie diet or modified macronutrient intake without vitamin supplementation for an extended period of time, there is a potential risk of vitamin B deficiency, thereby indicating the need for laboratory assessment of nutrients thought to be absent or impacted by restricted intake.

Clinical observation of the distribution of body fat along with other signs of malnutrition including visual assessment of hair, nails, and skin is appropriate (1).

Table 2 Common Preoperative Laboratory Tests to Assess Nutrition

A comprehensive metabolic panel to include:		
	Albumin	Calcium
	Total protein	Bilirubin
	Phosphorus	Glucose
A complete blood count:	Hemoglobin	Hematocrit
	MCV	MCH
Additional studies:	Glycosylated hemoglobin (HgbAIC)	
	Lipid panel	
	Vitamin B12	
	Homocysteine	
	Iron studies (ferritin, total iron, TIBC)	
	TSH	
	PTH	
	Vitamin D (25, hydroxyvitamin D)	

Table 3 Complications and Nutrition Management

Complication	Evaluation	Nutrition management
Anastomotic leak	Upper GI Clinical presentation	NPO; G-tube feed into remnant or TPN
Dehydration	Orthostatic blood pressure Electrolyte panel Elimination patterns Classic symptoms	Resucitation/IV fluids, 48–64 oz fluids/day; fluids may need the addition of sodium or other solute
Wound infection/ dehiscence	CBC with differential Clinical presentation	Protein/calorie adjustment, fluid adjustment, additional vitamin C, zinc, and arginine
Stricture/stomal stenosis	Gastric emptying study Vomiting	Clear liquid protein with gradual advancement; consider TPN if prolonged (dilatation after three months)
Marginal ulcer	History of nausea/ vomiting Epigastric pain Bloody emesis	Small frequent meals usually better tolerated after antibiotics; acid blocker or inhibitor
Persistent nausea and vomiting	Early: rule out leak Rule out pregnancy, stricture, ulcer and infection	Monitor thiamine status, 100 mg IV thiamine before IV glucose administration; ensure frequent feeds and limited simple carbohydrate; avoid lactose if necessary; adjust temperature of liquids.
Alopecia/hair loss	Hair loss Low Zn, total protein, albumin	Ensure protein intake; monitor lab values

Clinical evaluation of patients who are athletic or muscular is an important consideration in the use of BMI classifications Table 3.

Dietary intake and physical activity information can be collected using 24-hour recall, food frequency, or other diet and activity records. Intake questionnaires should include questions that allow the practitioner to uncover disordered eating patterns including anorexia nervosa, binge eating, and bulimia nervosa. While a history of disordered eating does not preclude surgery, it can be a trigger to address psychosocial or psychological needs and interventions in an attempt to improve surgical outcomes (7–9). Assessment of intake should identify food group omissions (such as dairy and starches/grains) or other dietary practices and customs that place the individual at risk for nutrient deficiency. A detailed history of weight-loss attempts including successes and failures is also an important component of pre-surgical nutrition assessment and documentation (10). The National Institutes of Health (NIH) guidelines for surgery recommend that only patients who demonstrate failed medical management of their obesity pursue surgical intervention (11). In a retrospective review of 181 subjects, Ray et al. (12) noted that multiple attempts at weight loss prior to surgery were correlated with improved outcomes. Specifically, the more attempts or "practice runs" a patient had before surgery, the more likely that he or she achieved surgical weight loss success (>50% EBW loss).

Some programs now require patients to lose a portion of EBW prior to surgery, a practice which was endorsed and recommended by an expert panel on weight-loss surgery despite a lack of objective evidence in support of such a requirement (13). Third-party payers may also require a defined period of conventional weight management prior to surgery to confirm that medical management has, in fact, failed. The specific criteria for insurance approval vary widely, and reflect a lack of consensus between surgeons and coverage authors regarding the validity of pre-surgical weight-loss requirements. While there may be a theoretical advantage in terms of surgical risks, there may also be behavioral change benefits that foster better outcomes. A recent report suggests that pre-surgical weight loss results in a decrease in liver size which would possibly make surgical exposure easier in a laparoscopic environment (14). The use of commercial products in a series of 100 patients found that an average weight loss of 17 kg was both achievable and safe (15). However, the most effective means by which such pre-surgical weight loss should be achieved and its correlate to long-term weight-loss maintenance remain unknown. It is well known that a 5–10% reduction in body weight significantly improves many comorbid conditions, and may result in at least a transient discontinuation of medications prescribed for polycystic ovarian syndrome (PCOS), hypertension, type 2 diabetes and dyslipidemia (16). One researcher observed that patients ($n = 40$) who were not required to control weight prior to surgery had an average weight gain of 4.3 kg, however this research has not been conducted to date in a randomized controlled setting (17). While weight-loss requirements are controversial, many programs propose that at minimum, weight maintenance should be encouraged. Other surgeons argue that a prolonged attempt at weight loss that delays surgical intervention may place patients with significant comorbid conditions at a greater risk than any benefit that would be achieved with minimal weight loss.

Finally, the patient's readiness to make the behavioral changes required with regard to diet and exercise must be evaluated and documented (18). This evaluation should include reasons for seeking surgical weight loss, a history of previous diet attempts, a review of the patient's support system, and an examination of the patient's attitude and beliefs with regard to lifestyle and physical activity. Many of the same challenges that patients experience with conventional weight-loss methods resurface after the initial phase of weight-loss surgery. It is therefore important to identify personal barriers for each individual and to provide anticipatory guidance whenever possible (1).

PRE-SURGICAL NUTRITION EDUCATION

During the preoperative process, nutrition education should include early and late dietary guidelines. While patients may be most concerned about the immediate post-operative diet phases and adjustment to food intolerances, considerable attention should be given to long-term strategies required for successful weight-loss maintenance. Patients must be well informed with regard to the diet implications for surgery including the possibility of chronic macro- and micronutrient malabsorption and failure to lose weight. Since most potential vitamin deficiencies can be prevented with consistent and adequate supplementation, the patients should be educated in this area and should agree to follow the prescribed dietary regimen, preferably by signing either a contract or by agreeing as part of the surgical consent process.

Self-monitoring techniques described in the literature as being useful in long-term weight-loss maintenance should be introduced and thoroughly explained to prospective patients. These include eating a low-fat diet, frequent self-monitoring of weight and intake, and high levels of physical activity (19). Patients may have difficulty keeping accurate food records or measuring portion sizes, and need coaching from the dietitian in order to employ these skills. The concept of "self care" such as that used as a tool for diabetes management can be similarly applied to weight-loss surgery. While it is important to assess the patient's understanding of the changes required to be successful postoperatively, the application of such principles demonstrates the ability to make lifestyle change.

POSTOPERATIVE DIET GUIDELINES

Many programs suggest a multi-phase approach to postoperative nutrition. One common progression employs clear liquids for one to three days with a gradual advancement to a high-protein full liquid diet for one to two weeks. Patients are then advanced to a pureed or semi-soft diet and finally to a regular diet by approximately eight weeks after surgery (20). The diet progression, while commonly used, is not supported by the nutrition or surgical literature as being more effective than solid foods with regard to weight loss or the prevention of complications after bariatric surgery. Some programs advocate rapid diet advancement to regular food.

A literature review by Heymsfield et al. found that meal replacements are an important consideration in medical weight loss (21). At 12 months after weight loss, the meal replacement group (n = 249) demonstrated a 7–8% weight loss while those who utilized a reduced-calorie meal plan were found to have a 3–7% weight loss (n = 239). Moreover, 74% of subjects in the meal replacement group had maintained >5% weight loss while only 33% of those on a low-calorie diet maintained a similar loss. Kawamura et al. studied pre-surgical patients placed on a modified protein fast that consisted of either a commercial liquid regimen or food products, and found that there were some clinical benefits of the liquid formula. These included changes in lipid profiles and measures of nitrogen balance (22). The long-term or post-surgical implications of using meal replacements are not known. Natural food products may be associated with early satiety and with an unpredictable macronutrient distribution. The use of whole foods relies upon patient knowledge and application to adhere to caloric and protein recommendations. The role of meal replacements in bariatric surgery warrants additional investigation.

Clinical practice recommendations for protein intake following surgery are consistent with those made for medically supervised modified protein fasts and for reduced calorie diets. Experts recommend 65 to 70 g/day during weight loss and very low calorie diets (VLCDs). The recommended dietary allowance (RDA) for protein ranges from 50 to 60 g/day for normal adults (23). Many programs recommend a range of 60–80 grams per day or 1.0 to 1.5 g/kg ideal body weight, although exact needs have yet to be defined. The use of 1.5 g/kg for Roux-en-Y patients beyond the early post-surgical phase is probably above metabolic requirements and prevents the consumption of other macronutrients in the context of volume restrictions. Following duodenal switch or BPD procedures, the amount of protein should be increased by ~30% to accommodate for malabsorption as will be later described (24).

One common myth is that only 30 g of protein can be absorbed per hour. While this is commonly found in both lay and some professional literature, there is no scientific basis for this claim. It is possible that from a volume stand-point, patients may only realistically consume 30 grams per meal during the first year. Supplements are commercially available that can be used to meet the protein needs after surgery. The highest quality proteins are whey protein isolates, ion exchange whey protein, whey hydrolysate, or whey peptides which contain high levels of branched-chain amino acids important to prevent lean tissue breakdown. Supplements that contain whey protein concentrate may contain significant amounts of lactose and should be avoided by individuals with intolerance. Meal replacement supplements typically contain higher levels of vitamins and minerals than simple protein supplements, as well as additional fiber.

Bariatric surgery patients follow VLCDs as a result of restrictive measures; most individuals will consume between 400 and 800 kcal in the early postoperative period. Very little is known about the long-term caloric needs of gastric bypass patients. A 1000- to 1200-calorie intake in one series ($n = 22$) was noted at one year (25). A gradual increase in calories over the first year postoperative resulted from the return of carbohydrate and lipid sources to the diet. A survey by Warde-Kamar et al. (26) found that the average daily caloric intake for 69 patients at least 18 months out from surgery was 1733, but ranged from 624 to 3486 calories. Correlates with caloric intake and weight maintenance were not provided. Changes in diet quality and caloric intake and their relationship to successful weight loss and maintenance are areas that require scientific research.

NUTRIENT ABSORPTION AND DEFICIENCY

The mechanisms by which surgical weight-loss procedures facilitate weight loss in the morbidly obese vary by procedure. In general, procedures are described as being malabsorptive, restrictive or a combination of the two. Studies have been published that address the impact of such procedures on acute and long-term nutritional status. These studies have attempted, for the most part, to indirectly determine the surgical impact on nutrition status by the evaluation of metabolic and laboratory markers rather than by evaluating actual absorption.

Nutrient deficiencies after gastric bypass can result from either primary or secondary malabsorption or from inadequate dietary intake. Malabsorptive procedures such as the duodenal switch are thought to cause weight loss primarily through the malabsorption of macronutrients; however, such primary malabsorption results in concomitant malabsorption of micronutrients. Similarly, there is thought to be a minimal amount of macronutrient malabsorption with combination procedures such as the RYGB. There are, however, specific micronutrients that appear to be malabsorbed postoperatively and present as deficiencies without adequate vitamin and mineral supplementation. Purely restrictive procedures such as the adjustable gastric band (AGB) may also result in micronutrient deficiencies related to changes in dietary intake. It is commonly accepted that because there is no alteration in the absorptive pathway, malabsorption does not occur as a result AGB procedures.

MALABSORPTIVE PROCEDURES

The duodenal switch involves bypassing a large section of the small intestine leaving only 75–100 cm in the common channel. The result is that protein, fat, and carbohydrate absorption is negatively impacted. Early work by Scopinaro et al. found that only 28% of ingested fat (24) and 75% of ingested protein (27) are absorbed after biliopancreatic diversion procedures. Subjects frequently report bouts of diarrhea and steatorrhea most notably related to fat malabsorption. It reasons that fat-soluble vitamins including vitamin A, vitamin D, vitamin E and to a lesser extent vitamin K are poorly absorbed after this procedure. Two bariatric surgery centers collaborated to review the incidence of fat-soluble vitamin deficiency after malabsorptive surgery in supplemented patients who were at least 12 months out from surgery. Their review found that the status of vitamin A, vitamin K, and vitamin D progressively declined over a period of up to four years. At four years, more than 50% of patients were deficient in these nutrients. (28). While this study confirms that deficiencies can exist, it does not measure dietary intake versus absorption. Neither pre-surgical vitamin status nor nutrient intake was measured for these patients making it unreasonable to imply a true causal relationship. Others have reported, for example, that low vitamin D levels may be associated with obesity per se. Buffington et al. found that in morbidly obese pre-operative females, 62% had low 25-hydroxyvitamin D levels before surgery (29). Pre-surgical status must be considered when evaluating the impacts of the procedure on postoperative nutrition status.

Those vitamins and minerals which rely on fat metabolism may also be affected when absorption is impaired. The decrease in gastrointestinal transit time may also result in secondary malabsorption of a wide range of micronutrients related to limited contact with the brush border. Micronutrient deficiency concerns most commonly reported relate to zinc, iron, vitamin B12, and folate. Slater et al. noted zinc levels were low in over 50% of post-surgical patients at one year and that this number remained similar four years out from surgery (28).

It is unclear as to whether intestinal adaptation occurs and to what degree it impacts both long-term weight maintenance and nutrition status. Adaptation is a compensatory response that follows an abrupt decrease in mucosal surface area that has been well studied in short-bowel patients who require bowel resection (30). The process includes both anatomic and functional changes that increase the gut's digestive and absorptive capacity. While these changes begin to take place in the early postoperative period, total adaptation may take up to three years to complete. Adaptation in gastric bypass has not been considered in absorption or metabolic studies. This consideration may be important even when determining early and late macro- and micronutrient intake recommendations. The impact of pancreatic enzyme replacement therapy on vitamin and mineral absorption in this population is also unknown. Malabsorptive procedures and the specific nutrient concerns are further described elsewhere.

ROUX-en-Y (RYGB)

RYGB is the most commonly performed bariatric surgical procedure in the United States (31). Retrospective analyses of patients who have undergone gastric bypass have revealed predictable nutrient deficiencies including iron, vitamin B12 and folate (25,32–34). Recent case reports have also shown that thiamine deficiency may occur with prolonged postoperative vomiting (35–38). Studies to measure absorption after measured and quantified intake are not found in the literature. It can be hypothesized that the bypassed duodenum and proximal ileum negatively impact nutrient assimilation. Bradley et al. studied patients who had undergone total gastrectomies, the procedure from which the RYGB evolved. The researchers found that the majority of nutritional status changes in patients were most likely due to changes in intake versus malabsorption. These balance studies were conducted in a controlled research setting (39).

Protein Considerations

Protein deficiency (albumin $<3.5\,g/dL$) is not as common following RYGB as it is with malabsorptive procedures. Brolin et al. reported that 13% of patients who underwent a distal RYGB as part of a prospective randomized study were found to have hypoalbuminemia at least two years after surgery. Those with short Roux-limbs ($<150\,cm$) were not found to have decreased albumin levels (40). In another prospective randomized study, protein deficiency was not found in patients who were a mean 43 months out from surgery (41). A retrospective study determined that hypoalbuminemia was negligible (albumin $>4.0\,g/dL$) with a peak incidence at one to two years postoperatively (42). The clinical practice of recommending 60–80 grams per day appears to satisfactorily meet the needs of postoperative patients.

Vitamin B$_1$ (Thiamine)

Several case reports have been noted in both adult and pediatric gastric bypass patients that allude to surgery-related changes in thiamin status (35–38,43). Thiamine is absorbed in the duodenum in an acid milieu and while malabsorption is possible, it is more likely that confounding issues cause occasional of thiamine status. Thiamine status is most readily measured by serum or plasma assays; however, these are less sensitive than erythrocyte transketolase assays in predicting thiamine stores (44). Clinical presentation of thiamine deficiency symptoms is an important observation when patients report frequent vomiting episodes which can lead to acute deficiency. Chang et al. have described acute post-gastric reductionn surgery (APGARS) neuropathy as a "polynutrition multisystem disorder characterized by protracted postoperative vomiting, hyporeflexia, and muscular weakness." In a survey of bariatric surgeons, the incidence was found to be 5.9 cases per 10,000 cases with thiamine deficiency noted in 40% of the cases (45). Late thiamine deficiency could potentially occur with severe restriction of foods high in B-vitamins in conjunction with the surgery and/or with poor compliance with supplementation recommendations. If frequent vomiting is occurring beyond that which is customary, eating disturbances such as bulimia nervosa should be explored along with possible alcohol abuse. Thiamine levels should be assessed preoperatively and then annually in the non-complicated patient.

Vitamin B12 (Cobalamin)

Vitamin B12 deficiency has been frequently reported following RYGB surgery (46–49). One recent study predicted that deficiency will most likely occur seven months after RYGB and 7.9 months after BPD, however non-surgica variables were not explored as many patients may have pre-surgical values near the lower end of the normal range (42). Experts have noted the significance of subclinical deficiency in the low-normal cobalamin range in non-gastric bypass patients who do not exhibit clinical evidence of deficiency. Methylmalonic Acid (MMA) assay is the preferred marker of B12 status, because metabolic changes often precede low cobalamin levels in the progression to deficiency. Serum B12 assays may miss as much as 25% to 30% of B12 deficiencies making it less reliable than MMA (50).

Reliance on red blood cell indices to identify anemias may not be clinically useful as a screen for anemia. Since gastric bypass patients have increased risks for both iron and vitamin B12 deficiencies, measures that are more sensitive than cell size should be employed. MMA and serum B12 levels should be monitored pre-operatively and then annually unless clinical evidence of deficiency exists.

Rhode et al. found that a dosage of 350–600 mcg per day of oral crystalline B12 prevented vitamin B12 deficiency in 95% of patients (51), while an oral dose of 500 mcg was sufficient to overcome an existing deficiency in a similar study (52). While the majority of vitamin B12 in normal adults is absorbed in the ileum in the presence of intrinsic factors, approximately 1% of supplemented B12 will be absorbed passively by surgical weight loss patients given an oral supplement. The vitamin B12 from food sources may be less absorbed in individuals who have had gastric bypass surgery, although boiling the food may enhance absorption. The use of IM injections for vitamin B12 is common but relies on patient compliance with return visits. In addition to using oral supplements, many patients use nasal spray and sublingual sources of vitamin B12.

Iron

Iron deficiency is also common after gastric bypass surgery. Brolin et al. reported that up to 51% of female patients in one series were iron deficient (52). Screening for iron status may include the use of serum ferritin levels. Such levels, however, should not be used to diagnose deficiency. Ferritin is an acute phase reactant and may fluctuate with age, inflammation and infection—including the common cold. Measuring serum iron along with total iron-binding capacity (TIBC) is preferred to determine iron status. Hemoglobin and hematocrit changes reflect late iron-deficient anemia and are less valuable in identifying early anemia. Serum iron along with TIBC should be measured at six months postoperatively since deficiency can occur rapidly, then annually in addition to analyzing a complete blood count (CBC).

Food choices are an important consideration in evaluating and treating iron deficiency since food sources of iron are more bio-available than non-food sources. Post-surgical meal consumption often includes less meat and meat products which are iron-rich foods. Vitamin C may enhance iron absorption of non-heme iron making it a worthy recommendation for inclusion in the diet (53). Women of reproductive age who have menstrual cycles, and adolescents may require additional supplementation of 50 mg of elemental iron per day, although the efficacy of such prophylactic treatment is unknown (52,54). The use of two adult multivitamins or two children's chewable vitamins is customary for low-risk patients. A history of anemia or a change in laboratory values may indicate the need for additional supplementation in conjunction with age and gender, and reproductive considerations.

Folate

While folate malabsorption could potentially occur after gastric bypass surgery, this has not been widely reflected in current research. The use of multivitamin supplements, which commonly contain 400 mcg of folate, appear adequate to correct low levels (52) and prevent folate deficiency. The supplementation of folate above 1000 mcg/day is not recommended due to its potential masking of vitamin B12 deficiency. Homocysteine (Hcy) is thought to be the most sensitive marker of folate status in conjunction with erythrocyte folate (50). The known role of folate status in the development of neural tube defects makes consistent supplementation and monitoring in fertile women an important consideration.

Metabolic Bone Markers

Several studies have attempted to determine the impact of gastric bypass procedures on bone health. These studies have included some components of absorption, but few have included the necessary components to evaluate the absorption of a pre-scribed and monitored diet in a metabolic setting. Calcium is absorbed preferentially in the duodenum which is facilitated by vitamin D in an acid environment. Goode et fal. found that post-menopausal women show evidence of secondary hyper-parathyroidism, elevated bone resorption, and patterns of bone loss after RYGB using urinary markers, consistent with bone degradation. Dietary supplementation with vitamin D and calcium did not affect these measures, but noted that greater supplementation may be beneficial (55).

Secondary elevated parathyroid hormone (PTH) and urinary bone marker levels consistent with increased bone turnover postoperatively were found in one small series ($n = 15$). The subjects were found to have significant changes in total hip, trochanter, and total body bone mineral density (56). Another series (57) found elevated PTH levels in 29% of gastric bypass patients (n = 110). The significance of elevated PTH levels is clearly an important area for future investigation as a component of bone health maintenance in post-surgical patients. Patients who have a history of anti-seizure or glucocorticoid medication use have an increased risk of metabolic bone disease; therefore, close monitoring of these individuals is appropriate.

Supplementation with calcium during all weight loss modalities is critical to preventing bone resorption (56). The preferred form of calcium supplementation is an area of debate in current clinical practice. Studies have found in non-gastric bypass post-menopausal female subjects that calcium citrate decreased markers of bone resorption, but there was no difference in calcium excretion or PTH as compared to calcium carbonate (57). A meta-analysis of calcium bioavailability suggested that calcium citrate is better absorbed than carbonate by 22% to 27% regardless of whether it was taken on an empty stomach or with meals (58). It is appropriate to advise calcium citrate supplementation despite limited evidence, since it could have potential benefit without additional risk.

POST-SURGICAL NUTRITION ASSESSMENT

Assessment of nutrition status in the early postoperative period, at two or three months, at six months, and then annually is recommended. Similar to the pre-surgical assessment, evaluation includes a review of anthropometric, biochemical, and clinical data.

Pre-surgical weight loss and current weight should be compared as a percent weight change and noted with the percent change in EBW. Medications should be reviewed, especially those used to treat hypertension and diabetes which have rapid resolution following surgery. Patients should be encouraged to review all medication requirements with their primary care physician. Although it is outside of the typical nutrition history, the use of contraception in women of child-bearing age should be noted with providing anticipatory guidance to avoid pregnancy for 12 to 18 months after surgery. Supplementation with vitamins should be recorded.

A review of the usual or actual intake should be collected in order to determine energy, protein, and fluid intake. Many patients will experience food intolerances and dumping syndrome. Early "dumping" occurs when undigested food or simple carbohydrates enter the jejunum in gastric bypass patients 10 to 15 minutes after eating. Symptoms include nausea, fullness, cramping, pain, and diarrhea within 15 minutes of eating as a result of a shift in fluid from the plasma and extracellular fluid into the jejunum as the body attempts to dilute the hypertonic jejunal content (59). Eventually, the shift in fluids may lead to decreases in circulating blood volume and cardiac output. Complaints then may also include feeling light-headed, dizziness, weakness, fainting, feeling warm, increased pulse rate, diaphoresis, or the presence of a cold sweat, which improve with lying recumbent.

Late dumping may occur also due to an insulin-induced hypoglycemic state resulting from a rapid release of insulin in response to a glycemic load. Insulin response is greater than the glucose demand in this condition frequently referred to as "rebound hypoglycemia." Small frequent meals consisting of both protein and complex carbohydrates will decrease the potential for late dumping. Treatment includes a carbohydrate source with protein such as reduced-fat milk or cheese with fruit.

The amount and type of physical activity should be noted along with the status of the patient's support system. Regression of habits in the patient's stage of change should be documented and addressed in the patient-driven education and plan of action.

NUTRITION AND SURGICAL COMPLICATIONS

Surgical complications after gastric bypass surgery may result in the inability of the patients to consume an oral diet. The use of gastric tubes placed into the remnant stomach at the time of the original surgery or during subsequent re-operation may be done. Gastrostomy feeding can be continued and can include the administration of medications and fluids. The long-term efficacy of such feeds remains questionable due to the common denervation that may accompany gastric bypass procedures. Feeding into the remnant offers the option of higher osmolarity feeds without restriction on feeding rates. Slow-drip enteral feeds into the gastric pouch via a nasogastric (NG) tube are typically not recommended, especially with intestinal complications including an ileus or peritoneal infection. NG enteral feeds into the gastric pouch should not be attempted until three months postoperatively and then should be placed only by interventional radiology. Prior to this time, risks exist for stomal stenosis or staple-line disruption. Close monitoring of such feeds is recommended as there is not a mechanism such as gastric residual to measure delayed gastric emptying, as would normally be used to monitor enteral feeds. The use of NG feeds into the pouch may be appropriate for feeding patients after a substantial period (after three months) in situations which are not related to gastrointestinal complications or gastric bypass such as trauma. The potential tolerance for feeds and appropriateness of feeding rates remains understudied and is a potential area for clinical nutrition research.

The use of total parenteral nutrition (TPN) is clinically indicated for surgical complications involving the gastrointestinal tract after gastric bypass surgery.

Recent literature suggests that permissive underfeeding in acute situations may have potential risk benefits including a reduction in morbidity and mortality (60). The adjustment of macronutrients, specifically the dextrose concentration of feeds to prevent hyperglycemia, is the primary goal rather than achieving caloric goals. Protein or amino acid administration should be given at 1.5 to 2.0 g/kg of IBW to prevent the breakdown of lean body stores and as a fuel source, since they do not play a role in infectious complications. Amino acids promote nitrogen retention and provide important Kreb cycle components, antioxidants, and factors for muscle and bowel anabolism. Despite inadequate energy in undernourished patients, nitrogen balance can remain positive with adequate protein administration (61). Fatty acids are usually not indicated during acute phase feedings. Fat as a fuel substrate is poorly utilized in the acute phase, and does not prevent the loss of lean body mass (62). Obese subjects in one randomized trial of 150 patients in the ICU found that reduced caloric intake was associated with less pneumonia, antibiotic use, and ventilator dependency (63).

The prolonged use of enteral nutrition or home TPN requires a revision of nutrition goals established in the acute care stetting, since metabolic changes are marked outside of the acute phase response. Weight loss after gastric bypass surgery during the administration of EN or TPN is not contraindicated as some might propose. Adequate wound healing can occur in a hypocaloric state if protein needs, fluids, and other components of wound healing such as arginine, zinc, and vitamin C are available. The provision of basal energy requirements and protein along with anabolic electrolytes, zinc, and selenium may be appropriate. Weekly or bi-weekly monitoring should include an evaluation of electrolytes, nutrition markers of protein status along with magnesium and phosphorous levels for TPN patients.

CONCLUSION

The role of nutrition education and medical nutrition therapy in bariatric surgery is becoming more evident as tools to enhance surgical outcome and long-term weight maintenance are explored. Micronutrient deficiencies can commonly be prevented with adequate supplementation and patient follow-up. Nutrition assessment is an important component of long-term patient care as well as when surgical complications occur.

REFERENCES

1. Position of the American Dietetic Association. Weight management. J Am Diet Assoc 2002; 102:1145–1155.
2. Dietel M. Recommendations for reporting weight loss. Obes Surg 2003; 13:159–160.
3. Buchwald H, Avidor Y, Braunwald E, et al. Bariatric surgery, a systematic review and meta-analysis. JAMA 2004; 292:1724–1737.
4. MacLean LD, Rhode BM, Samplais J, et al. Results of the surgical treatment of obesity. Am J Surg 1993; 165:155–159.
5. Kuczmarski RJ, Carrol MD, Flegal KM, et al. Varying body mass index cutoff points to describe overweight prevalence among U.S. adults: NHANES III (1988 to 1994). Obes Res 1997; 5:542–548.
6. Nieman DC, Trone GA, Austin MD. A new handheld device for measuring resting metabolic rate and oxygen consumption. J Am Diet Assoc 2003; 103(5):588.

7. Hsu LK, Sullivan SP, Benotti PN. Eating disturbances and outcome of gastric bypass surgery: a pilot study. Int J Disord 1997; 21:385–390.
8. Saunders R, Grazing A. High risk behavior. Obes Surg 2004; 14:98–102.
9. Malone M, Alger-Mayer S. Binge status and quality of life after gastric bypass surgery: a one-year study. Obes Res 2004; 12:473–481.
10. Marcus, E. Bariatric surgery: the role of the RD in patient assessment and management. SCAN's Pulse, a newsletter of the Sports, Cardiovascular and Wellness Nutrition Practice Group of the American Dietetic Association 2005; 18–20.
11. National Institutes of Health/National Heart Lung and Blood Institute, North American Association for the Study of Obesity. Practical Guide to the Identification, Evaluation and Treatment of Overweight and Obesity in Adults. National Institutes of Health, Bethesda, MD, 2000.
12. Ray EC, Nickels MW, Sayeed S, et al. Predicting success after gastric bypass: the role of psychosocial and behavioral factors. Surgery 2003; 134(4):555–563.
13. Executive Report of the Expert Panel on Weight Loss Surgery. The Commonwealth of Massachusetts, Betsy Lehman Center for Patient Safety and Medical Error Reduction, August 4, 2004. Available at www.mass.gov/dph/betsylehman/panel_summary.htm.
14. Fris, RJ. Preoperative low energy diet diminishes liver size. Obes Surg 2004; 1165–1170.
15. Martin LF, Tan TL, Holmes PA, et al. Can morbidly obese patients safely lose weight preoperatively? Am J Surg 1995; 169:245–253.
16. Franz MJ. Managing obesity in patients with comorbidities. J Am Diet Assoc 1998; 98:S39–S43.
17. Verselewel de Witt Hamer PC, Tuinebreijer WE. Preoperative weight gain in bariatric surgery. Obes Surg 1998; 8:300–301.
18. Rosal MC, Ebbeling CB, Lofgren I, et al. Facilitating dietary change: the patient-centered counseling model. J Am Diet Assoc 2001; 101:332–341.
19. Wing RR, Hill JD. Successful weight loss maintenance. Annu Rev Nutr 2001; 21:323.
20. Mattson AS. In: Foster GD, Nonas CA, eds. Surgical Treatment. Part B. Practical Applications in Managing Obesity: A Clinical Guide. The American Dietetic Association, 2004.
21. Heymsfield SB, Van Mierlo CA, van der Knaap HC, et al. Weight management using a meal replacement strategy: meta- and pooling analysis from six studies. Int J Obes Relat Metab Disord 2003; 27(5):537.
22. Kawamura I, Chen CC, Yamazaki K, et al. A clinical study of protein sparing modified fast (PSMF) administered preoperatively to morbidly obese patients: comparison of PSMF with natural food products to originally prepared PSMF. Obes Surg 1992; 2:33–40.
23. Dietary Reference Intake. National Academy of Science, Institute of Medicine, Food and Nutrition Board, September 5, 2002. Available at www.nal.usda.gov/fnic.
24. Scopinaro N, Adami GF, Marinari GM, et al. Biliopancreatic diversion. World J Surg 1998; 22:936–946.
25. Boylan LM, Sugerman HJ, Driskell JA. Vitamin E, vitamin B-6, vitamin B-12 and folate status of gastric bypass surgery patients. J Am Diet Assoc 1988; 88:579–585.
26. Warde-Kamar J, Rogers MR, Flancbaum L, et al. Caloric intake and meal patterns up to 4 years after Roux-en-Y gastric bypass surgery. Obes Surg 2004; 14:1070–1079.
27. Scopinaro N, Gianetta E, Adami GF, et al. Biliopancreatic diversion for obesity at eighteen years. Surgery 1996; 119:261–268.
28. Slater GH, Ren CJ, Seigel N, et al. Serum fat-soluble vitamin deficiency and abnormal calcium metabolism after malabsorptive bariatric surgery. J Gastrointest Surg 2004; 8:48–55.
29. Buffington C, Walker B, Cowan GS, et al. Vitamin D deficiency in the morbidly obese. Obes Surg 1993; 3(4):421–424.
30. O'Brien DP, Nelson LA, Huang FS, et al. Intestinal adaptation: structure, function and regulation. Semin Pediatric Surg 2001; 10:56–64.

31. Kim JJ, Tarnoff ME, Shikora SA. Surgical treatment for extreme obesity: evolution of a rapidly growing field. Nutr Clin Pract 2003; 18:109–123.
32. Halverson JD. Micronutrient deficiencies after gastric bypass for morbid obesity. Am Surg 1986; 52:594–598.
33. Avinoah E, Ovnat A, Charuzi I. Nutritional status seven years after Roux-en-Y gastric bypass surgery. Surgery 1992; 111:137–142.
34. Rhode BM, Shustik C, Christou NV, et al. Iron absorption and therapy after gastric bypass. Obes Surg 1999; 9:17–21.
35. Salas-Salvado J, Garcia-Lorda P, Cuatrecasas G, et al. Wernicke's syndrome after bariatric surgery. Clin Nutr 2000; 12:371–373.
36. Loh Y, Watson WD, Verma A, et al. Acute Wernicke's Encephalopathy following bariatric surgery: clinical course and MRI correlation. Obes Surg 2004; 14:129–132.
37. Chaves L, Faintuch J, Kahwage S, et al. A cluster of polyneuropathy and Wernicke–Korsakoff Syndrome in a bariatric unit. Obes Surg 2002; 12:328–334.
38. Sola E, Morillas C, Garzon S, et al. Rapid onset of Wernicke's Encephalopathy following gastric restrictive surgery. Obes Surg 2003; 13:661–662.
39. Bradley EL, Isaacs J, Hersh T, et al. Nutritional consequences of total gastrectomy. Ann Surg 1975; 182:415–429.
40. Brolin RE, LaMarca LB, Kenler HA, et al. Malabsorptive gastric bypass in patients with super-obesity. J Gastrointest Surg 2002; 6:195–203.
41. Brolin RE, Kenler HA, Gorman JH, et al. Long-limb gastric bypass in the superobese. A prospective randomized study. Ann Surg 1992; 215:387–395.
42. Skroubis G, Sakellaropoulos G, Pouggouras K, et al. Comparison of nutritional deficiencies after Roux-en-Y gastric bypass and biliopancreatic diversion with Roux-en-Y gastric bypass. Obes Surg 2002; 551–558.
43. Towbin A, Inge TH, Garcia VF, et al. Beriberi after gastric bypass surgery in adolescence. J Pediatr 2004; 145:263–267.
44. Shils ME et al., eds. Modern Nutrition in Health and Disease. 9th ed. Williams & Wilkins, 1999.
45. Chang CG, Adams-Huet B, Provost DA. Acute Post-Gastric Reduction Surgery Neuropathy (APGARS). Obes Surg 2004; 14:182–189.
46. Schilling RF, Gohdes PN, Hardie GH. Vitamin B12 deficiency after gastric bypass surgery for obesity. Ann Intern Med 1984; 101:501–502.
47. Amaral JF, Thompson WR, Caldwell MD, et al. Prospective hematologic evaluation of gastric exclusion surgery for morbid obesity. Ann Surg 1985; 201:186–193.
48. Crowley LV, Seay J, Mullin G. Late effects of gastric bypass for obesity. Am J Gastroenterol 1984; 79:850–860.
49. Halverson JD, Zuckerman GR, Koehle RE, et al. Gastric bypass for morbid obesity. Ann Surg 1981; 194:152–160.
50. Carmel R, Green R, Rosenblatt DS, et al. Update on cobalamin, folate and homocysteine [Review]. Hematology 2003; 62–81.
51. Rhode BM, Tamim H, Gilfix MB, et al. Treatment of Vitamin B12 deficiency after gastric bypass surgery for severe obesity. Obes Surg 1995; 5:154–158.
52. Brolin RE, Gorman JH, Gorman RC, et al. Are vitamin B12 and folate deficiency clinically important after Roux-en-Y gastric bypass? J Gastrointest Surg 1998; 2:436–442.
53. Rhode BM, Shustik C, Christou NV, et al. Iron absorption and therapy after gastric bypass. Obes Surg 1999; 9:17–21.
54. Brolin RE, Gorman JH, Gorman, et al. Prophylactic iron supplementation after Roux-en-Y gastric bypass: a prospective, double-blind, randomized study. Arch Surg 1998; 133:740–744.
55. Goode LR, Brolin RE, Chowdhury HA, et al. Bone and gastric bypass surgery: effects of dietary calcium and vitamin D. Obes Res 2004; 12:40–47.

56. Coates PS, Fernstrom JD, Fernstrom MH, et al. Gastric bypass surgery for morbid obesity leads to an increase in bone turnover and a decrease in bone mass. J Clin Endo and Metab 2004; 89:1061–1065.

57. Kenny AM, Prestwood KM, Biskup B, et al. Comparison of the effects of calcium loading with calcium citrate or calcium carbonate on bone turnover in postmenopausal women. Osteoporos Int 2004; 4:290–294.

58. Sakhaee K, Bhuket T, Adams-Huet B, et al. Meta-analysis of calcium bioavailability: a comparison of calcium citrate with calcium carbonate. Am J Ther 1999; 6:313–321.

59. Gastrointestinal disease. Manual of Clinical Dietetics. 6th edn. The American Dietetic Association, 2000.

60. Jeejeebhoy KN. Permissive underfeeding in the critically ill patient. Nutr Clin Pract 2004; 19:477–480.

61. Greenberg GR, Jeejeebhoy KN. Intravenous protein-sparing therapy in patients with gastrointestinal disease. JPEN 1979; 3:427–432.

62. Hart DW, Wolf SE, Herndon DN, et al. Energy expenditure and caloric balance after burn: increased feeding leads to fat rather than lean mass accretion. Ann Surg 2002; 235:152–161.

63. Ibrahim EH, Mehringer L, Prentice D, et al. Early versus late enteral feeding of mechanically ventilated patients: results of a clinical trail. JPEN 2002; 26:174–181.

7

Laparoscopic Vertical Banded Gastroplasty

J. K. Champion
Mercer University School of Medicine and Emory-Dunwoody Medical Center, Atlanta, Georgia, U.S.A.

Michael Williams
Emory-Dunwoody Medical Center, Atlanta, Georgia, U.S.A.

INTRODUCTION

Simple gastric restriction was introduced as a surgical method to achieve weight reduction for clinically severe obesity by Mason et al. in 1971 in the form of a horizontal gastroplasty (1). Over the next decade, as numerous attempts were made to modify the procedure, it became apparent that the horizontal orientation of the pouch, which incorporated the fundus, dilated significantly over time, and the outlet was resistant to stabilization efforts, both of which contributed to poor weight loss and frequent revisions (2).

The next significant modifications occurred in the early 1980s when a vertically oriented pouch was introduced along the lesser curve of the stomach where the sero-muscular fibers were less distensible, and the outlet was stabilized with a circumferential prosthetic band (3). In 1986 Mason described his final version of the "modern" vertical banded gastroplasty (VBG) that consisted of an undivided vertically oriented proximal gastric pouch, measured and calibrated to be less than 30 cc, with an outlet stabilized by an externally calibrated 1.5×5 cm circumferential prosthetic polypropylene mesh band (Fig. 1). In one widely adapted variation, Laws substituted a silastic ring for outlet stabilization in place of the mesh band which allowed the omission of the circular "key-hole" in the stomach (Fig. 2) (4). Despite Mason's repeated emphasis on the technical aspects of performing a VBG in a consistent standardized and calibrated manner, there was a wide variation in all aspects of the operation, which was the most popular weight-reduction procedure in the early 1990s. The VBG appealed to surgeons in search of a bariatric operation with lower morbidity than the intestinal or gastric bypass, but it was apparent that open bariatric surgery was associated with a significant wound morbidity in morbidly obese patients (5,6). As experience was gained with laparoscopic foregut surgery, it was a natural progression that a minimally invasive approach be expanded to bariatric surgery.

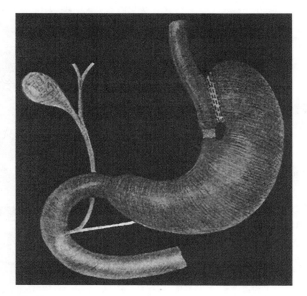

Figure 1   Mason's vertical banded gastroplasty.

A minimally invasive approach to perform a "Mason-like" VBG was first performed in 1993 and later reported by Chua and Mendiola in the United States, and by Lonroth et al. in Europe (7,8). These early series reported that a laparoscopic VBG which attempted to replicate the open technique was "technically feasible," but was challenging due to the limited instrumentation and difficulty in forming an accurate small proximal pouch secondary to the required manipulation of the circular stapler through the abdominal wall to form a "keyhole." In 1995, Champion introduced the concept of a "wedge VBG" that utilized a linear stapler to remove a

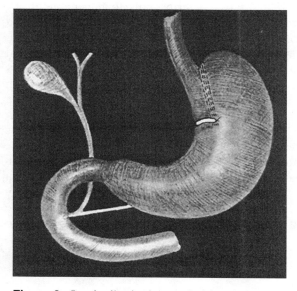

Figure 2   Law's silastic ring vertical banded gastroplasty.

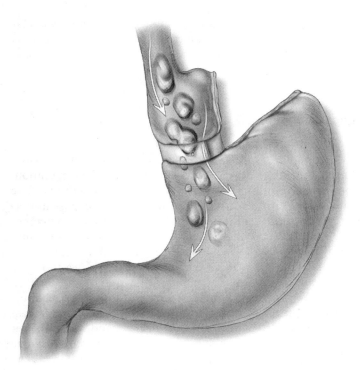

Figure 3 Champion's wedge vertical banded gastroplasty.

5×5 cm segment of fundus to form a calibrated proximal pouch of less than 30 cc in a simplified manner compared to the "Mason-like" approach (Fig. 3) (9). This approach simplified the procedure by eliminating the need for a circular stapler, permitted the entire operation to be performed through the trocars, and allowed a more accurate formation of the pouch. In addition, the technique was an excellent approach to performing a gastroplasty for a shortened esophagus associated with reflux. Instead of applying a prosthetic band around the distal pouch, the fundus can be wrapped around to form a fundoplication of the surgeon's choice.

This chapter describes the "wedge VBG" performed laparoscopically, and reports its early outcomes compared to the laparoscopic "Mason-like" VBG and historical open series.

METHODS

Indications for Surgery

Patients may be considered for weight-reduction surgery utilizing the National Institutes for Health (NIH) guidelines from the 1991 consensus conference. Surgery is an option if patients are 100 pounds or more over an ideal body weight or if their body mass index (BMI) is greater than or equal to 40. Patients with a BMI of 35 to 39 may be considered if they exhibit an associated comorbidity such as hypertension, diabetes mellitus, hyperlipidemia, or sleep apnea. Additional obesity-related comorbid conditions include, but are not limited to, osteoarthritis, urinary stress incontinence, gastro-esophageal reflux, venous insufficiency, pseudo-tumor cerebri, cardiovascular heart disease, and certain cancers. Females are at an increased risk for breast, uterine, cervical and ovarian cancer, or recurrence, and males are at an increased risk for colon and prostate malignancies.

Patient Selection for Laparoscopic VBG

The current "holy grail" in bariatric surgery is to be able to tailor the operation and identify pre-operatively which patients will be able to succeed with simple gastric restriction, and who will need a malabsorptive component added to their operation. The VBG has been demonstrated overall to be associated with less weight loss, late weight regain, and more revisions than the proximal or distal gastric bypass in randomized trials, but some patients do demonstrate excellent long-term outcomes (5,6,9–12). Sugerman et al. identified several subgroups who had poorer outcomes with a VBG in a randomized study, and they included sweet eaters, Afro-Americans, and super obese patients with a BMI >50 (5). In our own experience, we too have observed that African American patients or patients with an initial BMI >50 do not do as well with the VBG. We also discourage patients with diabetes mellitus, hyperlipidemia, severe gastroesophageal reflux disease (GERD), or an esophageal motility disorder from undergoing a VBG or adjustable gastric band due to better outcomes with a gastric bypass in our experience (Table 1). The laparoscopic approach to bariatric surgery has relative contra-indications which must be taken into consideration depending on the skill level of the bariatric surgeon as listed in Table 2. We discuss treatment options with risks, complications, alternatives, and anticipated outcomes with each patient, and leave the final decision to the patient's choice unless there is a contra-indication to the laparoscopic VBG in our opinion. An example would be a patient who is a sweet-eater, has a BMI of 60, and exhibits insulin-dependent diabetes mellitus. I personally would decline to perform a VBG in this patient, as I strongly feel a gastric bypass would be in this patient's best interest.

Operative Technique Wedge VBG

Patients are admitted the morning of surgery in a 23-hour stay. Sequential compression devices are applied to the legs, and Lovenox® 40 mg (Aventis, Bridgewater, New Jersey, U.S.A.) is administered subcutaneously for thromboprophylaxis. Antibiotic prophylaxis is given as Rocephin® 2 g (Roche, Nutley, New Jersey, U.S.A.) intravenously.

Table 1   Relative Contraindications to a VBG

BMI > 50
African Americans
Sweet eaters
Diabetes mellitus
Hyperlipidemia
GERD
Primary motility disorder

Abbreviations: GERD, gastroesophageal reflux disease.

Table 2   Relative Contraindications to a Laparoscopic Approach for VBG*

Android body habitus
Previous open upper abdominal incision
Weight >400 pounds
BMI >70
Hepatomegaly
Chronic obstructive pulmonary disease with CO_2 retention
Congestive heart failure with ejection fraction <30

*Depends on learning curve and skill of surgeon.

Patients are placed under general endotracheal anesthesia in a supine position with the surgeon and camera assistant on the patient's right and the first assistant and scrub nurse on the patient's left. A footboard is applied to the table, and the patient is securely strapped in place with appropriate padding of extremities to allow extreme reverse Trendelenburg positioning on a bariatric operating room (OR) table designed to lift up to 800 pounds.

After the abdomen is prepped and draped, a 12-mm incision is made 15 cm below the xiphoid process to the left of the midline over the rectus sheath, and an optical trocar with a zero degree laparoscope is utilized to enter the abdominal cavity under direct visualization without insufflation. Insufflation is begun at 15 cm and the abdomen carefully inspected to rule out any iatrogenic injury, or other abnormality. The remaining four 5-mm trocars and one 12-mm port are inserted as indicated in Figure 4. The 12-mm port for the stapler is inserted in the left upper abdomen, just below the costal margin in the anterior axillary line.

The patient is positioned in reverse Trendelenburg, and a 5-mm ratcheted allis clamp is passed through the xiphoid trocar under the left lobe of the liver,

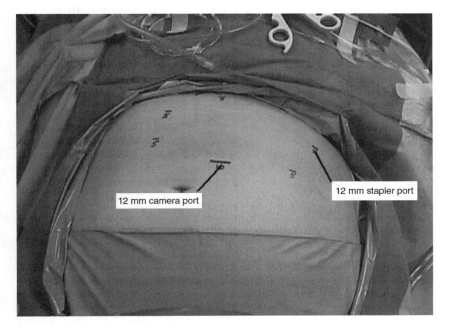

Figure 4   Trocar insertion sites.

and attached to the diaphragm just above the esophageal hiatus for retraction. The assistant retracts the fundus of the stomach laterally, and the surgeon takes down the peritoneal attachments along the left crus and angle of HIS with electrocautery. This helps define the angle of HIS formation and assists in applying the stapler later while forming the pouch. A measurement is then made 5 cm down from the angle of HIS along the lesser curve, and a peri-gastric window is created into the lesser sac directly alongside the gastric wall utilizing gentle blunt dissection and preserving the branches of the vagus nerve. This window will be used to position the band around the pouch at the end of the case, and is used as a landmark while stapling the pouch.

The dissection now proceeds horizontally from the window to the greater curve of the stomach, and the short gastric vessels are divided along the upper fundus all the way to the left crus and angle of HIS. We utilize bipolar cautery to obtain hemostasis, but any energy source, clips, or suture ligature is appropriate. A 50 Fr bougie is then positioned along the lesser curve of the stomach to serve as a template to form the pouch during stapling. The 12-mm linear stapler (Endo GIA-2, USSC, Norwalk, Connecticut, U.S.A.) with a 45-mm 3.5 load is inserted via the 12-mm port in the left subcostal position and applied transversely on the stomach beginning at the greater curve directly horizontal from the window on the lesser curve. The stapler is fired horizontally for two to three firings until the end of the stapler rolls off the bougie at the lesser curve. The stapler is now repositioned vertically alongside the bougie and fired repeatedly up through the angle of HIS, transecting and removing a 5×5 cm section of stomach. The transected segment can usually be withdrawn through the 12-mm port in the left upper abdomen without enlarging the port site. The staple line along the pouch is oversewn with a running 2–0 silk, since the patients are begun on liquids immediately post-op. The large bougie is removed and replaced with a 30 Fr bougie positioned across the outlet for placement of the band around the pouch to prevent inadvertent suture closure of the stoma. The outlet size is externally calibrated (approximately 12 mm) by the length of the band, not the internal bougie size.

A band is constructed from polypropylene mesh and is 1.5 cm by 7.0 cm. The band will be overlapped 1 cm on the ends to create a 5 cm band, so the band is marked with a stay suture 1 cm from each end to aid in the placement. The band is inserted via the left upper abdominal 12-mm port and positioned around the distal pouch through the window 5 cm below the gastro-esophageal (GE) junction. The band is overlapped 1 cm and sutured with two horizontal mattress sutures of 0 Ethibond (Ethicon Inc., Sommerville, New Jersey, U.S.A.) tied extracorporeally. The bougie is removed and an intra-operative esophagogastroscopy is performed to ensure proper pouch and stoma size and no leaks from the staple or suture lines. The band is then covered with an omental patch to prevent adherence to the underside of the liver which can result in torsion and a pseudo-obstruction of the outlet.

The abdomen is irrigated with saline and all trocars removed under direct visualization to rule out bleeding. Trocar sites are not closed at the fascia level unless the left upper abdominal 12-mm port site required enlargement for removal of the stomach specimen. Skin incisions are closed with 3–0 plain subcuticular sutures and steri-strips.

Postoperative Care

Patients are allowed a clear liquid diet immediately postoperative and are ambulated as soon as they arrive in their room. The following morning, a gastrograffin swallow is performed to rule out a staple line leak or outlet obstruction. If the patient tolerates liquids and oral pain medication, the vital signs are normalized and the gastrograffin swallow satisfactory, then the patient is discharged.

The postoperative diet is full liquids for two weeks, a soft diet of cooked fruits, vegetables, and fish for three weeks, and a regular diet at six weeks. Patients are instructed to have six small meals per day for the first six weeks, with three liquid protein supplements each counting as one meal. After six weeks the protein supplements are discontinued unless weight loss is excessive. Patients are placed on a multi-vitamin with iron and calcium supplement (1000 mg) daily for life.

Postoperative visits occur at three weeks, three months, six months, and one year, then annually for life. Two-day diet histories, vital signs, and weights and BMIs are checked at each visit. A comprehensive blood chemistry, complete blood count, serum iron, and serum vitamin B12 level is checked at six months and then yearly for life. Dietary counseling is required at each visit and patients are required to attend four support group meetings after surgery. Patients who appear to be behind the anticipated weight loss, or who are struggling with the dietary changes, are placed in an intense monthly dietary counseling and usually referred for psychological counseling to address stress and adaptation problems.

RESULTS

Long-term follow-up (10 years) is not available at present with the laparoscopic VBG, but intermediate five-year outcomes for both the "Mason-like" VBG and "Wedge" VBG have been reported to compare with historical results from the open VBG as listed in Table 3 (6,9,12,13). The incidences of chronic vomiting, gastro-esophageal reflux, and band erosion are listed in Table 4.

Utilizing evidence-based criteria, there has been one randomized prospective study comparing open to laparoscopic VBG utilizing a "Mason-like" technique, which created the pouch 9 cm below the gastro-esophageal junction utilizing a circular stapler window and naso-gastric tube as a stent, and partial division of the pouch with only one firing of a non-cutting 60-mm cartridge (14). Azagra et al. (14) demonstrated a significant reduction in incisional hernias from 15.8% to 0% ($p = 0.04$) and wound infections from 10.8% to 3.3% ($p = 0.04$) with the laparoscopic "Mason-like" approach compared to their similar open technique. Weight loss and BMI were reported as "similar" between groups, but absolute values were not

Table 3 Selective Outcomes for VBG with 5- to 10-Year Follow-Up

Author	Procedure/ follow-up	%EWL/BMI	SD	Revisions	%FU	Wound morbidity
Olbers $n = 139$	Lap VBG 5 yrs	50%/32	2.0% Undivided	8%	NR	NR
Champion $n = 58$	Lap VBG 7 yrs	49%/34	0% Divided	10.3%	100%	None
Balsinger $n = 71$	Open VBG 10 yrs	30%/39	2.8% Undivided-2 row Ta90	17%	99%	9% infection 23% hernia
Naslund $n = 198$	Open VBG 7 yrs	NR/34	9.5% Undivided-1 row Ta90	15%	89%	2.5% infection 7.5% hernia

Abbreviations: EWL, excess weight loss; SD, staple line disruption; FU, follow-up; NR, not reported.

Table 4 Morbidity Secondary to Banding the Pouch with Gastric Restriction

Author	Vomiting	GERD	Erosion
Olbers	7%	7%	0.7%
Champion	9%	3%	None
Balsinger	21%	16%	None
Naslund	7%	24%	1%

listed and follow-up was short. OR time, however, was significantly longer in the laparoscopic (150 minutes) compared to the open approach (90 minutes, $p = 0.001$).

OR time was not listed in Table 3, but averaged 148 minutes for Olbers, while our mean OR time was 60 minutes with the simplified "Wedge" approach. Melissas experienced a similar reduction in OR time when he switched from a laparoscopic "Mason-like" VBG (155 minutes) to a linear "wedge" VBG (115 minutes) (15).

DISCUSSION

A comparison between groups and techniques in bariatric surgery is difficult due to a lack of standardization of the technical operation and reporting of outcomes, and the lack of strong evidence-based studies utilizing randomized, prospective trials. Small changes in technical aspects of the VBG which are meant to improve outcomes will result in a negative outcome also, which may not be evident for a period of time. In addition, simple gastric restriction relies on a strong aftercare program provided by the surgeon's practice to improve outcomes.

Our own laparoscopic experience reproduced the reduction in wound morbidity seen in Azagra et al.'s randomized trial, and appears to be the principal benefit of the minimally invasive approach for a VBG. Incisional wound infections appear to be more common with the circular stapler employed with the "Mason" gastroplasty, as has been demonstrated comparing a pure linear stapler gastric bypass with a circular stapler approach (16). The large 2-cm incision required for the insertion of the circular device and the withdrawal of the anvil through the abdominal wall after firing across the stomach, which may contaminate the anvil, is believed to be the etiology of the increased infections.

In addition to a decrease in wound infections, we experienced a reduction in OR time with the "Wedge" technique utilizing only a linear stapler. We feel this reduction is due to the simplified construction of the pouch with a linear stapler and the elimination of the required abdominal wall closure associated with the circular stapler technique.

Upon close review of the literature, it appears that the percentage of excess weight loss is approximately 50% at five years in both the laparoscopic and open techniques, but there is a gradual decline and late weight regain as the follow-up continues out to 10 years in the open studies with longer monitoring. We have begun to see a similar decline and weight regain in our five-year cohort and it now averages only 40% EWL. Also revisions appear to be more frequent in the open groups, but they had much longer follow-up, and we anticipate the revision rates will be similar for the laparoscopic cohorts after 10 years. We currently have three pending revisions for poor weight loss which will increase our revision rate to 15.5% which is in line with the open reports in Table 3. A major concern is that the average reduction in BMI was only approximately 10 units, whether an open or laparoscopic VBG technique and the final BMI remained obese or morbidly obese for the average patient in our experience and in review of the literature (range 32–39).

Staple line disruption was not seen in our experience with a divided staple line, but Olbers et al. did experience a 2% incidence in their first 109 laparoscopic cases which they performed with an undivided four-row linear stapler (12). After converting to a divided technique, they did not experience any further staple line disruptions to date. We had one patient develop a contained leak six weeks post-op after prolonged retching associated with poorly chewed chicken causing an outlet obstruction, and we were able to manage this staple line disruption conservatively (Fig. 5). The modification of performing a divided pouch appears to eliminate staple line disruption without an increase in peritonitis secondary to staple line leaks, which is probably due to improved stapler design with newer six-row endoscopic devices.

What is the place for open VBG today? Our recommendation is a limited role for extremely obese patients who are not laparoscopy candidates, during the learning phase of the surgeon who lacks laparoscopic skills, as a conversion from a laparoscopic approach to manage a problem, or if another concomitant procedure requires addressing at the same time.

A selective and tailored approach to stratify patients to the least invasive bariatric operation appropriate for their weight and comorbidities would be the ideal we bariatric surgeons need to strive for in the future. Gastric restriction for weight loss has undergone modification over 30 years in an attempt to improve outcomes,

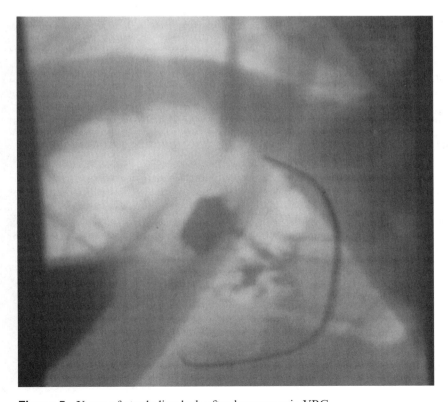

Figure 5 X-ray of staple line leak after laparoscopic VBG.

but the major variable remains the non-compliant patient and the inability to identify that person before surgery.

REFERENCES

1. Mason EE, Doherty C, Cullen JJ, Scott D, Rodriquez EM, Maher JW. Vertical gastro-plasty: evolution of vertical banded gastroplasty. World J Surg 1998; 22:919–924.
2. Dietel M. Overview of operations for morbid obesity. World J Surg 1998; 22:913.
3. Buchwald H, Buchwald JN. Evolution of operative procedures for the management of morbid obesity 1950–2000. Obes Surg 2002; 12:705–717.
4. Laws H. Standardized gastroplasty orifice. Am J Surg 1981; 141:393.
5. Sugerman HJ, Londrey GL, Kellum JM, Wolf L, Liszka T, Engle KM, Birkenhauer R, Starkey JV. Weight loss with vertical banded gastroplasty and Roux-en-Y gastric bypass for morbid obesity with selective versus random assignment. Am J Surg 1989; 157: 93–102.
6. Naslund E, Backman L, Granstrom L, Stockeld D. Seven year results of vertical banded gastroplasty for morbid obesity. Eur J Surg 1997; 163:281–286.
7. Chua TY, Mendiola RM. Laparoscopic vertical banded gastroplasty: the Milwaukee experience. Obes Surg 1995; 5:77–80.
8. Lonroth H, Dalenback J, Haglind E, Josefsson K, Olbe L, Olsen MF, Lundell L. Vertical banded gastroplasty by laparoscopic technique in the treatment of morbid obesity. Surg Laparosc Endosc 1996; 6:102–107.
9. Champion JK. Laparoscopic vertical banded gastroplasty. In: Cohen RV, Schiavon A, Schauer P, eds. Videolaparoscopic Approach to Morbid Obesity. San Paulo: Via Letera Med Publishers, 2002.
10. Sweet WA. Vertical banded gastroplasty: stable trends in weight control at 10 or more years. Obes Surg 1994; 4:149–152.
11. Fox SR, Oh KH, Fox K. Vertical banded gastroplasty and distal gastric bypass as primary procedures: a comparison. Obes Surg 1996; 6:421.
12. Olbers T, Lonroth H, Dalenback J, Haglind E, Lundell L. Laparoscopic vertical banded gastroplasty—an effective long-term therapy for morbid obesity patients? Obes Surg 2001; 11:726–730.
13. Balsinger BM, Poggio JL, Mai J, Kelley KA, Sarr MG. Ten and more years after vertical banded gastroplasty as primary operation for morbid obesity. J Gastrointest Surg 2000; 4:595–605.
14. Azagra JS, Goergen M, Ansay J, DeSimone P, Vanhaverbeek M, Devuyst L, Squelaert J. Laparoscopic gastric reduction surgery. Surg Endosc 1999; 13:555–558.
15. Melissas J, Schoretsanitis G, Grammatikakis J, Tsiftsis DD. Technical modification of laparoscopic vertical banded gastroplasty. Obes Surg 2003; 13:132–135.
16. Gonzalez R, Lin E, Venkatesh KR, Bowers SP, Smith CD. Gastrojejunostomy during laparoscopic gastric bypass: an analysis of three techniques. Arch Surg 2003; 138: 181–184.

8

Physiology of Laparoscopy in the Morbidly Obese

David Magner and Ninh T. Nguyen
Department of Surgery, University of California Irvine Medical Center, Orange, California, U.S.A.

With refinement of the laparoscopic approach to bariatric surgery, there has been a recent surge in the number of bariatric operations being performed in the United States. The increase in the public demand for bariatric surgery has sparked an interest in many surgeons to incorporate bariatric surgery into their practice. Physiologically, laparoscopic bariatric surgery is different from an open bariatric surgery because of the intraoperative use of carbon dioxide gas (CO_2) during pneumoperitoneum. Carbon dioxide pneumoperitoneum has been used clinically since the introduction of laparoscopic cholecystectomy in the late 1980s. The two main physiologic effects of pneumoperitoneum are systemic absorption of CO_2, and hemodynamic and physiologic alterations from the increased intra-abdominal pressure. Carbon dioxide is easily absorbed across the peritoneal surface into the systemic circulation and can lead to hypercarbia. Without ventilatory changes, hypercarbia can lead to eventual systemic acidosis. The increased intra-abdominal pressure at 15 mmHg during pneumoperitoneum has been shown to result in hemodynamic alteration including changes in femoral venous flow and renal, hepatic, and cardiorespiratory function (1–4). Morbidly obese patients often have many comorbid conditions that can predispose them to develop intraoperative complications associated with the use of pneumoperitoneum. Laparoscopic bariatric surgery, such as laparoscopic gastric bypass (GBP), is a complex operation and is often associated with a longer operative time than other commonly performed laparoscopic procedures. A longer operative time translates to longer exposure of these patients to the adverse physiologic effects of pneumoperitoneum. This chapter reviews our current understanding of the effects of pneumoperitoneum on CO_2 absorption and excretion, femoral venous flow, and hepatic, renal, and cardiorespiratory function.

EFFECTS OF CARBON DIOXIDE ABSORPTION
DURING PNEUMOPERITONEUM

Pneumoperitoneum can result in a systemic absorption of CO_2 and an alteration of acid–base balance. Absorption of CO_2 across the peritoneum into the systemic circulation is normally eliminated through the lungs because of the high solubility and diffusibility of CO_2. If intraoperative ventilation is impaired, CO_2 absorption can result in systemic and respiratory acidosis (5). To minimize intraoperative hypercapnia, close intraoperative monitoring should be performed using either end-tidal CO_2 ($ETCO_2$) level or arterial partial pressure of CO_2 ($PaCO_2$). The $ETCO_2$ level is an easily accessible parameter; however, it can underestimate the true level of $PaCO_2$ (6). The $ETCO_2$ levels normally increase by 15% of baseline (up to 40 mmHg) and $PaCO_2$ levels increase by 9% of baseline (from 38 mmHg to 42 mmHg) during pneumoperitoneum in the morbidly obese (7,8). Although $ETCO_2$ and $PaCO_2$ levels often increase during laparoscopy, these levels can be maintained in the upper part of normal range if appropriate ventilatory adjustments are performed.

During pneumoperitoneum, appropriate ventilatory changes should be performed to eliminate the increased CO_2 load and to prevent systemic acidosis. Ventilatory changes consist of increasing the minute ventilation. In a study of laparoscopic gastroplasty, minute ventilation was increased by 21% (9). Increase in minute ventilation is accomplished by increasing the respiratory rate. In a study of laparoscopic GBP, respiratory rate was increased by 25% to eliminate the increased CO_2 load (8). The measuring of the total volume of exhaled CO_2 through the lungs during pneumoperitoneum is a good indirect method for the quantification of the amount of CO_2 absorbed during laparoscopy. In non-obese patients, the estimated volume of CO_2 absorbed from the peritoneal cavity ranged from 38 to 42 mL/min during laparoscopy (10). In morbidly obese patients, the estimated volume of CO_2 absorbed from the peritoneal cavity ranged from 19 to 39 mL/min (8). Therefore, the absorption of CO_2 in morbidly obese subjects appears to be similar to that of non-obese subjects.

EFFECTS OF INCREASED INTRA-ABDOMINAL PRESSURE DURING
PNEUMOPERITONEUM

The normal intra-abdominal pressure of morbidly obese individuals can be as high as 9 to 10 mmHg (11,12). Typically, the intra-abdominal pressure is set at 15 mmHg during laparoscopy to provide adequate visualization of the operative field. Pneumoperitoneum therefore creates a state of acutely elevated intra-abdominal pressure.

Hemodynamic Changes and Cardiac Function

The increased intra-abdominal pressure during pneumoperitoneum has been shown to alter the mean arterial pressure and heart rate. Heart rate and mean arterial blood pressure often increase with pneumoperitoneum in both non-obese and obese individuals; however, obese individuals had a more pronounced increase in the heart rate level (13). The heart rate and mean arterial pressure increase after the initiation of pneumoperitoneum, and often remain elevated throughout the operation (14).

Clinical studies evaluating the effects of CO_2 pneumoperitoneum on cardiac function have documented variable results. Certain studies demonstrated a significant reduction in cardiac output with abdominal insufflation, while other studies demonstrated minimal change (15–18). In a study of laparoscopic cholecystectomy, cardiac index decreased by 30% with pneumoperitoneum (15,16). However, there is minimal change in cardiac function when laparoscopy is performed using the abdominal wall–lifting method rather than the pneumoperitoneum (19). Therefore, the increased intra-abdominal pressure is the major factor responsible for the alteration of cardiac function. In contrast to the results observed in non-obese subjects, cardiac output only decreased by 6% after the initiation of pneumoperitoneum in morbidly obese subjects (14).

Factors influencing cardiac function include preload, afterload, cardiac contractility, heart rate, and myocardial compliance. The increased intra-abdominal pressure can decrease the preload by impeding venous return. Therefore, a euvolemic preoperative volume status is very important to minimize any cardiac depression related to the increased intra-abdominal pressure. Cardiac depression has also been attributed to significant systemic acidosis. However, a moderate rise in $PaCO_2$ levels ($<45\,mmHg$) should not contribute to cardiac impairment. The increased intra-abdominal pressure can also cause cardiac depression by increasing the afterload. In one study, the systemic vascular resistance increased by 25% of baseline values after abdominal insufflation and decreased immediately with desufflation (20). Cardiac depression observed during pneumoperitoneum is often transient as the body compensates for the altered physiology. In a study of laparoscopic gastric bypass after a period of transient cardiac depression, cardiac output levels recovered and increased above baseline value by 2.5 hour after abdominal insufflation (14).

Hepatic Function

The increased intra-abdominal pressure has been shown to reduce portal venous flow and affect hepatic function. In a clinical study of laparoscopic cholecystectomy, a 53% reduction in portal blood flow was reported (21). A reduction in portal venous blood flow during pneumoperitoneum may lead to hepatic hypoperfusion and acute hepatocyte injury. The clinical implication of portal hypoperfusion is minimal except for a transient elevation of liver enzymes (22,23). In a study of morbidly obese subjects, an acute elevation of hepatic transaminases was observed after laparoscopic GBP; however, the elevation was only transient and returned to baseline by the third postoperative day (24). Other mechanisms for alteration of postoperative hepatic function include direct operative trauma to the liver and the use of general anesthetics. Direct operative trauma to the liver occurs during mechanical retraction of the left lobe of the liver. Certain anesthetic agents, metabolized through the liver, can be hepatotoxic and can contribute to hepatocyte injury. Despite the effects of increased intra-abdominal pressure on portal venous flow, pneumoperitoneum in the morbidly obese is considered safe in patients with normal baseline liver function. Further studies are needed to evaluate the safety of pneumoperitoneum in patients with pre-existing liver dysfunction (e.g., severe liver cirrhosis).

Intraoperative Pulmonary Mechanics

The increased intra-abdominal pressure during laparoscopy can also adversely affect the intraoperative pulmonary mechanics. Pneumoperitoneum in non-obese subjects can result in a decrease of respiratory compliance and an increase in airway pressure (25,26). In morbidly obese patients undergoing laparoscopic bariatric surgery, the increased intra-abdominal pressure can decrease the pulmonary compliance by

31–42% and can increase the airway pressure by 12–17% (8,9). Although pneumo-peritoneum alters the respiratory compliance and airway pressure, the pulmonary gas exchange is not affected (10). No significant changes in the physiologic dead space-to-tidal volume ratio or the alveolar-arterial oxygen gradient were observed in patients who underwent laparoscopic GBP (8).

Renal Function

The increased intra-abdominal pressure during laparoscopy has also been shown to alter renal function. Intraoperative oliguria and, occasionally, anuria have been documented during laparoscopy (27,28). The mechanism for oliguria during laparo-scopy is thought to be related to the acute increased intra-abdominal pressure. In a trial of laparoscopic vs. open GBP, intraoperative urine output decreased immedi-ately after abdominal insufflation in the laparoscopic group and remained 31–64% lower compared to the urine output in the open group (29). There are several mechanisms for diminished urine output during laparoscopy. Pneumoperitoneum has a direct pressure effect on the renal cortical blood flow (3), and also on the renal vasculature, resulting in reduced renal blood flow (30). In addition, intraoperative releases of certain hormones such as antidiuretic hormone, plasma rennin activity, and serum aldosterone may diminish urine output (31). Despite intraoperative oliguria, pneumoperitoneum is considered clinically safe. In a study of patients undergoing laparoscopic GBP, no significant changes in blood urea nitrogen or serum creatinine levels were observed in the perioperative period after laparoscopic GBP (30). Additionally, the creatinine clearance measured in patients who under-went laparoscopic GBP was in the normal range on both the first and the second postoperative days (12).

Venous Stasis

The true incidence of deep venous thrombosis after laparoscopic operation is unknown but venous stasis is a major consequence of laparoscopy. The increased intra-abdominal pressure and the reverse Trendelenburg position during laparoscopy have been shown to reduce femoral venous flow (32,33). The increased intra-abdominal pressure during laparoscopy has a direct compressive effect on the inferior vena cava and iliac veins and decreases lower extremity venous flow. By the force of gravity during reverse Trendelenburg position, the abdominal viscera produce a compressive effect on the iliac veins also resulting in decreased femoral venous flow. In a study of the morbidly obese subjects who underwent laparoscopic GBP, the increased intra-abdominal pressure and reverse Trendelenburg positioning indepen-dently resulted in a decrease in femoral peak systolic velocity (34). The presence of reverse Trendelenburg position during laparoscopy has an additive effect and further reduces femoral peak systolic velocity (34).

   The use of sequential compression devices (SCD) during laparoscopy has been shown to reverse the reduction in femoral venous flow during laparoscopy (35). Studies of non-obese patients have shown that the use of SCD during laparoscopic cholecystectomy was effective in reversing the reduced femoral peak systolic velocity to baseline values (32,35). In contrast, the use of SCD in morbidly obese subjects was only partially effective in augmenting the reduced femoral venous flow. In a study of laparoscopic GBP, a combination of abdominal insufflation and reverse Trendelenburg position decreased the femoral peak systolic velocity by 57% of the baseline; the reduced femoral systolic velocity level was only partially reversed with the use of SCD (34). The ineffectiveness of SCD in returning the femoral peak systolic velocity to baseline value in morbidly obese patients is attributed to the larger calves and thighs of these individuals (34), who may need higher compression pressure to augment the venous flow.

CONCLUSIONS

Altered physiology has been demonstrated during laparoscopy in the morbidly obese. The two main factors that result in adverse physiologic changes during laparoscopy are absorption of CO_2 and the increased intra-abdominal pressure. Absorption of CO_2 during pneumoperitoneum can lead to hypercapnia and alteration of the acid–base balance. The increased intra-abdominal pressure can reduce femoral venous flow, intraoperative urine output, portal venous flow, respiratory compliance, and cardiac index. Appropriate intraoperative changes should be instituted to minimize these physiologic changes. In addition, the surgeon should be aware that a decrease in the operative time is important to reduce the patient's exposure to CO_2 pneumoperitoneum and its adverse consequences. Despite the adverse physiologic changes during pneumoperitoneum, laparoscopic surgery in the morbidly obese is considered safe, but patients with a history of severe cardiac, renal, hepatic, or respiratory insufficiency may be at risk for complications.

REFERENCES

1. Jakimowics J, Stultiens G, Smulders F. Laparoscopic insufflation of the abdomen reduces portal venous flow. Surg Endosc 1998; 12:129–132.
2. Beebe DS, McNevin MP, Crain JM, Letourneau JG, Belani KG, Abrams JA, Goodale RL. Evidence of venous stasis after abdominal insufflation for laparoscopic cholecystectomy. Surg Gynecol Obstet 1993; 176:443–447.
3. Chiu AW, Chang LS, Birkett DH, Babayan RK. The impact of pneumoperitoneum, pneumoretroperitoneum, and gasless laparoscopy on the systemic and renal hemodynamics. J Am Coll Surg 1995; 181:397–406.
4. Hirvonen EA, Poikolainen EO, Paakkonen ME, Nuutinen LS. The adverse hemodynamic effects of anesthesia, head-up tilt, and carbon dioxide pneumoperitoneum during laparoscopic cholecystectomy. Surg Endosc 2000; 14:272–277.
5. Lindgren L, Koivusalo AM, Kellokumpu I. Conventional pneumoperitoneum compared with abdominal wall lift for laparoscopic cholecystectomy. Br J Anaesth 1995; 75: 567–572.
6. Sharma KC, Brandstetter RD, Brensilver JM, Jung LD. Cardiopulmonary physiology and pathophysiology as a consequence of laparoscopic surgery. Chest 1996; 110:810–815.
7. Demiroluk S, Salihoglu Z, Zengin K, Kose Y, Taskin M. The effects of pneumoperitoneum on respiratory mechanics during bariatric surgery. Obes Surg 2002; 12:376–379.
8. Nguyen NT, Anderson J, Fleming NW, Ho HS, Jahr J, Wolfe BM. Effects of pneumoperitoneum on intraoperative respiratory mechanics and gas exchange during laparoscopic gastric bypass. Surg Endosc 2004; 18:64–71.
9. Dumont L, Mattys M, Mardirosoff C, Vervloesem N, Alle JL, Massaut L. Changes in pulmonary mechanics during laparoscopic gastroplasty in the morbidly obese patient. Acta Scand Anaesth 1997; 41:408–413.
10. Tan PL, Lee TL, Tweed WA. Carbon dioxide absorption and gas exchange during pelvic laparoscopy. Can J Anaesth 1992; 39:677–681.

11. Sanchez NC, Tenofsky PL, Dort JM, Shen LY, Helmer SD, Smith RS. What is normal intra-abdominal pressure? Am Surg 2001; 67:243–248.

12. Nguyen NT, Lee SL, Anderson JT, Palmer LS, Canet F, Wolfe BM. Evaluation of intraabdominal pressure after open and laparoscopic gastric bypass. Obes Surg 2001; 11:40–45.

13. Fried M, Krska Z, Danzig V. Does the laparoscopic approach significantly affect cardiac functions in laparoscopic surgery? Pilot study in non-obese and morbidly obese patients. Obes Surg 2001; 11:293–296.

14. Nguyen NT, Ho HS, Fleming NW, Moore P, Lee J, Goldman CD, Cole CJ, Wolfe BM. Cardiac function during laparoscopic vs. open gastric bypass: a randomized comparison. Surg Endosc 2002; 16:78–83.

15. Westerband A, Van De Water JM, Amzallag M, Lebowitz PW, Nwasokwa ON, Chardavoyne R, Abou-Taleb A, Wand X, Wise L. Cardiovascular changes during laparoscopic cholecystectomy. Surg Gynecol Obstet 1992; 175:535–538.

16. McLaughlin JG, Scheeres DE, Dean RJ, Bonnell BW. The adverse hemodynamic effects of laparoscopic cholecystectomy. Surg Endosc 1995; 9:121–124.

17. D'Ugo D, Persiani R, Pennestri F, Adducci E, Primieri P, Pende V, De Cosmo G. Transesophageal echocardiographic assessment of hemodynamic function during laparoscopic cholecystectomy in healthy patients. Surg Endosc 2000; 14:120–122.

18. Dorsay DA, Greene FL, Baysinger CL. Hemodynamic changes during laparoscopic cholecystectomy monitored with transesophageal echocardiography. Surg Endosc 1995; 9:128–133.

19. Ninomiya K, Kitano S, Yoshida T, Bandoh T, Baatar D, Matsumoto T. Comparison of pneumoperitoneum and abdominal wall lifting as to hemodynamics and surgical stress response during laparoscopic cholecystectomy. Surg Endosc 1998; 12:124–128.

20. Declan Fleming RY, Dougherty TB, Feig BW. The safety of helium for abdominal insufflation. Surg Endosc 1997; 11:230–234.

21. Jakimowics J, Stultiens G, Smulders F. Laparoscopic insufflation of the abdomen reduces portal venous flow. Surg Endosc 1998; 12:129–132.

22. Halevy A, Gold-Deutch R, Negri M, Lin G, Shlamkovich N, Evans S, Cotania D, Scapa E, Bahar L, Sackier J. Are elevated liver enzymes and bilirubin levels significant after laparoscopic cholecystectomy in the absence of bile duct injury? Ann Surg 1994; 219:362–364.

23. Saber AA, Laraja RD, Nalbandian HI, Pablos-Mendez A, Hanna K. Changes in liver function tests after laparoscopic cholecystectomy: not so rare, not always ominous. Am Surg 2000; 66:699–702.

24. Nguyen NT, Braley S, Fleming NW, Lambourne L, Rivers R, Wolfe BM. Comparison of postoperative hepatic function after laparoscopic versus open gastric bypass. Am J Surg 2003; 186:40–44.

25. Lindgren L. Koivusalo AM, Kellokumpu I. Conventional pneumoperitoneum compared with abdominal wall lift for laparoscopic cholecystectomy. Br J Anaesth 1995; 75:567–572.

26. Galizia G, Prizio G, Lieto E, Castellano P, Pelosio L, Imperatore V, Ferrara I, Pignatelli C. Hemodynamic and pulmonary changes during open, carbon dioxide pneumoperitoneum and abdominal wall-lifting cholecystectomy. Surg Endosc 2001; 15:477–483.

27. Nishio S, Takeda H, Yokoyama M. Changes in urinary output during laparoscopic adrenalectomy. BJU Int 1999; 83:944–947.

28. McDougall EM, Monk TG, Wolf JS, Hicks M, Clayman RV, Gardner S, Humphrey P, Sharp T, Martin K. The effect of prolonged pneumoperitoneum on renal function in an animal model. J Am Coll Surg 1996; 182:317–328.

29. Nguyen NT, Perez RV, Fleming N, Rivers R, Wolfe BM. Effect of prolonged pneumoperitoneum on intraoperative urine output during laparoscopic gastric bypass. J Am Coll Surg 2002; 195:476–483.

30. Are C, Kutka M, Talamini M, Hardacre J, Mendoza-Sagaon M, Hanley E, Toung T. Effect of laparoscopic antireflux surgery upon renal blood flow. Am J Surg 2002; 183:419–423.

31. Ortega AE, Peters JH, Incarbone R, Estreda L, Ehoan A, Kwan Y, Spencer CJ, Moore-Jeffries E, Kuchta K, Nicoloff JJ. A prospective randomized comparison of the metabolic and stress hormonal responses of laparoscopic and open cholecystectomy. J Am Coll Surg 1996; 183:249–256.

32. Millard JA, Hill BB, Cook PS, Fenoglio ME, Stahlgren LH. Intermittent sequential pneumatic compression in prevention of venous stasis associated with pneumoperitoneum during laparoscopic cholecystectomy. Arch Surg 1993; 914–919.

33. Ido K, Suzuki T, Kimura K, Taniguchi Y, Kawamoto C, Isoda N, Nagamine N, Ioka T, Kumagai M, Hirayama Y. Lower-extremity venous stasis during laparoscopic cholecystectomy as assessed using color Doppler ultrasound. Surg Endosc 1995; 9:310–313.

34. Nguyen NT, Cronan M, Braley S, Rivers R, Wolfe BM. Duplex ultrasound assessment of femoral venous flow during laparoscopic and open gastric bypass. Surg Endosc 2001; 192:469–476.

35. Schwenk W, Bohm B, Fugener A, Muller JM. Intermittent pneumatic sequential compression (ISC) of the lower extremities prevents venous stasis during laparoscopic cholecystectomy. A prospective randomized study. Surg Endosc 1998; 12:7–11.

9

The Pathophysiology of Severe Obesity and the Effects of Surgically Induced Weight Loss

Harvey J. Sugerman
Department of Surgery, Virginia Commonwealth University, Richmond, Virginia, U.S.A.

INTRODUCTION

Severe obesity is associated with a large number of associated problems that have given rise to the term "morbid obesity" (Table 1). Although some consider this term to be perjorative, severe obesity is often associated with a number of problems that are truly morbid and incapacitating. The medical problems caused by obesity begin with the head and end with the toes and involve almost every organ in-between. Several of these problems contribute to the earlier mortality associated with obesity and include coronary artery disease, severe hypertension that may be refractory to medical management, impaired cardiac function, adult onset (Type II) diabetes mellitus, obesity hypoventilation and sleep apnea syndromes, cirrhosis, venous stasis and hypercoagulability leading to an increased risk of pulmonary embolism, and necrotizing panniculitis (1,2). Morbidly obese patients can also die as a result of difficulties in recognizing the signs and symptoms of peritonitis (3). There is an increased risk of prostate, uterine, breast, kidney, esophageal, and colon cancer. Premature death is much more common in the severely obese individual; one study noted a 12-fold excess mortality in morbidly obese men in the 25- to 34-year age group (4). Increased morbidity and mortality have been noted in several other studies (5–8).

A number of obesity-related problems may not be associated with death, but can lead to significant physical or psychological disabilities. These include degenerative osteoarthritis, pseudotumor cerebri (idiopathic intracranial hypertension), cholecystitis, skin infections, chronic venous stasis ulcers, stress overflow urinary incontinence, gastroesophageal reflux, sex hormone imbalance with dysmenorrhea, hirsutism, infertility, nephrotic syndrome, and non-alcoholic liver disease (NALD) or, in its more severe form, non-alcoholic steatohepatitis (NASH). Many morbidly obese patients suffer from severe psychological and social disabilities, including marked prejudice regarding employment (9,10).

Reprinted with permission from *Surgery for Obesity and Related Diseases 2005:1; 109–119*

Table 1 Morbidity and Comorbidity of Severe Obesity

Morbidity
Central obesity
  Metabolic complications (syndrome X)
    Non–insulin-dependent diabetes (adult onset/Type II)
    Hypertension
    Dyslipidemia: elevated triglycerides, cholesterol
    Cholelithiasis, cholecystitis
  Increased intra-abdominal pressure
    Stress overflow urinary incontinence
    Gastroesophageal reflux
    Venous disease: thrombophlebitis, venous stasis ulcers, pulmonary embolism
    Obesity hypoventilation syndrome
    Nephrotic syndrome
    Hernias (incisional, inguinal)
    Pre-eclampsia
    Pseudotumor cerebri
Respiratory insufficiency of obesity (Pickwickian syndrome)
  Obesity hypoventilation syndrome
  Obstructive sleep apnea syndrome
Cardiovascular dysfunction
  Coronary artery disease
  Increased complications after coronary bypass surgery
  Heart failure subsequent to:
    Left ventricular concentric hypertrophy—hypertension
    Left ventricular eccentric hypertrophy—obesity
    Right ventricular hypertrophy—pulmonary failure
    Prolonged Q–T interval with sudden death
Sexual hormone dysfunction
  Amenorrhea, hypermenorhea
  Stein-Leventhal or polycystic ovary syndrome: hirsutism, ovarian cysts
  Infertility
  Endometrial carcinoma
  Breast carcinoma
Other carcinomas: colon, renal cell, prostate
Infectious complications
  Difficulty recognizing peritonitis
  Necrotizing pancreatitis
  Necrotizing subcutaneous infections
  Wound infections, dehiscence
Pseudotumor cerebri (idiopathic intracranial hypertension)
Degenerative osteoarthritis
  Feet, ankles, knees, hips, back, shoulders
Psychosocial impairment
  Decreased employability, work discrimination

Comorbidity (From the top of the head to the tip of the toes and almost every organ
  in-between)
Head
  Brain
    Stroke
    Headaches

(Continued)

Table 1   Morbidity and Comorbidity of Severe Obesity (*Continued*)

Hypertension
Pseudotumor cerebri: headaches
    I Optic nerve:
        Visual field cuts
        Blindness
    III Oculomotor nerve palsy
    V Trigeminal nerve: Tic Doloreaux
    VII Facial nerve: Bell's palsy
    VIII Auditory nerve: pulsatile tinnitus
Eyes: diabetic retinopathy + pseudotumor complications
Mouth/throat
  Sleep apnea
Chest
  Breast cancer
  Obesity hypoventilation
    Heavy chest wall
    Elevated diaphragm
    Increased intra-thoracic pressure
    Decreased expiratory reserve volume
Heart
  Left ventricular hypertrophy
    Eccentric: increased cardiac output
    Concentric: increased peripheral vascular resistance
  Increased cardiac filling pressures (CVP, PAP, WP)
  Right heart failure
    Tricuspid insufficiency
Esophagus
  Acid reflux
  Asthma
  Adenocarcinoma
  Esophageal varices
Abdomen
  Gall bladder
    Cholecystitis
    Adenocarcinoma
  Liver
    Non-alcholic liver disease (NALD)
    Non-alcoholic steatohepatitis (NASH)
    Cirrhosis
    Type II diabetes mellitus
  Spleen
    Splenomegaly (portal hypertension)
    Hypersplenism (portal hypertension)
  Pancreas
    Type II diabetes mellitus
    Necrotizing pancreatitis
  Colon
    Adenocarcinoma
    Diverticulitis

(Continued)

Table 1 Morbidity and Comorbidity of Severe Obesity (*Continued*)

General
  Difficulty diagnosing peritonitis
  Hernia
    Incisional
    Inguinal
    Spighelian
  Wound infection
  "Apron"
    Peau d'Orange lymphatic stasis
Kidney
  Hypertension
  Proteinuria
  Renal cell carcinoma
Urinary bladder
  Stress incontinence
Ovaries/uterus
  Increased estradiol, androstenedione
  Polycystic ovary syndrome, Stein-Leventhal syndrome
    Infertility
    Dysmenorrhea
    Hirsutism
  Endometrial carcinoma
  Breast cancer
Prostate: adenocarcinoma
Anus
  Perianal abscesses
  Necrotizing panniculitis
Integument
  Necrotizing panniculitis
  Hirsutism
Increased risk of operative complications
  Colectomy
  Hysterectomy
  Kidney, liver transplantation
Spine
  Herniated disc
Upper extremities
  Shoulder girdle pain
  Edema
Lower extremities
  Osteoarthritis
    Hip arthralgia
    Knee arthralgia
  Venous stasis
    Edema
    Thrombophlebitis
    Stasis ulcers
    Pulmonary embolism
  Toes
    Diabetic neuropathy
    Diabetic ulcers

CENTRAL (ANDROID) VS. PERIPHERAL (GYNOID) FAT DISTRIBUTION

It has been noted that central obesity is associated with a higher mortality than peripheral obesity, commonly referred to as android versus gynoid obesity because of their relative prevalence in men and women, respectively. This has been attributed to the metabolically more active visceral adipose tissue than to the subcutaneous fat so that there is a greater rate of glucose production, Type II diabetes, and hyperinsulinism. Increased insulin secretion is thought to increase sodium reabsorption and, thus, cause hypertension (11–18). Central obesity also is associated with a greater production of cholesterol, primarily in the form of low-density lipoprotein, leading to a higher-than-normal incidence of atherosclerotic cardiovascular disease, and an increased incidence of gallstones. The increased visceral fat has been related to an increased waist:hip (W:H) ratio or, in more common terms, as the "apple" versus "pear" distribution of fat. Computerized axial tomographic (CAT) scans, however, have noted a much better correlation between anterior–posterior abdominal diameter and visceral fat distribution than with the W:H ratio (19,20), especially in women who may have both central and peripheral obesity. In this situation, the peripheral obesity "dilutes" the central obesity using a W:H ratio, so that either the waist circumference alone or the saggital abdominal diameter should be used as a measurement of central obesity.

A recent study documented an increased bladder pressure in morbidly obese women, which was associated with a high incidence of urinary incontinence (21). It is quite probable that much of the comorbidity of severe obesity is related to an increased intra-abdominal pressure (22) secondary to a central distribution of fat (Table 1) and that the urinary bladder pressure, a surrogate for intra-abdominal pressure, is highly correlated with the sagittal abdominal diameter or waist circumference. Animal studies (23) have documented a close relationship between urinary bladder pressure and directly measured intra-abdominal pressure. In addition to urinary incontinence, this increased intra-abdominal pressure is probably responsible for the increased venous stasis disease and venous stasis ulcers, gastroesophageal reflux, nephrotic syndrome secondary to increased renal venous pressure, incisional and inguinal hernias, and obesity hypoventilation syndrome secondary to a high-riding diaphragm and restrictive lung disease. This can also lead to an increased intra-pleural pressure which can then cause increased intracardiac pressure, so that severely obese patients with obesity hypoventilation syndrome may require high cardiac filling pressure to maintain an adequate cardiac output (23,24). It is also quite possible that increased intra-abdominal pressure is responsible for the high incidence of systemic hypertension in the morbidly obese, as well as the cause of "idiopathic" intracranial hypertension (23,25–27).

In a previous study (22), we noted a much higher intra-abdominal pressure in morbidly obese patients at the time of gastric bypass surgery than the five non-obese patients who were undergoing colectomy, ileal pouch anal anastomosis (IPAA) for ulcerative colitis. To realize how high these pressures can be in severe obesity, one needs to relate them to the pressures seen in patients with an acute abdominal compartment syndrome (28,29), where it is generally thought that a urinary bladder pressure of ≥ 20–25 cmH$_2$O is an indication to return the patient to the operating room for emergency laparotomy and abdominal decompression. Many severely obese patients have urinary bladder pressures well above 25 cmH$_2$O. Surgically-induced weight loss was associated with a significant decrease in sagittal abdominal diameter, urinary bladder pressures, and obesity co-morbidity (30).

HYPERTENSION

We hypothesize that obesity-associated hypertension is secondary to an increased intra-abdominal pressure rather than to increased insulin-induced sodium reabsorption. The presumed pathophysiology is related to the activation of the rennin–angiotensin–aldosterone system through one or a combination of three possible renal mechanisms. The first presumed mechanism is due to direct pressure on the renal veins leading to an increased glomerular capillary pressure, a capillary leak with either a microalbuminuria commonly seen in the morbidly obese or, on occasion, a large protein leak with development of the nephrotic syndrome (31,32). The increased glomerular pressure probably stimulates the juxta-glomerular apparatus (JGA) to increase renin secretion (33). A second mechanism relates to a direct pressure on the renal capsule, leading to a renal compartment syndrome and activation of the rennin–angiotensin–aldosterone system. The third possibility relates to the increased pleural pressure secondary to a rising diaphragm which impedes venous return to the heart, leading to a decrease in cardiac output and renal arterial pressure which again stimulates activation of the JGA to produce renin (23,34). Increased renin and aldosterone levels are seen in a porcine model of acutely increased intra-abdominal pressure (34). Activation of the rennin–angiotensin–aldosterone system leads to salt and water retention, commonly seen in the severely obese, and vasoconstriction. Surgically induced weight loss is associated with a clinically significant, long-lasting improvement in blood pressure with the elimination of anti-hypertensive medications in two-thirds to three-quarters of hypertensive patients or a marked decrease in their use (35–43). The Swedish Obesity Study (SOS) initially noted a significant improvement in both diabetes and hypertension in the surgically treated patients as compared to matched controls (36). However, the improvement in hypertension for the overall group was no longer present at eight years after surgery (38). Unfortunately, only 6% of the surgical patients in the SOS trial had a gastric bypass, 70% a vertical banded gastroplasty, and 24% a gastric banding. The gastric bypass patients had a significantly greater weight loss than either the gastroplasty or gastric banded patients, and also maintained a significant decrease in both systolic and diastolic pressures at five years after surgery (39).

CARDIAC DYSFUNCTION AND DYSLIPIDEMIA

Morbid obesity may be associated with cardiomegaly and impaired left-, right-, or biventricular function. Severe obesity may be associated with a high cardiac output and a low systemic vascular resistance leading to left ventricular hypertrophy. Obesity also is associated with hypertension, which leads to concentric left ventricular hypertrophy. This combination of obesity and hypertension with left ventricular eccentric and concentric hypertrophy may lead to left ventricular failure (44,45). Correction of morbid obesity improves cardiac function in these patients (24,46–49). Morbid obesity is also associated with an accelerated rate of coronary atherosclerosis. These patients often have hypercholesterolemia and a decreased high density (HDL) to low density lipoprotein (LDL) ratio. In the Nurses Study, women with a BMI $> 29 \, kg/m^2$ have a significantly increased incidence of myocardial angina and/or infarction (50,51). Surgically induced weight loss has been shown in several studies to significantly reduce triglyceride and LDL cholesterol levels, while increasing HDL levels (38,43,52–56). Respiratory insufficiency associated with morbid obesity can result in hypoxemic pulmonary artery vasoconstriction, which in severe cases may lead to right, or biventricular, heart failure associated with tricuspid valvular insufficiency. Correction of hypoxemia and hypercarbia with surgically induced weight loss will correct the elevated pulmonary artery and wedge pressures within three to nine months after surgery (24). Severe obstructive sleep apnea syndrome (SAS) may be associated with prolonged sinus arrest, premature ventricular contractions, and sudden death.

PULMONARY DYSFUNCTION

Respiratory insufficiency of obesity is associated with either obesity hypoventilation syndrome (OHS), SAS, or a combination of the two, commonly called the Pickwickian syndrome (24,57–64).

Obesity hypoventilation syndrome. This problem arises primarily from the increased intra-abdominal pressure in patients with central, abdominal obesity which leads to high-riding diaphragm (22,65). As a result, the lungs are squeezed, producing a restrictive pulmonary defect. A heavy, obese thoracic cage may also contribute to the pathophysiology secondary to a decreased chest wall compliance. These patients have a markedly decreased expiratory reserve volume, leading to alveolar collapse and arterio-venous shunting at end-expiration. They also have smaller reductions in all other lung volumes (59). They have hypoxemia and hypercarbia while awake and a blunted ventilator response to CO_2.

Chronic hypoxemia leads to pulmonary artery vasoconstriction. However, obesity hypoventilation patients often have both markedly elevated pulmonary artery pressures and pulmonary capillary wedge pressures, suggesting both right and left ventricular failure. Despite these high pressures, overt heart failure is unusual, even with pulmonary capillary wedge pressures as high as 40 mmHg (24). These pressures are increased as a result of a marked increase in pleural pressures secondary to the high-riding diaphragm and increased intra-abdominal pressure, so that the transatrial and transventricular pressures may be, in fact, normal (23). These findings have been noted in a porcine model of acutely increased intra-abdominal pressure. Thus, morbidly obese patients with OHS may not respond well to diuresis, and may need these elevated pressures to maintain an adequate cardiac output.

As a result of the increased inferior vena caval and pulmonary artery pressures, obesity hypoventilation patients are at risk for a fatal pulmonary embolism (57). Thus, right heart catheterization should be considered prior to obesity surgery and a prophylactic inferior vena caval filter inserted at the time of surgery in patients with a mean pulmonary artery pressure $\geq 40 \, mmHg$. Surgically induced weight loss (24,59,60,63) corrects hypoxemia, hypercarbia, and increased cardiac filling pressures associated with obesity hypoventilation syndrome.

Sleep apnea syndrome. Sleep apnea syndrome (SAS) is associated with central obesity and is due to both depression of the normal genioglossus reflex, possibly secondary to a large, heavy tongue, and deposition of fat within the hypopharynx with narrowing of the cervical airway (58). These patients snore loudly while asleep and suffer from severe daytime somnolence, with tendencies to fall asleep while driving or at work. The daytime somnolence is probably secondary to impaired stage III, IV, and REM sleep. The diagnosis of obstructive SAS is suggested by a history of severe daytime somnolence, frequent nocturnal awakening, loud snoring, and morning headaches and is confirmed with sleep polysomnography. This technique documents cessation of airflow during sleep associated with persistent respiratory efforts. Most of the apneic episodes are obstructive, but some are central. The latter is seen with central nervous system hypoxemia, analogous to the Cheynes-Stokes respirations seen at high altitudes. The severity of sleep apnea is usually determined by the respiratory disturbance index (RDI), which is a combination of apneic episodes (cessation of airflow for ≥ 10 seconds) and hypopneic episodes (diminution by 50% of airflow for ≥ 10 seconds) and is divided into mild (RDI ≤ 19), moderate (RDI 20–39) and severe (RDI ≥ 40). Moderate-to-severe sleep apnea should be treated with nocturnal nasal continuous positive airway pressure (nasal CPAP); if the patient cannot tolerate nasal CPAP and has severe sleep apnea, a tracheostomy should be considered at the time of obesity surgery. All patients with moderate-to-severe sleep apnea should be managed with intubation and mechanical ventilation in the intensive care unit, weaned, and on the morning after surgery, unless they also have obesity hypoventilation in which case they may have to be ventilated for several days until their arterial blood gases return to their preoperative values.

Patients with severe sleep apnea have difficulty staying awake during the day. This syndrome may be associated with sudden death and should always be considered in trauma victims who have fallen asleep while driving. We have seen many patients with severe sleep apnea who are in occupations which are incompatible with this syndrome: taxi-cab and interstate truck drivers and state prison guards! Surgically induced weight loss corrects or markedly improves sleep apnea syndrome, permitting removal of their tracheostomy tube or discontinuation of nasal CPAP (59–64).

In a series from the Medical College of Virginia, 12.5% of the patients who underwent gastric surgery for morbid obesity had respiratory insufficiency (59). Of the affected individuals, 51% had sleep apnea syndrome alone, 12% had obesity hypoventilation syndrome alone, and 37% had both. Of these, 64% were men in contrast to only 14% of the entire group of patients who underwent surgery for obesity. Patients with respiratory insufficiency were significantly more obese than those without pulmonary dysfunction. However, obesity is not the only factor causing respiratory dysfunction or insufficiency, since many patients who underwent surgery for morbid obesity and who did not have a clinically significant pulmonary problem, weighed more than the patients with respiratory insufficiency. Most of the obese patients with respiratory dysfunction had an additional pulmonary problem, such as sarcoidosis, heavy cigarette use, recurrent pulmonary embolism, myotonic dystrophy, or idiopathic pulmonary fibrosis. Obstructive SAS and OHS are associated with a high mortality and serious morbidity; weight reduction will correct both (24,59–64).

DIABETES

Obesity is a frequent etiologic factor in the development of Type II adult onset diabetes mellitus. Morbidly obese patients can be very resistant to insulin due to the marked down-regulation of insulin receptors. The tendency toward hyperglycemia manifested by obese patients is another risk factor for coronary artery disease as well as for fatal subcutaneous infections. Gastric surgery–induced weight loss, performed

Table 2 Decreases in Obesity Comorbidity after Weight-Loss Surgery

Comorbidity	References
Type II diabetes mellitus	38,40,42,66–79
Systemic hypertension	35–43
Obstructive sleep apnea	59–64
Obesity hypoventilation	24,59,60,63
Cardiac dysfunction	24,45–49
Pseudotumor cerebri	27,110
Venous stasis disease	81
Gastroesophageal reflux	90–92
Asthma	98,99
Dyslipidemia	38,43,52–56
Stress urinary incontinence	21
Polycystic ovary syndrome	102
Pregnancy outcomes	104–107
Fatty liver disease	122–125
Musculoskeletal pain	85–87
Health-related quality of life	126–130
Psychological status	131–136
Mortality	70,137

both open and laparoscopically, is associated with resolution of the diabetes (38,40,42,66–79) in 85% of patients and this effect is long-lasting (Table 2). Pories and colleagues have found that the earlier the patients with Type II diabetes mellitus undergo weight reduction gastric bypass surgery, the greater is their likelihood to have complete resolution of their diabetes (67,68). In another study, it was noted that patients without diabetes or hypertension are significantly younger by five years than those with either diabetes or hypertension, and are significantly younger by another five years than those with both diabetes and hypertension (42). Furthermore, the more weight the patients lost, the more they were likely to correct their diabetes and hypertension (42). These data support the earlier operations in morbidly obese diabetic patients before their diabetes-related complications develop (neuropathy, retinopathy, renal insufficiency). Peripheral insulin resistance, primarily in the skeletal muscle, is present in morbidly obese patients and may resolve with surgically induced weight loss. There are data suggesting that Type II diabetes mellitus could be a disease of the foregut (69). The gastric bypass operation has been found to decrease the progression and mortality of non–insulin-dependent diabetes mellitus when compared to a matched control group of patients who either chose not to have surgery or were unable to obtain insurance coverage (70).

VENOUS STASIS DISEASE

Morbidly obese patients have an increased risk for deep venous thrombosis, venous stasis ulcers, and pulmonary embolism. Low levels of antithrombin III may increase their risk of blood clots (80). The increased weight within the abdomen raises the intra-abdominal pressure and therefore, the inferior vena caval pressure with an increased resistance to venous return, leading to the pretibial bronze edema, lower extremity venous stasis ulcers, and tendency toward deep venous thrombosis.

A similar mechanism may be responsible for the increased risk of pulmonary embolism in patients with right heart failure secondary to hypoxemic pulmonary artery vasoconstriction. Venous stasis ulcers can be incapacitating and extremely difficult to treat in the morbidly obese; weight reduction may be the critical factor, as skin grafts, pressure stockings, medicated rigid compression boots, and wound care are often ineffective. Surgically induced weight loss reduces intra-abdominal pressure and permits healing of these stasis ulcers (81).

DEGENERATIVE JOINT DISEASE

The increased weight in the morbidly obese leads to early degenerative arthritic changes of the weight-bearing joints, including the knees, hips, and spine. Many orthopedic surgeons refuse to insert total hip or knee prosthetics in patients weighing over 250 pounds because of an unacceptable incidence of prosthetic loosening (82). There is a high risk of complications in obese patients following intramedullary nailing of femoral fractures (83). Severe obesity is a common problem in patients requiring intervertebral disc surgery (84). Weight reduction following gastric surgery for obesity permits subsequent successful joint replacement (85) and is associated with decreases in musculoskeletal and lower back pain (86,87). In some instances, the decrease in pain following weight loss obviates the need for joint or intervertebral disc surgery.

GASTROESOPHAGEAL REFLUX AND ASTHMA

Morbidly obese patients frequently suffer from gastroesophageal reflux disease (GERD). Although one study did not find a relationship to severe obesity (88), others have (89). This is also probably secondary to an increased intra-abdominal pressure. The lower esophageal sphincter may be normal in these patients, but the increased intra-abdominal pressure can overcome a normal sphincter pressure. Surgically induced weight loss has corrected this problem (90–92). GERD resolves promptly following gastric bypass for obesity as neither acid nor bile can reflux into the esophagus after this procedure. Some studies have noted an increased GERD following vertical banded gastroplasty (93–95) which resolves following conversion to gastric bypass (94,95). An antireflux procedure (e.g., Nissen fundoplication) is probably inappropriate in a severly obese patient, as gastric surgery-induced weight loss not only corrects acid and bile reflux but also improves additional co-morbidity usually present in these individuals. The increase risk of GERD in obese individuals increases their risk of esophageal adenocarcinoma, and the epidemic of obesity may be one explanation for the marked increase in the incidence of this cancer (96,97). Two studies have documented improvement in asthma following surgically induced weight loss, presumably due to the prevention of nocturnal gastroesophageal reflux and tracheobronchial aspiration or spasm (98,99).

URINARY INCONTINENCE

Severely obese women often have stress overflow urinary incontinence. Some men with central obesity also complain of urinary urgency, although incontinence in men is rare. Significantly increased urinary bladder pressures have been noted in women with this problem (21). Surgically induced weight loss is associated with a correction of urinary incontinence in 95% of patients, often within a few months of surgery, and this is associated with a significant decrease in urinary bladder pressure when measured one year after surgery. The rapid resolution of this vexing problem, often within one to two months after surgery, may be related to a rapid decrease in the intra-abdominal and urinary bladder pressures following obesity surgery-induced weight loss as a result of the relationship between wall tension and volume of a sphere according to LaPlace's Law, where pressure is proportional to the radius to the fourth power. This is best thought of as a tense balloon that rapidly loses tension when a small amount of air escapes.

FEMALE SEXUAL HORMONE DYSFUNCTION

Women often suffer from sexual dysfunction due to excessive levels of both the virilizing hormone, androstenedione, and the feminizing hormone, estradiol. These may produce infertility, hirsutism, ovarian cysts (Stein-Leventhal or polycystic ovary syndrome), hypermenorrhea, and a significantly increased risk of breast and endometrial carcinoma. Polycystic ovary syndrome has also been found to be associated with Type II diabetes and, in mild cases, may improve with metformin treatment (100,101). Surgically induced weight loss often returns sex hormone levels to normal, increasing fertility and menstrual regularity (102). It is thought that there may be a higher incidence of neural tube defects in infants born to women during the rapid weight loss that occurs after surgery (103), probably due to deficient folic acid levels. Thus, birth control is strongly recommended for one year after surgically induced weight loss procedures. Surgery has permitted pregnancies in previously infertile morbidly obese women. Increased weight also increases the risk of complications of pregnancy including the higher incidence of pre-eclampsia seen in obese women, problems with delivery, and an increased risk of venous thrombosis and pulmonary embolism. Surgically induced weight loss is associated with decreased pregnancy-related complications, including pre-eclampsia, and reduces the frequency of cesarean section (104–107).

PSEUDOTUMOR CEREBRI

Pseudotumor cerebri, also known as idiopathic intracranial hypertension, may be associated with morbid obesity. The problem is almost always seen in women. Symptoms include severe headache which is usually worse in the morning, bilateral pulsatile auditory tinnitus, and visual field cuts. Severely increased intracranial pressure (ICP) can lead to permanent blindness. Additional cranial nerves that can be involved include the Vth (Tic Doloreaux), the VIth (oculomotor nerve paralysis), and the VIIth (Bell's palsy). Studies suggest that pseudotumor cerebri is secondary to an increased intra-abdominal pressure leading to an increased pleural pressure and decreased venous drainage from the brain, with a consequent cerebral venous engorgement and an increased ICP. Increased ICP occurs in an acute porcine model of increased intra-abdominal pressure which is prevented by median sternotomy (25,26). Patients with impending blindness should undergo emergent optic nerve fenestration (108). In the past, pseudotumor cerebri has been treated with ventriculo-peritoneal or lumbar-peritoneal cerebrospinal fluid (CSF) shunts. There is a high incidence of shunt occlusion (109), and in some instances patients can have continued headache and auditory tinnitus despite a patent shunt. These failures are probably secondary to shunting from one high-pressure system to another. Patients may also develop major neurological complications following insertion of ventriculo-peritoneal or lumbo-peritoneal shunts. Surgically induced weight loss decreases CSF pressures, relieves headache and tinnitus (27,110), and is the procedure of choice rather than CSF-peritoneal shunting. The rapid resolution of headache, tinnitus, and other pseudotumor cerebri symptoms is probably a result of the rapid decrease in intra-abdominal pressure. It is difficult to understand, however, why this syndrome is almost entirely restricted to women, since men with central obesity also have increased intra-abdominal and pleural pressures.

MALIGNANCY RISK WITH OBESITY

In addition to uterine carcinoma, there is also a significantly increased risk of breast, prostate, kidney, esophageal, and colon cancers in the morbidly obese (96,97,111–114). The increased risk of breast, uterine, and prostate cancers is probably secondary to the high levels of sex hormones seen in these patients. As previously mentioned, the increased incidence of GERD in the morbidly obese, a probable consequence of increased intra-abdominal pressure, is probably responsible for the increased incidence of esophageal adenocarcinoma. The causes for the increased incidences of colon and renal cell cancers are unknown.

HERNIA RISK WITH OBESITY

Severe obesity is also associated with a significantly increased risk of all types of hernias. This is also probably secondary to the increased intra-abdominal pressure associated with central obesity. A significantly higher incidence of incisional hernia has been noted following open gastric bypass surgery for morbid obesity than after total colectomy, proctectomy, and stapled IPAA for ulcerative colitis, in patients 60% of whom were taking approximately 30 mg of prednisone and had incisions on the lower mid-abdomen to above the umbilicus, both of which are thought to increase the risk of hernia (115). Reduced risk of incisional hernias and other wound-related complications are significant advantages of the laparoscopic approach for obesity surgery. We have seen bilateral Spigelian hernias in one of our morbidly obese patients who also developed an incisional hernia. Repair of incisional hernias in morbidly obese patients has a high risk of recurrence and should probably be reinforced with a polypropylene mesh (115).

INFECTIOUS PROBLEMS ASSOCIATED WITH MORBID OBESITY

There is a higher incidence of fulminant diverticulitis (116,117), necrotizing pancreatitis (118), and necrotizing paniculitis (119) in severely obese patients. This is probably due to the increased retroperitoneal and subcutaneous fat, as well as diabetes, which provides an ideal growth medium for bacteria.

NALD/NASH

NALD is also associated with Type II diabetes mellitus. The exact pathophysiology is unknown. It is presumably secondary to the increased glycogen deposition in the liver with subsequent conversion to fat (120). Increased fatty infiltration produces markedly enlarged livers which can make bariatric surgery much more difficult and dangerous, and may prevent a successful laparoscopic procedure because of the difficulty in elevating the left lobe of the liver from the gastroesophageal tissues. The increased fat in the liver may be metabolized to free fatty acids which may be quite toxic to tissues, and be responsible for the development of NASH and the subsequent development of severe cirrhosis (88). There is a serious concern that NASH may overtake a combination of hepatitis A, B, and C as the primary cause for liver failure and the need for liver transplantation, if the epidemic of severe obesity remains unchecked (121). Surgically induced weight loss has been found to significantly decrease the severity of hepatic steatosis (122–125).

QUALITY OF LIFE

Severe obesity is associated with a marked reduction in the quality of life. Several studies have documented an improvement in the quality of life following surgically induced weight loss (126–130). Psychological profiles document significant psychological impairment in the morbidly obese which also improves following surgically induced weight loss (10,131–136). However, there may also be an increased risk of suicide if the individual believes that severe obesity was the total cause of their emotional impairment which does not resolve following major weight loss after surgery. Lastly, the morbidly obese are at risk of facing prejudice from many people, including physicians, but more economically importantly, from employers (137,138).

MORTALITY

Three studies have documented a decrease in mortality following bariatric surgery. One noted a significantly decreased mortality (1% vs. 4.5%) in diabetic patients who underwent gastric bypass as compared to diabetic patients who, for insurance or personal reasons, did not undergo surgery for obesity (70). A study from Canada noted an 89% reduction in long-term mortality (0.7% vs. 6.2%, $p < 0.001$) in patients who underwent surgery for obesity from 1983 to 2002 [194 vertical banded gastroplasty (35% subsequently converted to gastric bypass) and 841 gastric bypass] when compared to an age- and sex-matched non-operated cohort (139). Furthermore, the surgical patients also had a significantly decreased rate of developing new medical conditions (cardiovascular, cancer, endocrine, infectious diseases, psychiatric, and digestive), and this was associated with a significant decrease in the cost of care so that the operation was amortized at 3.5 years (139). A study from the State of Washington also noted a significant decrease in the mortality of patients who underwent obesity surgery, especially of those with obesity co-morbidities (140). However, this study also noted that surgeons who had performed ≤ 19 procedures had a significantly greater probability of causing patient death than those who had performed ≥ 20 procedures (140). The SOS has not yet reported a significantly decreased mortality in the surgical patients as compared to the control cohort, but 94% of the surgical patients in this study underwent a purely gastric restrictive procedure and have not lost as much weight as the 6% of patients who underwent a gastric bypass operation, and this could be a reason for the absence of a mortality benefit to date (41).

CONCLUSIONS

There are overwhelming amounts of data documenting a profound improvement in the co-morbidities associated with severe obesity. A recent meta-analysis noted a marked improvement in diabetes, hypertension, hyperlipidemia, and sleep apnea following surgically induced weight loss (141). If impaired quality of life, psychiatric dysfunction, social ostracism, and difficulties obtaining employment are included, then it is highly probable that all severely obese patients suffer from a significant obesity-related morbidity.

REFERENCES

1.   Sjöström LV. Morbidity of severely obese subjects. Am J Clin Nutr 1992; 55:508S–515S.
2.   Sjöström LV. Mortality of severely obese subjects. Am J Clin Nutr 1992; 55:516S–523S.
3.   Mason EE, Printen KJ, Barron P, et al. Risk reduction in gastric operations for obesity. Ann Surg 1979; 190:158–165.
4.   Drennick EJ, Bale GS, Seltter F, et al. Excessive mortality and causes of death in morbidly obese men. JAMA 1980; 243:443–445.
5.   Folsom AR, Kaye SA, Sellers TA, Hong CP, Cerhan JR, Potter TD, et al. Body fat distribution and 5-year risk of death in older women. JAMA 1993; 269:483–487.
6.   VanItalie TB. Obesity: adverse effects on health and longevity. Am J Clin Nutr 1979; 32:2723–2733.
7.   Lew EA, Garfinkel L. Variations in mortality by weight among 750,000 men and women. J Chronic Dis 1979; 32:563–568.
8.   Kral JG. Morbid obesity and health related risks. Ann Intern Med 1985; 103:1043–1046.
9.   Sarlio-Lahteenkorva S, Stunkard A, Rissanen A. Psycosocial factors and quality of life in obesity. Int J Obes Relat Metab Disord 1995; 19:1S–5S.
10. Stunkard AJ, Wadden TA. Psychological aspects of severe obesity. Am J Clin Nutr 1991; 55:532S–534S.
11. Kissebah A, Vydelingum N, Murray R, et al. Relation of body fat distribution to metabolic complications of obesity. J Clin Endocrinol Metab 1982; 54:254–257.
12. Reaven GM. Syndrome X: 6 years later. J Intern Med Suppl 1994; 736:13–22.
13. Kvist A, Chowdhury B, Grangard U, Tylen U, Sjostrom L. Total and visceral adipose tissue volumes derived from measurements with computed tomography in adult men and women: predictive equations. Am J Clin Nutr 1988; 48:1351–1361.
14. Gillum RF. The association of body fat distribution with hypertension, hypertensive heart disease, coronary heart disease, diabetes and cardiovascular risk factors in men and women aged 18–79 years. J Chronic Dis 1987; 40:421–428.
15. Micciolo R, Bosello O, Ferrari P, Armellini F. The association of body fat location with hemodynamic and metabolic status in men and women aged 21–60 years. J Clin Epidemiol 1991; 44:591–608.
16. Björntorp P. Abdominal obesity and the metabolic syndrome. Ann Med 1992; 24: 465–468.
17. Johnson D, Prud'homme D, Després JP, Nadeau A, Tremblay A, Bouchard C. Relation of abdominal obesity to hyperinsulinemia and high blood pressure in men. Int J Obes 1992; 16:881–890.

18. Mauriege P, Després JP, Marcotte M, Ferland M, Tremblay A, Nadeau A, et al. Abdominal fat cell lipolysis, body fat distribution, and metabolic variables in premenopausal women. J Clin Endocrinol Metab 1990; 71:1028–1035.
19. Sjöström L. A computer-tomography based multicompartment body composition technique and anthropometric predictions of lean body mass, total and subcutaneous adipose tissue. Int J Obes 1991; 15(suppl 2):19–30.
20. Lemiuex S, Prud'homme D, Tremblay A, Bouchard C, Després J-P. Anthropometric correlates to changes in visceral adipose tissue over 7 years in women. Int J Obes 1996; 20:618–624.
21. Bump RC, Sugerman HJ, Fantl JA, et al. Obesity and lower urinary tract function in women: effects of surgically induced weight loss. Am J Obstet Gynecol 1992; 167:392–397.
22. Sugerman H, Windsor A, Bessos M, Wolfe M. Abdominal pressure, sagittal abdominal diameter and obesity co-morbidity. J Int Med 1997; 241:71–79.
23. Ridings PC, Bloomfield GL, Blocher CR, Sugerman HJ. Cardiopulmonary effects of raised intra-abdominal pressure before and after volume expansion. J Trauma 1995; 39:1071–1075.
24. Sugerman HJ, Baron PL, Fairman RP, Evans CR, Vetrovec GW. Hemodynamic dysfunction in obesity hypoventilation syndrome and the effects of treatment with surgically induced weight loss. Ann Surg 1988; 207:604–613.
25. Bloomfield GL, Ridings PC, Blocher CS, Marmarou A, Sugerman HJ. Effects of increased intra-abdominal pressure upon intracranial and cerebral perfusion pressure before and after volume expansion. J Trauma 1996; 40:936–943.
26. Bloomfield GL, Ridings PC, Blocher CR, Sugerman HJ. Increased pleural pressure mediates the effects of elevated intra-abdominal pressure upon the central nervous and cardiovascular systems. Crit Care Med 1997; 25:496–503.
27. Sugerman HJ, Felton WL, Sismanis A, Salvant JB, Kellum JM. Effects of surgically induced weight loss on pseudotumor cerebri in morbid obesity. Neurology 1995; 45:1655–1659.
28. Harman PK, Kron IL, McLachlan HD, et al. Elevated intra-abdominal pressure and renal function. Ann Surg 1982; 196:594–599.
29. Iberti TJ, Lieber CE, Benjamin E. Determination of intra-abdominal pressure using a transurethral bladder catheter: clinical validation of the technique. Anesthesiology 1989; 70:47–50.
30. Sugerman H, Windsor A, Bessos M, Kellum J, Reines H, DeMaria E. Effects of surgically induced weight loss on urinary bladder pressure, sagittal abdominal diameter and obesity co-morbidity. Int J Obes Relat Metab Disord 1998; 22:230–235.
31. Valensi P, Assayag M, Busby M, Paries J, Lormeau B, Attali J-R. Microalbuminuria in obese patients with or without hypertension. Int J Obes Relat Metab Disord 1996; 20:574–579.
32. Weisinger JR, Kempson RL, Eldridge FL, Swenson RS. The nephrotic syndrome: a complication of massive obesity. Ann Intern Med 1974; 81:440–447.
33. Doty JM, Saggi BH, Sugerman HJ, Blocher CR, Pin R, Fakhry I, Gehr T, Sica D. The effect of increased renal venous pressure on renal function. J Trauma 1999; 47:1000–1004.
34. Bloomfield GL, Blocher CR, Sugerman HJ. Elevated intra-abdominal pressure increases plasma renin activity and aldosterone levels. J Trauma 1997; 42:997–1004.
35. Alaud-din A, Meterissian S, Lisbona R, MacLean LD, Forse RA. Assessment of cardiac function in patients who were morbidly obese. Surgery 1990; 108:809–818.
36. Foley EF, Benotti PN, Borlase BC, Hollingshead J, Blackburn GL. Impact of gastric restrictive surgery on hypertension in the morbidly obese. Am J Surg 1992; 163:294–297.
37. Carson JL, Ruddy ME, Duff AE, Holmes NJ, Cody RP, Brolin RE. The effect of gastric bypass surgery on hypertension in morbidly obese patients. Ann Intern Med 1994; 154:193–200.

38. Sjostrom CD, Lissner L, Wedel H, et al. Reduction in incidence of diabetes, hypertension and lipid disturbances after intentional weight loss induced by bariatric surgery: the SOS Intervention Study. Obes Res 1999; 7:477–484.

39. Ben-Dov I, Grossman E, Stein A, Shachor D, Gaides M. Marked weight reduction lowers resting and exercise blood pressure in morbidly obese subjects. Am J Hypertens 2000; 13:251–255.

40. Sjostrom CD, Peltonen M, Wedel H, et al. Differentiated long-term effects of intentional weight loss on diabetes and hypertension. Hypertension 2000; 36:20–25.

41. Sjostrom CD, Peltonen M, Sjostrom L. Blood pressure and pulse pressure during long-term weight loss in the obese: the Swedish Obese Subjects (SOS) Intervention Study. Obes Res 2001; 9:188–195.

42. Sugerman HJ, Wolfe LG, Sica DA, Clore JN. Diabetes and hypertension in severe obesity and effects of gastric bypass-induced weight loss. Ann Surg 2003; 237:751–756.

43. Frigg A, Peterli R, Peters T, Ackermann C, Tondelli P. Reduction in co-morbidities 4 years after laparoscopic adjustable gastric banding. Obes Surg 2004; 14:216–223.

44. Messerli FH, Sundgaard-Riise K, Reisin ED, et al. Disparate cardiovascular effects of obesity and arterial hypertension. Am J Med 1983; 74:808–811.

45. Alpert MA, Terry BE, Kelly DL. Effect of weight loss on cardiac chamber size, wall thickness and left ventricular function in morbid obesity. Am J Cardiol 1985; 55:783–786.

46. Alpert MA, Lambert CR, Panayiotou H, Terry BE, Cohen MV, et al. Relation of duration of morbid obesity to left ventricular mass, systolic function, and diastolic filling, and effect of weight loss. Am J Cardiol 1995; 76:1194–1197.

47. Karason K, Wallentin I, Larsson B, Sjostrom L. Effects of obesity and weight loss on left ventricular mass and relative wall thickness: survey and intervention study. Br Med J 1997; 315:912–916.

48. Karason K, Wallentin I, Larsson B, Sjostrom L. Effects of obesity and weight loss on cardiac function and valvular performance. Obes Res 1998; 6:422–429.

49. Kanoupakis E, Michaloudis D, Fraidakis O, Parthenakis F, Vardas P, Melissas J. Left ventricular function and cardiopulmonary performance following surgical treatment of morbid obesity. Obes Surg 2001; 11:552–558.

50. Manson JE, Colditz GA, Stampfer MJ, et al. A prospective study of obesity and risk of coronary heart disease in women. N Engl J Med 1990; 322:882–889.

51. Manson JE, Willett WC, Stampfer MJ, et al. Body weight and mortality among women. N Engl J Med 1995; 333:677–685.

52. Gleysteen JJ. Results of surgery: long-term effects on hyperlipidemia. Am J Clin Nutr 1992; 55:591S–593S.

53. Buffington CK, Cowan GS Jr, Smith H. Significant changes in the lipid-lipoprotein status of premenopausal morbidly obese females following gastric bypass surgery. Obes Surg 1994; 4:328–335.

54. Wolf AM, Beisiegel U, Kornter B, Kuhlmann HW. Does gastric restriction surgery reduce the risks of metabolic diseases? Obes Surg 1998; 8:9–13.

55. Busseto L, Pisent C, Rinaldi D, Longhin PL, Segato G, De Marchi F, Foletto M, Favretti F, Lise M, Enzi G. Variation in lipid levels in morbidly obese patients operated with Lap-Band® adjustable gastric banding system: effects of different levels of weight loss. Obes Surg 2000; 10:569–577.

56. Brolin RE, Bradley LJ, Wilson AC, Cody RP. Lipid risk profile and weight stability after gastric restrictive operations for morbid obesity. J Gastrointest Surg 2000; 4:464–469.

57. MacGregor MI, Block AJ, Ball WC. Topics in clinical medicine. Serious complications and sudden death in the Pickwickian syndrome. Hopkins Med J 1970; 189:279–295.

58. Guilleminault C, Partinen M, Quera-salva MA, Hayes B, Dement WC, Nino-Murcia G. Determinants of daytime sleepiness and obstructive sleep apnea. Chest 1986; 94:32–37.

59. Sugerman HJ, Fairman RP, Baron PL, Kwentus JA. Gastric surgery for respiratory insufficiency of obesity. Chest 1986; 90:82–91.

60. Sugerman HJ, Fairman RP, Sood RK, et al. Long-term effects of gastric surgery for treating respiratory insufficiency of obesity. Am J Clin Nutr 1992; 55:597S–601S.

61. Charuzi I, Ovnat A, Peiser J, et al. The effect of surgical weight reduction on sleep quality in obesity-related sleep apnea syndrome. Surgery 1985; 97:535–538.

62. Charuzi I, Lavie P, Peiser J, Peled R. Bariatric surgery in morbidly obese sleep-apnea patients: short and long-term follow-up. Am J Clin Nutr 1992; 55:594S–596S.

63. Boone KA, Cullen JJ, Mason EE, Scott DH, Doherty C, Maher JW. Impact of vertical banded gastroplasty on respiratory insufficiency of severe obesity. Obes Surg 1996; 6:454–458.

64. Rasheid S, Banasiak M, Gallagher SF, Lipska A, Kaba S, Ventimiglia D, Anderson WM, Murr MM. Gastric bypass is an effective treatment for obstructive sleep apnea in patients with clinically significant obesity. Obes Surg 2003; 13:58–61.

65. Hackney JD, Crane MG, Collier CC, Rokaw S, Griggs DE. Syndrome of extreme obesity and hypoventilation: studies of etiology. Ann Intern Med 1959; 51:541–552.

66. Herbst CA, Hughes TA, Gwynne JT, et al. Gastric bariatric operation in insulin-treated adults. Surgery 1984; 95:201–204.

67. Pories WJ, MacDonald KG, Morgan EJ, Sinha MK, Dohm GL, Swanson MS, et al. Surgical treatment of obesity and its effect on diabetes: 10-y follow-up. Am J Clin Nutr 1992; 55:582S–585S.

68. Pories WJ, Swanson MS, MacDonald KG, Long SB, Morris PG, Brown BM, et al. Who would have thought it? An operation proves to be the most effective therapy for adult-onset diabetes mellitus? Ann Surg 1995; 222:339–350.

69. Hickey MS, Pories WJ, MacDonald KG Jr, et al. A new paradigm for type 2 diabetes mellitus: could it be a disease of the foregut? Ann Surg 1998; 227:637–643.

70. MacDonald KG Jr, Long SD, Swanson MS, Brown BM, Morris P, Dohm GL, Pories WJ. The gastric bypass operation reduces the progression and mortality of non-insulin dependent diabetes mellitus. J Gastrointest Surg 1997; 1:213–220.

71. Pories WJ, Albrecht RJ. Etiology of type II diabetes mellitus: role of the foregut. World J Surg 2001; 25:527–531.

72. Neve HJ, Soulsby CT, Whiteley GS, Kincey J, Taylor TV. Resolution of diabetes following vertical gastroplasty in morbidly obese patients. Obes Surg 1993; 3:75–78.

73. Castagneto M, De Gaetano A, Mingrone G, Tacchino R, Nanni G, Capristo E, Benedetti G, Tataranni PA, Greco AV. Normalization of insulin sensitivity in obese patients after stable weight reduction with biliopancreatic diversion. Obes Surg 1994; 4:161–168.

74. Luyckx FH, Scheen AJ, Desaive C, Dewe W, Gielen JE, Lefebvre PJ. Effects of gastroplasty on body weight and related biological abnormalities in morbid obesity. Diabetes Metab 1998; 24:355–361.

75. Sjostrom CD, Lissner L, Wedel H, Sjostrom L. Reduction in incidence of diabetes, hypertension and lipid disturbances after intentional weight loss induced by bariatric surgery: the SOS Intervention Study. Obes Res 1999; 7:477–484.

76. Dixon JB, O'Brien PE. Health outcomes of severely obese type 2 diabetic subjects 1 year after laparoscopic adjustable gastric banding. Diabetes Care 2002; 25:397–398.

77. Schauer PR, Burguera B, Ikramuddin S, Cottan D, Gourash W, Hamad G, Eid GM, Mattar S, Ramanathan R, Barinas-Mitchel E, Rao RH, Kuller L, Kelley D. Effect of laparoscopic Roux-en-Y gastric bypass on type 2 diabetes mellitus. Ann Surg 2003; 238:467–484.

78. Polyzogopoulou EV, Kalfarentzos F, Vagenakis AG, Alexandrides TK. Restoration of euglycemia and normal acute insulin response to glucose in obese subjects with type 2 diabetes following bariatric surgery. Diabetes 2003; 52:1098–1103.

79. Giusti V, Suter M, Heraief E, Gaillard RC, Burckhardt P. Effects of laparoscopic gastric banding on body composition, metabolic profile and nutritional status of obese women: 12-months follow-up. Obes Surg 2004; 14:239–245.

80. Chan P, Lin TH, Pan WH, Lee YH. Thrombophilia associated with obesity in ethnic Chinese. Int J Obes Relat Metab Disord 1995; 19:756–759.

81. Sugerman HJ, Kellum JM, DeMaria EJ. Risks and benefits of gastric bypass in morbidly obese patients with severe venous stasis disease. Ann Surg 2001; 234:41–46.
82. Winiarsky R, Barth P, Lotke P. Total knee arthroplasty in morbidly obese patients. J Bone Joint Surg Am 1998; 80(12):1770–1774.
83. McKee MD, Waddekk JP. Intramedullary nailing of femoral fractures in morbidly obese patients. J Trauma 1994; 36:208–210.
84. Bostman OM. Body mass index and height in patients requiring surgery for lumbar intervertebral disc herniation. 1993; 18:851–854.
85. Parvizi J, Trousadale RT, Sarr MG. Total joint arthroplasty in patients surgically treated for morbid obesity. J Arthroplasty 2000; 15(8):1003–1008.
86. Peltonen M, Lindroos AK, Torgerson JS. Musculoskeletal pain in the obese: a comparison with the general population and long-term changes after conventional and surgical obesity treatment. Pain 2003; 104:549–557.
87. Melissas J, Volakakis E, Hadjipavlou A. Low-back pain in morbidly obese patients and the effect of weight loss following surgery. Obes Surg 2003; 13:389–393.
88. Zacchi P, Mearin F, Humbert P, et al. Effect of obesity on gastroesophageal resistance to flow in man. Dig Dis Sci 1991; 36:1473–1480.
89. Rigaud D, Merrouche M, LeMod G, et al. Facteurs de reflux gastro-oesophagien acide dans l'obesite severe. Gastroenterol Clin Biol 1995; 19:818–825.
90. Deitel M, Khanna RK, Hagen J, Ilves R. Vertical banded gastroplasty as an antireflux procedure. Am J Surg 1988; 155:512–514.
91. Smith SC, Edwards CB, Goodman GN. Symptomatic and clinical improvement in morbidly obese patients with gastroesophageal reflux disease following Roux-en-Y gastric bypass. Obes Surg 1997; 7:479–484.
92. Frezza EE, Ikramuddin S, Gourash W, Rakitt T, Kingston A, Luketich J, Schauer P. Symptomatic improvement in gastroesophageal reflux disease (GERD) following laparoscopic Roux-en-Y gastric bypass. Surg Endosc 2002; 16:1027–1031.
93. Naslund E, Granstrom L, Melcher A, Stockeld D, Backman L. Gastro-oesophageal reflux before and after vertical banded gastroplasty in the treatment of obesity. Eur J Surg 1996; 162:303–306.
94. Kim CH, Sarr MG. Severe reflux esophagitis after vertical banded gastroplasty for treatment of morbid obesity. Mayo Clin Proc 1992; 67:33–35.
95. Sugerman HJ, Kellum JM Jr, DeMaria EJ, Reines HD. Conversion of failed or complicated vertical banded gastroplasty to gastric bypass in morbid obesity. Am J Surg 1996; 171:263–269.
96. Wei JT, Shaheen N. The changing epidemiology of esophageal adenocarcinoma. Semin Gastroinetest Dis 2003; 14:112–127.
97. Macgregor A, Greenberg RA. Effect of surgically induced weight loss on asthma in the morbidly obese. Obes Surg 1993; 3:15–21.
98. Engel LS, Chow WH, Vaughan TL, Gammon MD, et al. Population attributable risks of esophageal and gastric cancers. J Natl Cancer Inst 2003; 17:1404–1413.
99. Dixon JB, Chapman L, O'Brien P. Marked improvement in asthma after Lap-Band® surgery for morbid obesity. Obes Surg 1999; 9:385–389.
100. Nestler JE, Jakubowicz DJ, Evans WS, Pasquali R. Effects of metformin on spontaneous and clomiphene-induced ovulation in the polycystic ovary syndrome. N Engl J Med 1998; 338:1876–1880.
101. Nestler JE, Jakubowicz DJ, Reamer P, Gunn RD, Allan G. Ovulatory and metabolic effects of D-chiro-inositol in the polycystic ovary syndrome. N Engl J Med 1999; 340:1314–1320.
102. Deitel M, Toan BT, Stone EM, et al. Sex hormone changes accompanying loss of massive excess weight. Gastroenterol Clin North Am 1987; 16:511–515.
103. Robert E, Francannet C, Shaw G. Neural tube defects and maternal weight reduction in early pregnancy. Reprod Toxicol 1995; 9:57–59.

104. Friedman D, Cunco S, Valenzano M, Marinari GM, Adami GF, Gianetti E, Traverso E, Scopinaro N. Pregnancies in an 18-year follow-up after biliopancreatic diversion. Obes Surg 1995; 5:308–313.
105. Wittgrove AC, Jester L, Wittgrove P, Clark GW. Pregnancy following gastric bypass for morbid obesity. Obes Surg 1998; 8:461–464.
106. Dixon JB, Dixon ME, O'Brien PE. Pregnancy after Lap-Band surgery: management of the band to achieve health weight outcomes. Obes Surg 2001; 11:59–65.
107. Skull AJ, Slater GH, Duncombe JE, Fielding GA. Laparoscopic adjustable banding in pregnancy: safety, patient tolerance and effect on obesity-related pregnancy outcomes. Obes Surg 2004; 14:230–235.
108. Liu GT, Volpe NJ, Schatz NJ, Galetta SL, Farrar JT, Raps EC. Severe sudden visual loss caused by pseudotumor cerebri and lumboperitoneal shunt failure. Am J Ophthalmol 1966; 122:129–131.
109. Rosenberg ML, Corbett JJ, Smith C, et al. Cerebrospinal fluid diversion procedures in pseudotumor cerebri. Neurology 1993; 43:1071–1072.
110. Sugerman HJ, Felton WL III, Sismanis A, et al. Gastric surgery for pseudotumor cerebri associated with severe obesity. Ann Surg 1999; 21:682–685.
111. Bayderdorffer E, Mannes GA, Ochsenkuhn T, Kopcke W, Wiebecke B, Paumgartner G. Increased risk of 'high-risk' colorectal adenomas in overweight men. Gastroenterol 1993; 104:137–144.
112. Garfinkel L. Overweight and cancer. Ann Intern Med 1985; 103:1034–1036.
113. Snowdon DA, Phillips R, Choi W. Diet, obesity, and risk of fatal prostate cancer. Am J Epidemiol 1984; 120:244–250.
114. Yu MC, Mack TM, Hanisch R, Cicioni C, Henderson BE. Cigarette smoking, obesity, diuretic use, and coffee consumption as risk factors for renal cell carcinoma. JNCI 1986; 77:351–356.
115. Sugerman HJ, Kellum JM Jr, Reines HD, DeMaria EJ, Newsome HH, Lowry JW. Greater risk of incisional hernia with morbidly obese than steroid-dependent patients and low recurrence with prefascial polypropylene mesh. Am J Surg 1996; 171:80–84.
116. Schauer PR, Ramos R, Ghiatas AA, Sirinek KR. Virulent diverticular disease in young obese men. Am J Surg 1992; 164:443–448.
117. Konvolinka CW. Acute diverticulitis under age forty. Am J Surg 1994; 167:562–565.
118. Funnell IC, Bornman PC, Weakley SP, Terblanche J, Marks IN. Obesity: an important prognostic factor in acute pancreatitis. Br J Surg 1993; 80:484–486.
119. Nauta RJ. A radical approach to bacterial panniculitis of the abdominal wall in the morbidly obese. Surgery 1990; 107:134–139.
120. Harrison SA, Kadakia S, Lang KA, Schenker S. Nonalcoholic steatohepatitis: what we know in the new millennium. Am J Gastroenterol 2002; 97:2714–2724.
121. Hui JM, Kench JG, Chitturi S, et al. Long-term outcomes of cirrhosis in nonalcoholic steatohepatitis compared with hepatitis C. Hepatology 2003; 38:420–427.
122. Ranlov I, Hardt F. Regression of liver steatosis following gastroplasty or gastric bypass for morbid obesity. Digestion 1990; 47:208–214.
123. Silverman EM, Sapala JA, Appelman HD. Regression of hepatic steatosis in morbidly obese persons after gastric bypass. Am J Clin Pathol 1995; 104:23–31.
124. Luyckx FH, Desaive C, Thiry A, Dewe W, Scheen AJ, Gielen JE, Lefebvre PJ. Liver abnormalities in severely obese subjects: effect of drastic weight loss after gastroplasty. Int J Obes Relat Metab Disord 1998; 22:222–226.
125. Kral JG, Thung SN, Biron S, Hould FS, et al. Effects of surgical treatment of the metabolic syndrome on liver fibrosis and cirrhosis. Surgery 2004; 135:48–58.
126. Rand CS, Macgregor A, Hankins G. Gastric bypass surgery for obesity: weight loss, psychosocial outcome, and morbidity one and three years later. South Med J 1986; 79(12):1511–514.
127. Kral JG, Sjostrom LV, Sullivan MB. Assessment of quality of life before and after surgery for severe obesity. Am J Clin Nutr 1992; 55(suppl 2):611S–614S.

128. Schauer PR, Ikramuddin S, Gourash W, et al. Outcomes after laparoscopic Roux-en-Y gastric bypass for morbid obesity. Ann Surg 2000; 232(4):515–529.

129. Nguyen NT, Goldman C, Rosenquist CJ, et al. Laparoscopic versus open gastric bypass: a randomized study of outcomes, quality of life, and costs. Ann Surg 2001; 234:279–291.

130. Dixon JB, O'Brien PE. Changes in comorbidities and improvements in quality of life after LAP-BAND placement. Am J Surg 2002; 184:51S–54S.

131. van Gemert WG, Severijas RM, Gree JW, Groenman N, Soeters PB. Psychological functioning of mobidly obese patients after surgical treatment. Int J Obes Relat Metab Disord 1998; 22:393–398.

132. Wadden TA, Sarwer DB, Womble LG, Foster GB, McGuckin BG, Schimmel A. Psychological aspects of obesity and obesity surgery. Surg Clin North Am 2001; 81:1001–1024.

133. Maddi SR, Fox SR, Khoshaba DM, Harvey RH, Lu JL, Persico M. Reduction in psychopathology following bariatric surgery for morbid obesity. Obes Surg 2001; 11:680–685.

134. Papageorgiou GM, Papakonstantinou A, Mamplekou E, Terzis I, Melissas J. Pre- and postoperative psychological characteristics in morbidly obese patients. Obes Surg 2002; 12:534–539.

135. Dixon JB, Dixon ME, O'Brien PE. Depression in association with severe obesity: changes with weight loss. Arch Intern Med 2003; 163:2058–2065.

136. Herpertz S, Kleimann R, Wolf AM, Langkafei M, Scaf W, Hebebrand J. Does obesity surgery improve psychosocial functioning? A systematic review. Int J Obes Relat Metab Disord 2003; 27:1300–1314.

137. Klesges RC, Klem ML, Hanson CL, Eck LH, Ernst J, O'Laughlin D, Garrott A, Rife R. The effects of applicant's health status and qualifications on simulating hiring decisions. Int J Obes 1990; 14:527–535.

138. Pingitore R, Dugoni BL, Tindale RS, Spring B. Bias against overweight job applicants in a simulated employment interview. J Appl Psychol 1994; 79:909–917.

139. Christou NV, Sampalis JS, Lieberman M, Look D, Auger S, McLean PA, MacLean LD. Surgery decreases long-term mortality in morbidly obese patients. Ann Surg 2004; 240:416–424.

140. Flum DR, Dellinger EP. Impact of gastric bypass operation on survival: a population-based analysis. 2004 ; 199:543–551.

141. Buchwald H, Avidor Y, Braunwald E, et al. Bariatric surgery. A systematic review and meta-analysis. JAMA 2004; 292:1724–1737.

10

Techniques of Laparoscopic Gastric Bypass

Benjamin E. Schneider and Daniel B. Jones
Harvard Medical School, Beth Israel Deaconess Medical Center, Boston, Massachusetts, U.S.A.

Ninh T. Nguyen
Department of Surgery, University of California Irvine Medical Center, Orange, California, U.S.A.

INTRODUCTION

Obesity has been recognized as a growing national and international epidemic. Weight-related health complications contribute to a tremendous cost to society as well as to the obese patient (1). It is now estimated that being overweight is second only to tobacco as a leading cause of death in the United States (2). The gastric bypass has undergone numerous modifications since its conception by Mason and Ito (3). This evolution ultimately led to the application of laparoscopic techniques described first by Wittgrove and Clark in the 1990s (4,5). When compared to the open approach, patients undergoing laparoscopic gastric bypass benefit from a lower incidence of incisional hernia, wound infection, and pulmonary complications, as well as from diminished pain, shorter hospitalization, and a more rapid return to the activities of daily living and work (6,7).

MATERIALS AND METHODS: LAPAROSCOPIC GASTRIC BYPASS TECHNIQUE

Patient Positioning and Operating Room Set-up

Patients are admitted the day of surgery after an overnight fast. Generally, patients receive a first-generation cephalosporin (8). Subcutaneous heparin and lower extremities sequential compression devices may be employed as prophylaxis against thromboembolism. The patient is positioned supine on the operative table; a cushioned bean bag and footboard may be used for added security. Following the establishment of general endotracheal anesthesia, an oro-gastric tube and a Foley catheter decompress the stomach and bladder. The arms are abducted and secured on padded arm boards. Video monitors are placed on either side of the patient's head. The surgical team is situated such that the surgeon stands on the patient's right along with the camera operator. The first assistant stands to the left side of the patient.

Port Placement

Pneumoperitoneum is established via a Veress needle placed in the left subcostal site. Insufflation with carbon dioxide to a pressure of 15 mm Hg creates a working space. Some surgeons find the addition of a second insufflator helpful to maintain adequate pneumoperitoneum. Six port sites are selected (Fig. 1). The first trocar is placed with the aid of a direct viewing dissector at the left mid-clavicular position (Visiport, U.S. Surgical Corporation). The remaining port sites consist of a 12-mm trocar at the right flank, through which a liver retraction device is placed. A 5-mm right subcostal and a 12-mm right mid-clavicular trocar serve as the surgeon's working ports. A 12-mm supra-umbilical port is used for the placement of the 30° angled laparoscope. A left 5-mm subcostal and a 12-mm mid-clavicular trocar represent the first assistant's working ports. It is often necessary to take down the falciform ligament using an ultrasonic sheers in order to achieve an optimal port placement as well as to allow a smooth insertion of the surgeon's instruments.

Dissection and Creation of the Mesocolic Window

Ultimately, the Roux limb may be brought up to the gastric pouch in three ways: (1) antecolic, antegastric; (2) retrocolic, antegastric; and (3) retrocolic, retrogastric. Arguably, the more direct retrocolic, retrogastric route may be preferable in that the least tension exists at the gastrojejunostomy. Proponents of the antecolic, antegastric method cite simplicity as well as the theoretically lower likelihood of serious

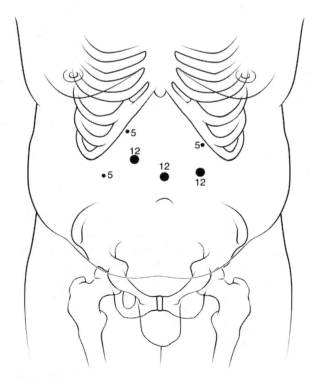

Figure 1 Trocar configuration.

internal hernia formation as the Peterson's defect is very large, and that mesocolic defect is avoided altogether. Currently, we favor a retrocolic, antegastric Roux route. In order to create a retrocolic tunnel, the gastrocolic ligament is identified and opened using an ultrasonic dissector, thus giving access to the lesser sac. The transverse mesocolon is then elevated from above and again using ultrasonic sheers, opened to create a mesocolic window to the right of the ligament of Treitz. Some surgeons prefer to elevate the greater omentum and transverse colon, identify the ligament of Treitz, and create the mesocolic window instead from below.

Creation of the Roux-en-Y

With the omentum and transverse colon lifted cephalad, the ligament of Treitz is identified and the jejunum is run for a distance of 40 to 50 cm. At this point, a suture is placed to mark the proximal bowel, which will represent the biliopancreatic limb. Distal to the suture, the jejunum is divided using an endoscopic gastrointestinal anastomosis (GIA) 60-mm stapler (2.5-mm staples). The associated mesentery is divided using a 45-mm endoscopic GIA stapler (2.0-mm staples). Care is taken with this maneuver to align the stapler perpendicular to the direction of the bowel in order to avoid ischemia at the end of either limb. Next, the distal "Roux limb" is run for a distance of 75 cm. The limbs are approximated with a long traction suture, which will later be used to help sleeve the bowel onto the endo GIA when creating the jejunojejunostomy. Each limb is opened with an ultrasonic sheers and a jaw of a 60-mm endoscopic GIA stapler (2.5-mm staples) is placed within each. This creates a side-to-side jejunojejunostomy. The enteric defect created after deploying the stapler is approximated with interrupted stay sutures placed in a transverse fashion. An additional load of the endo GIA (2.5-mm stapler, 60-mm length) is used to close the defect. Alternatively, the enteric defect may be closed by a hand-sewn technique. The mesenteric defect associated with the jejunojejunostomy is closed using either a running or an interrupted silk suture to reduce the likelihood of internal hernias. An interrupted suture is placed approximating the cut end of the biliopancreatic limb to the alimentary limb as a so-called "anti-obstruction stitch." The Roux limb is then placed through the mesocolic window, with care taken to avoid twisting of its mesentery (Fig. 2). The omentum and transverse colon are reflected caudally. The patient is placed in reverse Trendelenberg position and a liver retraction paddle is used to elevate the left lobe of the liver.

Creation of the Gastric Pouch

A small gastric pouch, approximately 30 mL in size, is fashioned based upon the lesser curvature. Particularly early in the surgeon's learning curve, the pouch may be sized with the aid of a 20-cc intra-gastric balloon placed by the anesthesiologist and withdrawn to the gastroesophageal junction (Fig. 3). The site of the gastric pouch division is selected; a retrogastric tunnel is created by first opening the gastro-hepatic ligament, entering the lesser sac, and identifying any retro-gastric adhesions. Next, an ultrasonic scalpel is used to create a peri-gastric window, thus preserving the Vagus nerve and left gastric artery. Similarly, the angle of His is mobilized using an ultrasonic dissector to free the peritoneal attachments.

The gastrojejunostomy may be performed in a variety of manners ranging from an entirely hand-sewn to a linear- or a circular-stapled anastomosis. To many, the circular route using an end-to-end anastomosis (EEA) stapler is preferable as it is

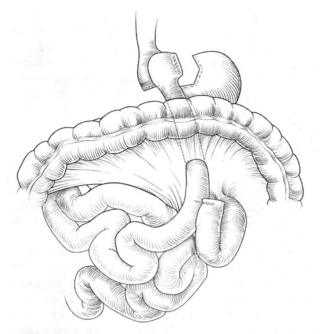

Figure 2 Retrocolic Roux limb.

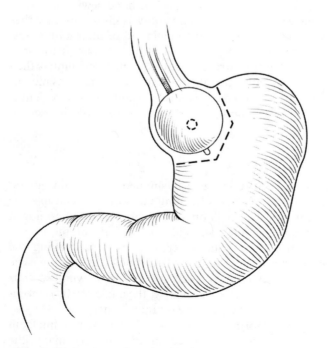

Figure 3 Intragastric balloon at gastroesophageal junction.

simple to perform and assures a consistent anastomotic apperature. Although several techniques to place an EEA anvil had been described, we favor the transgastric route as it avoids the risk of anvil dislodgement in the esophagus or hypopharyngeal perforation, which may occur with transoral insertion (9–12). First, a gastrotomy is performed on the anterior wall of the stomach approximately 5 cm distal to the intended pouch. A suture is tied to the 21-mm EEA anvil and a loop is made at the end. The left mid-clavicular port is removed and the facial defect dilated to allow placement of the 21-mm EEA anvil. The port is replaced and, if necessary, a suture is placed to control any port site leak. A modified 45-cm ("Jones Perforator") Maryland grasper with sharpened tips, is used to grasp the looped end of the suture affixed to the EEA anvil. By placing the grasper through the gastric defect, the suture is brought out through the anterior gastric wall at the intended site of the gastrojejunostomy (Fig. 4). The suture is pulled anteriorly allowing the spike of the anvil to follow through the gastric wall. At this point, the gastric tube is removed and the pouch is fashioned around the anvil using successive firings of the laparoscopic linear stapler (3.5-mm staples) (Fig. 5). The gastrotomy is closed using a linear stapler.

Alternatively, the EEA anvil may be placed via any number of transoral techniques. In general, the divided gastric pouch is created as previously described. Next, endoscopy is performed advancing into the gastric pouch. A venous catheter is used to introduce a wire into the gastric pouch. This is retrieved using an endoscopic snare. This pull-wire is then attached to the EEA anvil in a manner similar to that used for a percutaneous endoscopic gastrostomy tube. The wire is used to pull the

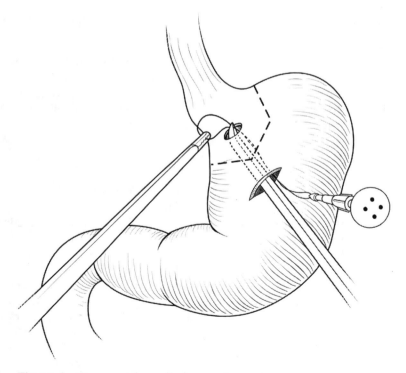

Figure 4 Trans-gastric anvil placement.

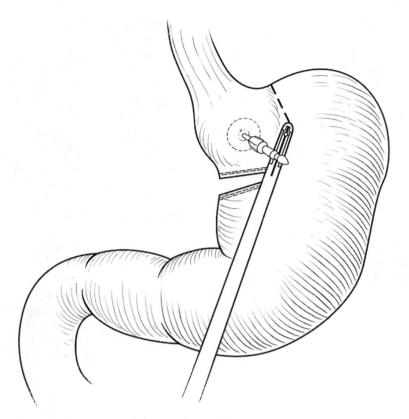

Figure 5 Creation of the gastric pouch.

anvil into the pouch in an antegrade fashion. At times, the balloon of the endotracheal tube must be deflated, and the patient's head and jaw lifted anteriorly in
order to navigate the anvil into the distal esophagus. Although the transoral technique
has proven to be reliable, a number of surgeons have reported significant complications
including esophageal perforation and gastric wall injuries (13–15).

Creation of the Gastrojejunostomy

The left mid-clavicular 12-mm port is removed and the shaft of the EEA stapler
introduced into the abdomen. The suture attached to the anvil is removed and the
end of the Roux limb is opened using an ultrasonic dissector. The EEA shaft is then
sleeved into the Roux limb, the spike is advanced through the wall of the jejunum
and then removed. The Roux mesentery is inspected to avoid kinking as the anvil
and shaft are mated and deployed (Fig. 6). The distal open end of the Roux limb
is then excised using a linear stapler (2.5-mm staples); several vicryl sutures are
placed over the anastomosis to help reduce tension. Under direct visualization, the
nasogastric tube is then carefully advanced into the pouch. Atraumatic graspers
are then used to occlude the Roux limb as 60 cc of methylene blue saline is injected
into the nasogastric tube to rule out obvious gastrojejunal anastomotic leak. Any
leaks are oversewn. Alternatively, an endoscope may be placed to evaluate the
anastomosis by insufflating air under a saline-flooded operative field.

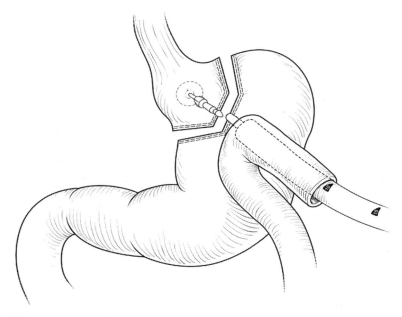

Figure 6 Gastrojejunostomy created with EEA.

Closure of Mesenteric Defects

Any redundant Roux limb is reduced below the mesocolic window; the omentum and transverse colon are reflected cephalad to allow for the visualization of both the Peterson's and the mesocolic defect. Silk sutures are placed in an interrupted fashion closing both the Peterson's defect and the mesocolon (Fig. 7). If a running stitch is to be used, care must be taken to avoid excessively narrowing the waist of the mesocolic window and causing a Roux limb obstruction. The facia at the left mid-clavicular port is closed with a vicryl suture placed with a facial closure device. Pneumoperitoneum is released. The trocar sites are irrigated, anesthetized with 0.25% Bupivacaine, and the skin closed with running absorbable sub-cuticular sutures.

Postoperative Management

Prophylaxis against thrombo-embolism using sequential compression devices and subcutaneous heparin is continued. Postoperative early ambulation is encouraged. Pain is controlled with a patient controled analgesia (PCA). An upper gastrointestinal contrast study (Gastrografin) is obtained on postoperative day one to detect gastrointestinal leak at the proximal anastomosis (16,17). Patients are subsequently begun on a liquid diet, which is advanced to a high-protein liquid supplement prior to discharge. The length of stay ranges from two to four days in a large series. We do not routinely perform cholecystectomy at the time of gastric bypass, favoring selective cholecystectomy in those patients with preoperatively diagnosed stones (18). Patients who have not undergone cholecystectomy are prescribed Ursodiol to reduce the incidence of gallstone formation (19). All patients receive multivitamin supplements and are followed lifelong to avoid malnutrition and vitamin deficiencies (20).

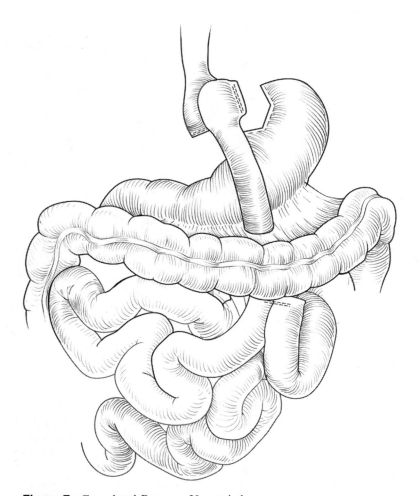

Figure 7 Completed Roux-en-Y gastric bypass.

DISCUSSION

The laparoscopic gastric bypass has increasingly become the standard therapy for patients undergoing bariatric surgery in the United States. Comparisons to open bypass demonstrate similar reduction in excess weight (68–80%), resolution of comorbidities, and complications (6,7). By employing minimally invasive techniques, surgeons are able to reduce wound complications and improve recovery.

REFERENCES

1. Wolf AM, Colditz GA. Current estimates of the economic cost of obesity in the United States. Obes Res 1998; 6:97–106.
2. Mokdad AH, Marks JS, Gerberding JL. Actual causes of death in the United States, 2000. JAMA 2004; 291:1238–1245.
3. Mason EE, Ito C. Gastric bypass. Ann Surg 1969; 179:329–339.

4. Wittgrove AC, Clark G, Tremblay LJ. Laparoscopic gastric bypass, Roux-en-Y: preliminary report of five cases. Obes Surg 1994; 4:353–357.
5. Wittgrove AC, Clark G. Laparoscopic gastric bypass, Roux-en-Y 500 patients: technique and results, with 3–60 month follow-up. Obes Surg 2000; 10:233–239.
6. Schneider BE, Villegas L, Blackburn GL, Mun EC, Critchlow JF, Jones DB. Laparoscopic gastric bypass surgery: outcomes. J Laparoendosc Adv Surg Tech 2003; 13(4): 247–255.
7. Nguyen NT, Goldman C, Rosenquist CJ, Arango A, Cole CJ, Lee SJ, Wolfe BM. Laparoscopic versus open gastric bypass: a randomized study of outcomes, quality of life, and costs. Ann Surg 2001; 234(3):279–291.
8. Pories WJ, van Riji AM, Burlingham BT, Fulghum RS, Meelheim D. Prophylactic cefazolin in gastric bypass surgery. Surgery 1981; 90:426–432.
9. Nguyen NT, Wolfe BM. Hypopharyngeal perforation during laparoscopic Roux-en-Y gastric bypass. Obes Surg 2000; 10:64–67.
10. Scott DJ, Provost DA, Jones DB. Laparoscopic Roux-en-Y gastric bypass: transoral or transgastric anvil placement? Obes Surg 2000; 10:361–365.
11. Wittgrove AC, Clark G. Laparoscopic gastric bypass: endostapler transoral or transabdominal anvil placement. Obes Surg 2000; 10:376.
12. Wittgrove AC, Clark G. Combined laparoscopic/endoscopic anvil placement for the performance of the gastroenterostomy. Obes Surg 2001; 11:565–569.
13. Wittgrove AC, Clark G. Laparoscopic gastric bypass: endostapler transoral or transabdominal anvil placement. Obes Surg 2000; 10:376.
14. Scott DJ, Provost DA, Jones DB. Laparoscopic Roux-en-Y gastric bypass: transoral or transgastric anvil Placement? Obes Surg 2000; 10:361–365.
15. Nguyen NT, Wolfe BM. Hypopharyngeal perforation during laparoscopic Roux-en-Y gastric bypass. Obes Surg 2000; 10:64–67.
16. Sims TL, Mullican MA, Hamilton EC, Provost DA, Jones DB. Routine upper gastrointestinal Gastrografin swallow after laparoscopic Roux-en-Y gastric bypass. Obes Surg 2003; 13:66–72.
17. Hamilton EC, Sims TL, Hamilton TT, Mullican MA, Jones DB, Provost DA. Clinical predictors of leak after Roux-en-Y gastric bypass. Surg Endosc 2003; 17:679–684.
18. Villegas L, Schneider B, Provost D, Chang C, Scott D, Sims T, Hill L, Jones DB. Is routine cholecystectomy required during laparoscopic gastric bypass? Obes Surg 2004; 14:60–66.
19. Sugerman H, Brewer WH, Shiffman ML, Brolin RE, Fobi MAL, Linner JH, MacDonald KG, Martín LF, Oram-Smith JC, Popoola D, Schirmer BD, Vickers FF. A multicenter, placebo-controlled, randomized, double-blind, prospective trial of prophylactic ursodiol for the prevention of gallstone formation following gastric-bypass-induced rapid weight loss. Am J Surg 1995; 169:91–97.
20. Kelly J, Tarnoff M, Shikora S, Thayer B, Jones DB, Forse RA, Fanelli R, Lautz D, Buckley F, Munshi I, Coe N. Best care recommendations for surgical care in weight loss surgery. Obesity Research 2005; 13:227–233.
21. Jones DB, DeMaria E, Provost DA, Smith CD, Morgenstern L, Schirmer B. Optimal management of the morbidly obese patient: SAGES appropriateness conference statement. Surg Endosc 2004; 18(7):1029–1037.
22. Schneider BE, Provost DA. Bariatric Surgical Techniques. In: Jones DB, WU JS, Soper NJ, eds. Principles and Procedures. 2nd ed. St. Louis: Marcel Dekkar, 2004.

11

Outcome of Laparoscopic Gastric Bypass

Corrigan L. McBride
Department of Surgery, University of Nebraska Medical Center, Omaha, Nebraska, U.S.A.

Harvey J. Sugerman
Department of Surgery, Virginia Commonwealth University, Richmond, Virginia, U.S.A.

Eric J. DeMaria
Department of Surgery, Duke University, Durham, North Carolina, U.S.A.

INTRODUCTION

Since Wittgrove et al. published the first report of five cases of laparoscopic gastric bypass for morbid obesity (1) in 1994, there have been additional reports supporting the feasibility of the operation. There have been multiple variations in the technical methodologies published, especially of gastrojejunostomy. Additional controversies have surfaced regarding the routing of the Roux limb (retrocolic vs. antecolic), necessity for drains, and the need for a routine postoperative upper gastrointestinal (UGI) contrast study. The experience with laparoscopic gastric bypass has continued to evolve at a number of centers around the world, but primarily in the United States. Both case series and prospective randomized clinical trials have been published. In those papers where the data have been published in multiple forms, the data will be reviewed as a cumulative series.

LITERATURE REVIEW—CASE SERIES

The initial case series by Wittgrove et al. in 1994 described the feasibility of performing a laparoscopic gastric bypass. Their technique included a ~15-cc lesser curvature-based gastric pouch, a 75-cm Roux limb with a retrocolic, retrogastric passage, and a circular stapled anastomosis (1). In 1996, Lonroth et al. also published a report of their first six patients demonstrating the possibility of performing a laparoscopic gastric bypass (2).

   In 1998, Lonroth reviewed his experience with 35 patients (3). The gastroenterostomy was created using a linear stapled technique with suture closure of the anterior wall. The reconstruction in the first 10 patients was an omega-loop gastroenteric

anastomosis. The remainder of the series had a retrocolic Roux-en-Y gastroenterostomy. There were three conversions: one was for accidental perforation of the
stomach and two because of difficult exposure from a large left hepatic lobe. In the first
15 patients followed for more than one year, there was a 67% loss of excess body
weight (EBW) (4). In 12 patients who were followed for more than two years
from surgery, there was a 70% loss of EBW (3). In the first 35 patients attempted by
Lonroth et al., four patients had bleeding requiring transfusion, one of these patients
had laparoscopic exploration and blood evacuation, and two other patients also
required reoperation for anastomotic leaks. One patient had a diagnostic laparoscopy
for a suspected leak, which was negative. One patient had an open re-exploration for
ileus at six weeks (3) and was found to have an internal hernia (4). There were four
postoperative pneumonias. One patient developed a marginal ulcer with perforation
at 2.5 years. There was no operative mortality (3,4).

In 1999, De la Torre and Scott published their initial experience with laparoscopic Roux-en-Y gastric bypass (5). Their technique included the creation of the
gastric pouch using a 16-Fr balloon-upped jejunostomy catheter to size the gastric
pouch. A biliopancreatic limb of 15 to 20 cm was anastomosed 75 to 150 cm distally
on the Roux limb. The Roux limb was passed retrocolic, but antegastric. The gastrojejunostomy was created with a 21-mm circular stapler on the anterior wall of the
gastric pouch. The anvil was placed into the stomach trans-abdominally prior to
the creation of the gastric pouch. In the first 50 patients, there was one conversion
to an open procedure secondary to extensive intra-abdominal adhesions. The mean
hospitalization was 3.8 days. There were two complications in the first three months
of follow-up, including a trocar site wound infection and an intra-abdominal abscess
from a presumed leak, which was treated with percutaneous drainage. Of the
patients who were employed, the average return to work was 11.9 days. At three
months postoperatively there was an average loss of 23 kg, which represented an
average loss of 38.5% of EBW. No long-term follow-up is available on these patients.

In 2000, Matthews et al. published the combined results of 48 patients from
two centers (6). The mean preoperative BMI was 52.3 kg/m^2. They created a gastric
pouch of 15 to 20 cc, a biliopancreatic limb of 25 to 40 cm, and a Roux limb of 60 to
100 cm. The Roux was passed either retrocolic or antecolic. The gastrojejunostomy
was created with a 21-mm or a 25-mm circular stapler. The anvil was passed trans-
orally on the end of a nasogastric tube. There were three (6.3%) conversions to open
technique (one for a shortened jejunal mesentery and two for inadequate visualization). There were six (12.5%) postoperative complications including one (2.1%)
gastrojejunal anastomotic leak. The remaining postoperative complications were
not presented in the publication. In eight patients, prior to this series, with hand-sewn
anastomosis, two (25%) had gastrojejunal anastomotic leaks. Thirteen (27.1%)
patients developed stomal stenosis at the gastrojejunostomy requiring one or more
endoscopic balloon dilatations. Twenty-seven patients had one-year follow-up; the
mean weight loss was 115 lbs, with a decrease in BMI of 18.5 kg/m^2.

Because of a shared concern of passage of the circular stapler anvil down the
esophagus, Teixeira et al., developed an alternate technique where the anvil was
placed in the gastric pouch trans-abdominally (7). The post of the anvil was passed
out the posterior wall of the gastric pouch. The 100- to 150-cm Roux limb was passed
retrocolic, retrogastric and anastomosed to the posterior gastric wall. They reported
on their first 18 patients to demonstrate the feasibility of this new technique. There
were no conversions to open surgery. The mean hospital stay was four days. One
patient required readmission for an intra-abdominal abscess. In addition there were

two wound infections and one urinary tract infection for an overall complication rate of 14% and a major complication rate of 3.5 %. There were no anastomotic leaks, no reoperations nor mortality.

Schauer et al. reported on 275 patients in 2000 (8). They described the creation of the gastric pouch using a Baker tube for sizing in the first 100 patients. A 30-cm biliopancreatic limb was created with a 75-cm Roux limb for morbidly obese patients (BMI $<50\,kg/m^2$) and a 150-cm Roux limb for superobese patients (BMI $\geq 50\,kg/m^2$). The Roux limb was passed retrocolic and retrogastric. For the first 150 cases, they utilized an end-to-end EEA stapled anastomosis. In the later 125 cases, a linear stapled technique was used. There were three (1.1%) patients who underwent conversion to open surgery. The indications for conversion were EEA stapler malfunction, mesenteric bleeding, and massive subcutaneous emphysema. In 42% of patients a concomitant procedure was performed, with the most common being laparoscopic cholecystectomy in 17% of patients. Nine (3.3%) patients had a total of 17 major complications early in their postoperative course, including four leaks resulting in peritonitis or abscess. There was one death, due to pulmonary embolism (PE), for a mortality of 0.4%. Seventy-five minor complications occurred in the first 30 days affecting 27% of patients. There were four leaks listed as major complications and eight "subclinical leaks" which were asymptomatic or contained. Therefore, the total leak rate was 4.4% for this series. Twenty-seven patients (9.8%) required a surgical intervention subsequent to their laparoscopic gastric bypass. In the first 50 patients without a bowel preparation the infection rate was 22%, but following the institution of a preoperative bowel preparation it fell to 10%. In patients having the linear stapled gastrojejunal anastomosis the wound infection rate was 1.5%. The excess weight loss at 24 and 30 months was 83% and 77%, respectively. For the 104 patients at one-year follow-up, co-morbidities were improved or resolved for the majority of patients who had them preoperatively. Specifically hypercholesterolemia improved or resolved in 96% of patients, gastroesophageal reflux disease (GERD) in 96%, hypertension (HTN) in 88%, sleep apnea in 93%, and diabetes in 100%. Ninety-five percent of patients reported a better or greatly improved quality of life.

Wittgrove and Clark published their 30- to 60-month follow-up for their first 500 patients in 2000 (9). Their technique remained as previously described. Eighty percent of patients lost $\geq 50\%$ of their EBW at follow-up. This loss was maintained in patients followed for 60 months. Diabetic patients, in general, lost less weight than non-diabetics. The patients had 1752 preoperative co-morbidities. These were decreased by 96% following surgery. Specifically, GERD was eliminated in 98% of patients. All diabetic patients were off medication for blood sugar control. In patients with elevated HgbA1c preoperatively who were not on medication, three of 64 patients had persistently elevated HgbA1c postoperatively. Sleep apnea and hypertension were resolved in 98% and 92%, respectively. In the first 300 patients the leak rate was 3%. It decreased to only 1% in the last 200 patients. Of the 11 patients with a leak, nine required reoperation (two open and seven laparoscopic). Four patients in the first 300 required reoperation for bleeding. The stomal stenosis rate was 1.6%. There were four major and 21 minor wound infections.

There are few comparisons between open and laparoscopic gastric bypass. One of the earliest was published by Nguyen et al. in 2000 (10). They reported the results of 35 patients who had undergone laparoscopic gastric bypass and 35 patients who had an open gastric bypass procedure in an earlier time period. A gastric pouch of 15 to 20 cc was created, and the gastrojejunal anastomosis was performed using a circular 21-mm stapler. The Roux limb was based on the patients' BMI (75 cm for BMI $<50 \, kg/m^2$ and 150 cm for BMI $\geq 50 \, kg/m^2$). Seventeen laparoscopic patients had one-year follow-up available. The mean percentage of EBW loss (%EBWL) was 69% and the mean length of stay was four days. Two patients had postoperative bleeding requiring transfusion. One patient had narrowing at the jejunojejunostomy, which required laparoscopic revision. One patient required more than 72 hours of ventilator support. The stomal stenosis rate was 20%. There was no deep vein thrombosis, PE, leak, conversion, or mortality.

In the largest series of laparoscopic gastric bypass with Roux-en-Y published to date, Higa et al. published the results and complications of their 1040 patients (11). They had previously published a report of their first 400 patients (12). Their technique included a proximal lesser-curve gastric pouch of 20 to 30 cc, a Roux limb of 100 to 150 cm, and a totally hand-sewn gastrojejunostomy sized at 32 Fr. The mean BMI was $47.8 \, kg/m^2$ (range, 35–78 kg/m^2). Two hundred seventy-six patients had a BMI $>50 \, kg/m^2$. The average one-year EBW loss was 70%. There was one operative death from the PE and four late deaths for the first year mortality of 0.5%. The total complication rate was 14.7% with the most prevalent being gastro-jejunal stomal stenosis (4.9%). Other complications comprising $>1\%$ frequency included internal hernia (2.5%), gallstone (1.4%), NSAID-induced marginal ulcer (1.4%), and staple line failure (1.0%).

A larger series by Rutledge describes the results of a "mini-gastric bypass" in 1274 patients (13). This technique has been controversial because of its loop recon-struction. The technique included creation of a lesser-curvature gastric pouch and an antecolic gastrojejunal loop anastomosis. The mean BMI was $47 \pm 7 \, kg/m^2$. Patients had a mean weight loss of 68% at 12 months and 77% at two years. Obesity co-morbidities resolved in 70% to 90% of the patients after surgery. The initial complication rate was 26%, however this decreased to $<4\%$ in the final 200 patients of the series. There was one hospital death (0.08%). Other complications reported included deep vein thrombosis (0.08%), PE (0.16%), leaks (1.6%), postoperative hernia rate (0.17%), marginal ulcer (1.8%), and esophagitis (0.47%). Four patients required revision for severe nausea with excessive weight loss, with anastomosis of the distal gastric pouch to the bypassed stomach. The mean operative time was 36.9 minutes and the mean length of stay was 1.5 days. The use of a loop reconstruction has caused much controversy in the bariatric community. Finally this publication has been criticized for not addressing alkaline reflux gastritis. Furthermore, Rutledge used clinic visits, mail or e-mail for the follow-up data presented. This also has been criticized by multiple leading bariatric surgeons (14).

There is limited data regarding the use of laparoscopic gastric bypass as a reoperative surgery. De Csepel et al. described their series of seven women who had had previous open restrictive procedures that required revision (15). The average BMI prior to their original bariatric surgery was $51.1 \, kg/m^2$ and prior to revision was $42.4 \, kg/m^2$. Vertical banded gastroplasty (VBG) was revised by partitioning the stomach proximal to the VBG staple line with the linear cutting staplers. Adjus-table gastric bands were divided and removed followed by the creation of a gastric pouch with linear cutting stapler. The mean operative time was four hours and 20 minutes with a length of stay of 4.1 days. There were two complications in these seven patients: the first was a diaphragmatic injury that required a thoracostomy tube and the second was a gastric remnant dilatation requiring a percutaneous gas-trostomy tube. There was no follow-up on these patients published regarding weight loss. In comparison, this group has published the results of their primary series in an abstract form (16).

In May 2002, our experience was published which included 281 laparoscopic Roux-en-Y gastric bypass procedures (17). The series included only patients who had a totally laparoscopic procedure, as opposed to the hand-assisted technique. The paper described the evolution of our technique, especially the changes in the creation of gastrojejunostomy. The gastrojejunostomy was initially created using a circular stapler in 15 patients, changed to a linear stapled anastomosis with a stapled closure of the enterotomy in 102 patients, and then a linear stapled anastomosis with a sewn closure of the enterotomy with circumferential oversewing of the anastomosis in 164 patients and a two-layer entirely sewn anastomosis in 12 patients. The enteroenterostomy was created in a stapled end-to-side fashion and the Roux limb was retrocolic, retrogastric.

There were eight conversions to open surgery. Ninety-four percent of patients had a proximal gastric bypass (30-cm biliopancreatic limb, 50-cm Roux limb), while the remainder had a long limb gastric bypass (75 cm/150 cm). Seventy-five percent of patients were discharged within three days. The mean length of stay was 4.0 ± 9 days with a median of two days. There were no wound infections, and only two port site incisional hernias in patients with a totally laparoscopic gastric bypass procedure. There were three wound infections and two incisional hernias in patients who had laparotomy for complications after their gastric bypass. There were five (1.8%) internal hernias that required surgery. There were 12 leaks at the gastrojejunal anastomosis, one from the staple line of the excluded stomach and one from the jejunojejunostomy. Seven leaks (6.8%) occurred in 102 patients with the single layer linear stapled anastomosis, which led to conversion to the two-layered anastomosis with only three (1.8%) leaks in the subsequent 164 patients. One-year follow-up was available for 69 patients (72% of patients for at least one year from surgery). The mean BMI decreased from 48.3 ± 5.2 to 30.5 ± 5.1. The average percent of weight lost was $70 \pm 15\%$. The resolution of co-morbidity one or more years after surgery was seen in 52% of patients with hypertension, 93% in diabetes requiring medication, 95% for GERD, 76% for orthopedic/joint pain problems and 88% of stress urinary incontinence.

LITERATURE REVIEW—PROSPECTIVE, RANDOMIZED CLINICAL TRIALS

Two centers have published results from prospective randomized clinical trials (PRCT). Westling and Gustavsson randomized 51 patients between laparoscopic and open gastric bypass (18). Their goal was to randomize 60% of patients to laparoscopic and 40% to open surgery to allow for any open conversions. The same technique and staplers were used in both open and laparoscopic operations. The patients and staff were blinded to the surgical procedure using sham dressings that were the same for all patients in size and "blood stained." The laparoscopic group had a 23% conversion rate, primarily for bleeding. The laparoscopic surgery took longer than open surgery. The laparoscopic group (excluding conversion) had less pain, required less parenteral narcotics, a shorter hospital stay, and faster return to work. There was a single mortality secondary to malignant hyperthermia. There were five with a stricture of the Roux limb at the mesocolon defect and one internal hernia, all laparoscopic patients. There was one leak and one PE in the laparoscopic group, and one incisional hernia in the open group. Ninety-two percent of patients were "very satisfied" at one year regardless of the operative approach. Weight loss was similar in the two groups with postoperative BMI being $27 \pm 4 \, kg/m^2$ in the laparo-scopic group and $30.6 \pm 4 \, kg/m^2$ in the open group (NS). The authors did not feel that laparoscopic gastric bypass was beneficial over open surgery because of the high incidence of open conversions and Roux limb obstruction. They acknowledged that they were in their learning curve during this study, and that their conversion and obstruction rates were much higher than the prospective series by other surgeons. They advocated additional PRCT.

Nguyen et al. conducted a PRCT in which 155 patients with a BMI of 40 to $60 \, kg/m^2$ were randomized between laparoscopic and open gastric bypass (19). The laparoscopic technique was previously described (10). In the later portion of the series, a trans-abdominal placement of the anvil was used. Additional modifica-tions of the technique included closure of the mesenteric defects and placement of an anti-obstruction stitch at the jejuno-jejunostomy as described by Brolin (20). The open gastric bypass also used a trans-abdominally placed circular stapler anvil. The gastric pouch was created with linear cutting staplers. The Roux limb was retro-colic, retrogastric in both groups. All patients had a gastrograffin contrast study on the second postoperative day. If no leak or obstruction was observed in the study, patients were started on a clear liquid diet and discharged when oral fluids were tolerated.

The two groups were similar from the standpoint of age, sex ratio, mean BMI $(47.6 \text{ vs. } 48.4 \, kg/m^2)$, preoperative co-morbidities, or American Society of Anesthesio-logis (ASA) class. In the laparoscopic group there were two conversions to open surgery. The estimated blood loss was three times greater in the open group with two splenic cap-sule tears. One open-group patient was excluded from analysis because of an iatrogenic injury to the spleen that required splenectomy, and the gastric bypass was not done. Three (3.9%) of the open-group patients required intraoperative transfusion, while none were required in the laparoscopic group. Median length of stay was shorter in the laparoscopic group (three vs. four days, $p < 0.01$). There were no operative deaths.

There was no difference in need for early reoperation or major complication rate. Major complications included anastomotic leak (one in each group), gastric outlet obstruction (one in the open group), hypopharyngeal injury (one in the laparoscopic group), jejunojejunostomy obstruction (three in the laparoscopic group), PE (one in the open group), respiratory failure (one in the open group), GI bleeding (one in the laparoscopic group), wound infection (two in the open group), and retained lapa-rotomy sponge (one in the open group). Minor complications were similar between groups. There was a higher mean %EBWL at three and six months in the laparoscopic group. This had equalized at one-year follow-up with the %EBWL $68 \pm 15\%$ for the laparoscopic and $62 \pm 14\%$ for the open group. Quality of life was evaluated using the SF-36 assessment tool. The preoperative SF-36 scores were significantly lower than the U.S. norms in both groups in seven of eight domains (only mental health showed no difference). At one-month follow-up, the SF-36 scores were significantly better for the laparoscopic group. By three months, the SF-36 scores of the laparoscopic group were at the U.S. norms. By six months the SF-36 scores of the laparoscopic and open groups were at the U.S. norms and were not significantly differ-ent from each other. The operative costs were greater for the laparoscopic group than for the open gastric bypass group; however, the nursing costs and the total hospital service costs were lower for the laparoscopic group, so that there was no significant difference in the total costs for the two groups.

In addition to the outcomes, quality of life, and cost data summarized above, Nguyen et al. looked at pulmonary function, postoperative pain, and systemic coagulation and fibrinolysis for a subgroup of patients (21,22). Preoperative pulmonary spirometry testing was obtained in 70 patients randomized between laparoscopic and open gastric bypass, and was repeated on postoperative day (POD) 1, 2, 3, and 7. Patients were also asked to record their pain on a visual analog scale (VAS). Patient-controlled analgesia was used in all patients for the first two postoperative days and the amount of morphine used recorded. A subset of patients had a chest radiograph on POD 1 for comparison to preoperative studies. The patients were well matched for age, gender, preoperative BMI, and pulmonary history. A similar number of patients were on opiates preoperatively for chronic pain issues. Postoperatively there were no pulmonary infections in either group. One patient in the open group had a respiratory failure requiring prolonged ventilation and one had a PE. None of the laparoscopic group required postoperative mechanical ventilation. Laparoscopic patients had less impairment of pulmonary function postoperatively for the first three days. By one week, all the laparoscopic groups' pulmonary function had returned to baseline, but only one patient in the open group had. Laparoscopic patients had lower VAS pain scores, required less morphine, and had lower frequency of hypoxia and segmental atelectasis on chest radiograph.

In the first 70 patients accrued in the PRCT, coagulation and fibrinolytic laboratory studies were looked at preoperatively, and at 1-, 24-, 48-, and 72 hours postoperatively. In addition, all patients had a lower extremity duplex preoperatively and again between PODs 3 and 5. Plasminogen levels decreased, while thrombin–antithrombin complex, prothombin fragments 1 and 2, and fibrinogen increased postoperatively in both groups. D-dimer levels increased in both groups with the levels significantly higher in the open group compared to the base line. Antithrombin III and protein C levels were decreased in both groups with a significant decrease in the laparoscopic group. There was one postoperative DVT and one PE in the open group and none in the laparoscopic group. Their conclusion was that the laparoscopic gastric bypass induces a hypercoagulable state similar to that of the open gastric bypass.

DISCUSSION

Laparoscopic gastric bypass has been shown to be a feasible procedure. Currently there are 13 authors and/or centers that have published their experience. The average BMI has ranged from 42 to $55 \, \text{kg/m}^2$. The available published operating room time (ORT) for the Roux-en-Y reconstruction range from 60 to 277 minutes. In the two PRCT, the ORT was significantly longer for laparoscopic surgery than open. The mean or median length of stay ranges from 1.6 to 4.0 days. In the two PRCT, the length of stay was significantly decreased, with decreased narcotic requirements in the laparoscopic group. Except for a single study where the surgeons acknowledged that they were in the learning curve, the conversion to open rate was 1.0% to 8.5%, and most authors with larger series have seen their conversion rate decreasing with time (Table 1).

In addition to being feasible, the laparoscopic gastric bypass is effective. The weight loss, for centers reporting at least one-year follow-up, ranges from 68% to 82% EBWL (Table 2). This compares favorably to the 62% average EWL reported by Sugerman et al. for open gastric bypass patients (23). Open gastric bypass has a

Table 1 Laparoscopic Gastric Bypass Series

Author	N	BMI	ORT	Conversions	Early complications	Late complications	Mortality	LOS (days)
Champion et al. (24)	63	50	NI	1.6%	4.7%	6.3%	1 (1.5%)	NI
De la Torre et al. (5)	50	43.6	199	2%	4%	NI	0	3.8
DeMaria et al. (17)	281	48.1	234	8 (2.8%)	7.3%	16.8%	0	2 days median
Gagner et al. (16)	52	55	277	0	15.0	4	0	4.0
Higa et al. (12)	400	46	60–90	3%	2.5%	12.8%	0	1.6[a]
Higa et al. (11)	1040	47.8	60				5 (0.5%)	1.9
Lonroth and Dalenback (4)	32	42	NI	4.3%	28.1%	6.2%	0	NI
Matthews et al. (6)	48	52.3	231	6.3%	12.5%		0	4
Nguyen et al. (R) (19)	155	47.6	225	2 (2.5%)	15.2%	18.9%	0	3 days median
Nguyen et al. (CS) (10)	35	51	246		5.7	20%	0	4.0
Rutledge (13)	1274	47	36.9		5.2	2.5%	1 (0.08%)	1.5
Schauer et al. (8)	275	48	260	3 (1.0%)	3.3%	27.0%	1 (0.3%)	2.6 median
Schweitzer et al. (25)	33	46	NI	NI	NI	NI	0	
Texiera et al. (7)	28	47	240	0	14%	NI	0	4
Westling and Gustavsson (18)	30	42	245	7 (23%)	20%	23%	1 (3.3%)	4
Wittgrove and Clark (9)	500		90		10.4%	22.2%	0	2.5

Abbreviations: BMI, Body mass index; ORT, operating room time; LOS, length of hospital stay (days); CS, case series; R, prospective, randomized controlled trials.

Table 2 Percent Excess Weight Loss After Laparoscopic Gastric Bypass

Author	3 mo	6 mo	12 mo	24 mo	36 mo	60 mo
Champion et al. (24)		56	82			
De la Torre et al. (5)	38%					
DeMaria et al. (17)	70		70			
Higa et al. (12)			69			
Higa et al. (11)			70			
Lonroth (3) and Lonroth and Dalenback (4)			67	70		
Nguyen et al. (R) (19)			68			
Nguyen et al. (CS) (10)			69			
Rutledge (13)		51	68	77		
Schauer et al. (8)		52.8	68.8	83.2	77 @ 30 mo	
Schweitzer et al. (25)			75			
Wittgrove and Clark (9)		60	77	~81	~74	~80

Abbreviations: CS, case series; R, prospective, randomized controlled trials.

recidivism rate of 10% to 15% of EBW. There is limited long-term follow-up for the laparoscopic gastric bypass.

Four series have published data regarding the efficacy of laparoscopic gastric bypass in resolving co-morbidities (Table 3). Diseases improved by weight loss after laparoscopic gastric bypass included diabetes mellitus resolved in 92% to 100% of the affected patients, hypertension in 52% to 92%, gastroesophageal reflux disease in 77% to 98%, and sleep apnea in 90% to 98%.

The weight loss and health benefits come with a price and that is the early and the late complications, including mortality. Sugerman et al. reviewed the complications in patients with at least five-year follow-up (23). Table 4 compares the complications between that open series (23), the open arm of Westling and Gustavsson's PRCT (18) and Nguyen et al.'s (19) PRCT, and the laparoscopic case series reviewed, focusing on the complications of anastomotic leak, wound infections and mortality. Laparoscopic series leak rates range from 1.0% to 5.1% with the frequency decreasing as surgeons' experience and progress on the "learning curve." It should be noted that in the two laparoscopic series with leak rates >2% (8,17), patients had routine

Table 3 Percent Improvement or Resolution of Obesity Comorbidities After Laparoscopic Gastric Bypass

Author	Diabetes mellitus	HTN	GERD	Sleep apnea	Elevated cholesterol/ lipids	Joint pain	Stress urinary incontinence
DeMaria et al. (17)	93	52	95			76	88
Rutledge (13)	92	90	77	90	93/100	72	81
Schauer et al. (8)	100	88	96	93	96/86	88	89
Wittgrove and Clark (9)	98	92	98	98	97/99	90	97

Abbreviations: HTN, hypertension; GERD, gastroesophageal reflux disease.

Table 4 Complications After Open Gastric Bypass Compared to Laparoscopic Gastric Bypass

Author	Leak/ fistula/ abscess	DVT/PE	SBO	Bleeding	Stomal stenosis	Hernia	MI/CVA	Pulmonary comp	Wound infection	Marginal ulcer
Sugerman et al. (23)	1.2%				14.6%	7%			15.8%	13.3%
Westling and Gustavsson (18)	1 (4.7%)	0	0		0	1 (4.7%)	0	0	3 (14.3%)	2 (9.5%)
Nguyen et al. (R) (19)	2 (2.9%)	1 (1.3%)	0	0	2 (2.9%)	6 (7.9%)	0		6 (7.9%)	
Champion et al. (24)	2 (3.0)	1 (1.5)	1 (1.5)	0	4 (6.3)	0	0	0	0	1 (1.6%)
De la Torre et al. (5)	1 (2.0%)	0	0	0	0	0	0	0	1 (2%)	
DeMaria et al. (17)	14 (5.1%)	3 (1.1%)	4 (1.5%)		18 (6.6%)	5 (1.8%)	0	1 (0.3%)	3 (1.1%)	14 (5.1%)
Gagner et al. (16)	5 (5.8%)	0	0	1 (1.9%)	NI	2 (3.8)	0	0		
Higa et al. (12)	8 (2.0%)c	NI/0	14 (3.5%)	2 (0.3%)	21 (5.25%)	0	0	0	0	4 (1.0%)
Higa et al. (11)	10 (1.0%)	2 (0.2%)/ 3 (0.3%)	<1%	6 (0.6%)	51 (4.9%)	3 (0.3%)	0	1 (0.1%)	1 (0.1%)	14 (1.4%)
Lonroth (3) and Lonroth and Dalenback (4)	2 (6.3%)	0	1 (3.1%)	4 (12.5%)	NI	NI	NI	4 (12.5%)	NI	1 (3.1%)
Matthews et al. (6)	1 (2.1%)				13 (27.1%)		0			

Study										
Nguyen et al. (CS) (10)	0	0	1 (2.8%)	1 (2.8%)	7 (20%)	0	0	1 (2.8%)	1 (2.8%)	0
Nguyen et al. (R) (19)	1 (1.2%)	1 (1.2%)/0	3 (3.8%)	4 (5%)	9 (11.4%)	0	0	0	1 (1.2%)	
Rutledge (13)	0.16%	0.08%/0.16%	1 (0.08%)			0.17%	0			1.8%
Schauer et al. (8)	12 (4.4%)		4 (1.5%)	9 (3.3%)					22% > 1.5% with change in technique 3%	
Schweitzer et al. (25)							0			
Westling and Gustavsson (18)	0	0/1 (3.3%)	6 (20%)	0	0	0	0	1 (3.3%)	0	3 (10%)
Wittgrove and Clark (9)	11 (2.2%)		3 (0.6%)	4 (0.8%)	8 (1.6%)		1 (0.2%)	7 (1.4%)	5%	

Abbreviations: CS, case series; R, prospective, randomized controlled trials.

Gastrograffin UGI. Not all patients with a leak required reoperation. Schauer et al. (8) subcategorized his leaks into four (1.5%) major (those that caused peritonitis or intra-abdominal leak and required reoperation) and eight (2.9%) minor (asymptomatic or contained that did not require surgery). Similarly DeMaria et al. (17) reported that four of the 12 leaks were managed non-operatively with intravenous nutrition and the operatively placed closed-suction drain. Seven of the 12 had laparoscopic repair of the leak, drainage, and insertion of a gastrostomy tube. Two patients required a laparotomy subsequent to the laparoscopic repair and three patients required laparotomy as their initial surgical procedure for leak. The wound complication rate is favorable for laparoscopic gastric bypass with fewer wound-related complications compared to Sugerman's (23) open series (wound infection 0–5% vs. 15.8%, incisional hernia 0–3.8% vs. 7%). Unfortunately there have been deaths following laparoscopic gastric bypass. Nine deaths have occurred in five series. Five of these deaths were due to PE, one from asthma, one from suicide, one from bowel perforation, and one from malignant hyperthermia. The predominance of PE re-enforces the importance of DVT/PE prophylaxis in this patient population.

There are only two prospective randomized clinical trials between open and laparoscopic gastric bypass; however, there are multiple case series available. The PRCT and the case series show comparable weight loss, resolution of co-morbidities, and complication profile as compared to long-term open gastric bypass data. These comparisons suggest that laparoscopic gastric bypass is an equivalent operation to the open gastric bypass. Because of the shorter hospital stay, decreased narcotic requirements, and decreased wound complications, it may even surpass open gastric bypass for the treatment of the morbidly obese patient.

REFERENCES

1. Wittgrove AC, Clark G, Tremblay L. Laparoscopic gastric bypass, Roux-en-Y: preliminary report of five cases. Obes Surg 1994; 4:353–357.
2. Lonroth H, Dalenback J, Haglind E, Lundell L. Laparoscopic gastric bypass: another option in bariatric surgery. Surg Endosc 1996; 10:636–638.
3. Lonroth H. Laparoscopic gastric bypass. Obes Surg 1998; 8:563–565.
4. Lonroth H, Dalenback J. Other laparoscopic bariatric procedures. World J Surg 1998; 22:964–968.
5. De la Torre RA, Scott JS. Laparoscopic Roux-en-y gastric bypass: a totally intra-abdominal approach—technique and preliminary report. Obes Surg 1999; 9:492–498.
6. Matthews BD, Sling RF, DeLegge MH, Ponsky JL, Heniford BT. Initial results with a stapled gastrojejunostomy for the laparoscopic isolated Roux-en-y gastric bypass. Am J Surg 2000; 179:476–481.
7. Teixeira JA, Borao FJ, Thomas TA, Cerabona T, Artuso D. An alternative technique for creating the gastrojejunostomy in laparoscopic Roux-en-y gastric bypass: experience with 28 consecutive patients. Obes Surg 2000; 10:240–244.
8. Schauer PR, Ikramuddin S, Gourash W, Ramanathan R, Luketich J. Outcomes after laparoscopic Roux-en-y gastric bypass for morbid obesity. Ann Surg 2000; 232:515–529.
9. Wittgrove AC, Clark GW. Laparoscopic gastric bypass, Roux-en-Y 500 patients: techniques and results with 3–60 month follow up. Obes Surg 2000; 10:233–239.
10. Nguyen NT, Ho HS, Palmer LS, Wolfe BM. A comparison study of laparoscopic versus open gastric bypass for morbid obesity. J Am Coll Surg 2000; 191:149–157.
11. Higa KD, Boone KB, Ho T. Complications of the laparoscopic Rou-en-y gastric bypass: 1,040 patients—what have we learned? Obes Surg 2000; 10:509–513.

12. Higa KD, Boone KB, Ho T, Davies OG. Laparoscopic Roux-en-y gastric bypass for morbid obesity: technique and preliminary results of our first 400 patients. Arch Surg 2000; 135:1029–1034.

13. Rutledge RR. The mini-gastric bypass: experience with the first 1,274 cases. Obes Surg 2001; 11:276–280.

14. Mini gastric bypass controversy. Letter to the Editor and response by R.R. Rutledge. Obes Surg 2001; 11:773–777.

15. De Csepel J, Nahouraii R, Gagner M. Laparoscopic gastric bypass as a reoperatrive bariatric surgery for failed open restrictive procedures: initial experience in seven patients. Surg Endosc 2001; 15:393–397.

16. Gagner M, Garcia-Ruiz A, Arca MJ, Heniford BT. Laparoscopic isolated gastric bypass for morbid obesity [abstr]. Surg Endosc 1999; 19(suppl 1):S6.

17. DeMaria EJ, Sugerman HJ, Kellum JM, Meador JG, Wolfe LG. Results of 281 consecutive laparoscopic Roux-en-y gastric bypasses to treat morbid obesity. Ann Surg 2002; 235:640–645.

18. Westling A, Gustavsson S. Laparoscopic vs. open Roux-en-y gastric bypass: a prospective randomized trial. Obes Surg 2001; 11:284–292.

19. Nguyen NT, Goldman C, Rosenquist J, Arango A, Cole CJ, Lee SJ, Wolfe BM. Laparoscopic versus open gastric bypass: a randomized study of outcomes, quality of life and costs. Ann Surg 2001; 234:279–291.

20. Brolin RE. The antiobstruction stitch in stapled Roux-en-Y enteroenterostomy. Am J Surg 1995; 169:355–357.

21. Nguyen NT, Lee ST, Goldman G, Fleming N, Arango A, McFall R, Wolfe BM. Comparison of pulmonary function and postoperative pain after laparoscopic versus open gastric bypass: a randomized trial. J Am Coll Surg 2001; 192:469–477.

22. Nguyen NT, Owings JT, Gosselin R, Pevec WC, Lee SJ, Goldman C, Wolfe BM. Systemic coagulation and fibrinolysis after laparoscopic and open gastric bypass. Arch Surg 2001; 136:909–916.

23. Sugerman HJ, Kellum JM, Engle KM, Wolfe L, Starkey JV, Birdenhauer R, Fletcher P, Sawyer M. Gastric bypass for treating severe obesity. Am J Clin Nutr 1992; 55: 560S–566S.

24. Champion JK, Hunt T, DeLisle N. Laparoscopic vertical banded gastroplasty and Roux-en-Y gastric bypass in morbid obesity [abstr]. Obes Surg 1999; 9:123.

25. Schweitzer MA, DeMaria EJ, Sugerman HJ. Laparoscopic gastric bypass. Surg Rounds 2000:371–378.

12

Changing Intestinal Absorption for Treating Obesity

**Picard Marceau, Simon Biron, Frédéric Simon Hould,
Stéfane Lebel, and Simon Marceau**
Department of Surgery, Laval Hospital, Laval University, Quebec, Canada

INTRODUCTION

To understand the impact of bariatric surgery, one must keep in mind that morbid obesity is a disease, a disease that creates an intolerable infirmity, and a disease for which the sole efficient treatment is surgical. Surgery is needed, not so much because the amount of weight to be lost is so important but because the treatment needs to be maintained for life. Losing weight, for these patients, is difficult but it can be done successfully by various means. Maintaining weight loss, on the other hand, is practically impossible without surgical help. As soon as food intake exceeds what is necessary for the basic metabolism, fat will accumulate. These patients have lost their normal capacity for disposing excess calories in ways other than storage as fat. Normally weight tends to remain stable despite the great variability in food intake (1). This is due to complex mechanisms (2–4) by which extra calories are disposed of in ways other than storage. These mechanisms are faulty in these patients. For each and every day, if calorie intake exceeds the minimum energy expenditure, which is about 1300 kcal for these patients after surgery (5–7), fat will reaccumulate and progressively morbid obesity will recur. The restriction of food needs to be permanently so severe that it is not possible for these people. To blame someone for not succeeding is totally unfair. In our societal environment with its strong cultural norm of at least three meals a day, constant incentives to eat, and the heavy accent on food attractiveness, it is impossible to go through life without exceeding basic needs unless it is forcefully imposed by mechanical means or by induced aversion. The only other approach would be to decrease intestinal absorptive capacity.

It took such a long time for health professionals to recognize the fact that severe obesity was a serious disease requiring more than counselling and goodwill for cure. In the 1960s, surgery was seen solely as an esthetical measure and accepted only in the absence of significant medical problems (8). Twenty years later, the "Task Force of the American Society for Clinical Nutrition" (9), because of the link between obesity and many other diseases, moved the comorbidities from contra-indications to indications for preventing surgery. The presence of diabetes, hypertension, and

153

cardiovascular disease became indications for surgery. It took another 10 years for the "NIH Consensus Conference" (10) to recognize morbid obesity as a disease in itself because of its detrimental effect on quality of life and its poor prognosis. The disease itself, without comorbidities, needed to be treated by surgery. Today with our better knowledge of the detrimental effects of obesity and superior technical options, the role of surgery is growing (11). It is now considered as a possible preventive measure in patients with a familial history of morbid obesity or type II diabetes. Until wider indications are accepted (12), BMIs above $40 \, kg/m^2$ without comorbidities and above $35 \, kg/m^2$ with comorbidities would remain the point of reference for surgery.

There are two surgical strategies: One is forcing the restriction of food, the other is changing intestinal absorption. To be free from the stigma of morbid obesity, a patient, hoping to lose appropriate weight, is willing to accept imposed restraint and the deprivation of the ability to eat normally for ever, even without a guarantee of success. This in itself is a powerful testimony of the enormous suffering of these patients. The restriction of food, by itself, in order to be succesful, must be so severe and permanent that with time, it is outsmarted and fails to sustain weight loss despite the major compromises it imposes on quality of life. To prevent the recurrence of morbid weight gain, food intake must be maintained below about 1300 kcal/day. The heavier the patient initially and the longer the follow-up, the greater the failure rate with this approach. For better permanent weight loss, it has been progressively recognized that changing the intestinal absorption may be necessary (13).

This will be a brief review of the role of malabsorptive procedures in the treatment of morbid obesity, and a presentation of what to expect with this approach in terms of its positive and negative impacts on these patients.

DEVELOPMENT OF BARIATRIC SURGERY

Initial Malabsorptive Attempt (Intestinal Bypass)

The first popular attempt to treat morbid obesity by surgery was aimed at changing intestinal absorption. This was in the 1970s and was initiated by academic surgeons. The goal was to decrease absorption using only one mechanism, that is by shortening the gut. The food passage was limited to only a short segment of intestine including a piece of both jejunum and ileum. The great majority of intestine (more than 90%) was bypassed and left aside, unused, and usually connected to the colon. These procedures were called "intestinal bypass" or "jejunoilial bypass (JIB)." This experiment turned out to be a fiasco. After a period of encouraging results, delayed malnutrition occurred, and liver damage appeared sometimes culmunating in cirrhosis. Most of the estimated 25,000 patients with this type of surgery in North America had to be returned to normal anatomy and regained their initial morbid weight. This negative experience caused skepticism and fear of any attempt at changing intestinal absorption. From then on, malabsorptive procedures were discredited and forbidden in the United States. No procedure with a malabsorptive component was to be considered, unless proven to be safe after a long-term surveillance.

Restrictive Phase

For the next 20 years priority was given to restrictive procedures, which, even today, remain the most popular approach. There were three successive periods of restrictive procedures: (1) gastroplasty, (2) gastric bypass, and (3) gastric banding.

Gastroplasty

Gastroplasty consists in creating a pouch at the beginning of the stomach (varying in size from 15 to 30 mL) with an obstructive outlet of 1–1.5 cm in size, the goal being to prevent food intake, hoping that filling the small pouch would create rapid satiety. Whether it creates aversion rather than satiety is debatable. Patients' efforts to overcome the obstruction and compensate with liquid food is a strong argument against the postulated mechanism of decreased appetite. The procedure worked in an insufficient number of patients and weight loss was unsatisfactory in most, particularly in heavier patients. After a long period of debate about its technical aspects, the procedure was progressively abandoned.

Gastric Bypass

Gastric bypass includes a gastroplasty, that is the creation of the same little gastric pouch, but instead of being left in continuity with the stomach, this pouch was directly anastomosed to the small intestine. In so doing, it bypassed the rest of the stomach and duodenum. This operation was shown to be more efficient than gastroplasty, probably due to the added aversion to sweet liquids from the dumping created by the gastroenterostomy (14). Weight loss was better but many patients remained morbidly obese. This approach has saved lives, cured a lot of comorbidities, and satisfied a great number of patients. But these patients can no longer eat normally for the rest of their lives. Food intake must be kept below ~1300 kcal/day, otherwise morbid obesity will recur.

Gastric Banding

Gastric banding consists in creating the same gastric pouch as in a gastroplasty but with the use of an appropriate prosthesis. The procedure is simpler, safer, and less costly. A new device was conceived that would enable changing the size of the pouch outlet when needed, by simply deflating or inflating the band. This is the most popular procedure in Europe, where its use has exploded in the last few years. An American multicentered prospective study has rated this procedure very negatively (15). However, the device was accepted for its general use by the U.S. Food and Drug Administration.

The negative aspects of this procedure are many. Its mechanism is clearly by aversion and not by influencing satiety or appetite. It works better when the device is placed to obstruct the esophagus itself, which hardly relates to normal satiety. With time, the obstruction of the esophagus can produce esophageal dilatation and motility disorders, whose long-term consequences have not been evaluated. An earlier experience with a somewhat similar device placed at the same place for preventing esophageal reflux turned out to be disastrous and required removal after some years because of its migration (16). Finally this approach has the same limitations as successful gastroplasty. It does not sufficiently reduce weight in heavier patients and does not cure most comorbidities. It is premature to know whether this device is here to stay. It may be indicated in some patients but it cannot be the answer for the great majority of patients with morbid obesity.

Past experience has shown that restrictive procedures at large often fail to maintain weight loss and many patients return to morbid weight with the additionnal handicap of not being able to eat normally. Patients surrender the pleasure of eating often without being freed from morbid obesity.

Biliopancreatic Diversion Phase

During the past 20 years, when the dominant focus was on restrictive procedures, the malabsorptive approach was being explored in only a few centers. For obtaining a better quality of life, investigators continued to work on reducing intestinal absorption rather than forcing abnormal food restriction. The main reason for the failure of previous intestinal approaches had been found to be the non-functional intestinal segment. This "blind loop" allowed detrimental bacterial colonization. In the midst of the controversy and despite strong opposition, Scopinaro and his Italian team proposed a new concept for changing intestinal absorption, based on the diversion of bile and pancreatic juice which had the advantage of not leaving any blind loop (17,18). They showed the procedure to be relatively safe and effective (19).

Today, for all practical purposes, there is only one accepted approach for changing food absorption and it is by diverting bile and pancreatic juice so as to limit its digestive role. This is called biliopancreatic diversion (BPD). This approach has been used in many ways different from those proposed by Scopinaro's group, and today BPD refers to an anatomophysiological change rather than a specific procedure. Among the proposed changes, in the construction of a BPD, there is one called the "duodenal switch" that has become increasingly popular and will be the focus of this presentation (Fig. 1).

BILIOPANCREATIC DIVERSION

BPD refers to a relatively simple and reversible procedure. The normal entry of bile into the intestine at its very beginning is diverted by conveying it through a bypassed segment of bowel to a delayed entry nearer the end of the bowel. The length of intestine used for conveying bile will determine the length of intestine left for the passage of food. In doing so, intestinal absorptive surface is shortened, the absorption particularly of high caloric fat is reduced, and bile turnover is respected. No resection is needed and no blind loop is left behind.

Removing bile from its normal entry just beyond the stomach has an unfortunate side effect. It compromises the role of bile at this level as a buffer of gastric acid. As a result, to prevent peptic ulcer, acid secretion must be reduced by some means when bile diversion is performed. It can be achieved by gastric bypass or gastric resection.

The mechanism of action of BPD differs greatly from earlier intestinal bypass (JIB) in the following ways: (1) the reduced absorption is directed particularly toward fat; (2) food passage is three to four times greater than with JIB; (3) there is no blind loop; and (4) bile turnover remains intact since most of the intestinal length remains available for its reabsorption.

As mentioned earlier, the concept of BPD and the credit for the demonstration of its safety and efficiency in bariatric surgery belongs to Scopinaro et al. (17,18). After animal and human experimentation, they concluded that it was best (1) to leave an alimentary tract of 250 cm in contact with food, (2) to reintroduce bile at 50 cm from the ileocecal valve, and (3) to decrease gastric acid by a distal gastrectomy with a gastroileostomy (20). Results were excellent as far as weight loss and quality of life were concerned (21), and this was confirmed by others (22,23) including ourselves (24).

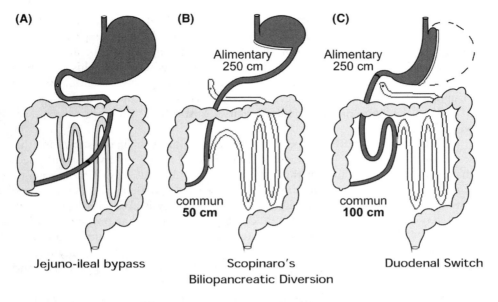

(A) Jejuno-ileal bypass

(B) Scopinaro's Biliopancreatic Diversion

(C) Duodenal Switch

Malabsorptive procedures

Figure 1 This is a schematic view of 3 described procedures meant to decrease intestinal absorption. In **(A)** "jejuno-ileal bypass" (now abandoned) food is allowed to go through a variable length of jejunum (15–60 cm) and ileum (10–50 cm) and the greater part of the intestine remains unused. In "biliopancreatic diversion" all intestinal segments remain functional, food absorption surface is two to three times longer than in a jejuno-ileal bypass, and the bile continues to go through most of the intestine. In **(B)** "BPD Scopinaro's type" the distal two-third of the stomach is removed, 250 cm of intestine is used for food absorption, and bile is reintroduced at 50 cm above the ileocecal valve. In **(C)** "BPD duodenal switch type" bile is reintroduced at 100 cm above the ileocecal valve and the distal gastrectomy is replaced by a sleeve gastrectomy to better preserve normal gastric function.

To decrease side effects, particularly diarrhea, changes were introduced. One change brought a major improvement. Distal gastrectomy was replaced by a sleeve gastrectomy with a duodenal switch. This was inspired by DeMeester (25), who, in looking for a treatment of alkaline reflux gastritis, showed in the dog that preservation of a piece of duodenum better protects against peptic ulcer. The best way to leave a piece of duodenum was by a sleeve gastrectomy. In doing so, normal gastric function was better protected. Preserving the antrum, the pylorus, and a piece of duodenum with their nerves would prevent dumping. It would assure a better role to the stomach as a gate keeper of food, an initiator of protein digestion, and as a trigger of satiety. Furthermore, leaving a piece of duodenum, which further decreases the risk of ulcer, allows leaving the stomach for better protein digestion.

Another modification from the original description was the lengthening of the common tract. It was found that, with an American diet, a common channel of 100 cm instead of 50 cm was better tolerated, decreased the side effects, and improved protein metabolism.

The ideal construction for a BPD is not yet established. A BPD has three components, and each of them, the length of the alimentary tract, the length of the common tract, and the size of the gastric remnant, have an impact on both weight loss and side effects. Whether its construction should be tailored to patient characteristics such as age, size, BMI, etc., is not yet known. Our own 10 years' experience with more than a thousand patients using the same standard procedure for all does not suggest the need for an individualized approach. We hypothesize that this is because the length of the alimentary tract does not need to be very precise. It should only be short enough to create a temporary "short gut syndrome" and recuperation will occur within the limit of individual capacity. Absorption will improve to meet individual needs.

Because results of BPD depend on the particular type of construction, this presentation will focus on the "duodenal switch" type unless otherwise mentioned. We have used this procedure for the last 12 years on 1354 patients. BPD is a major operation with a mortality and morbidity comparable to that of other bariatric operations except for simple banding. Operative mortality is around 1% (14/1354), hospital stay is a median of five days, and complication rate that prolongs hospital stay is about 15%. A progressive unrestricted diet is allowed and resumed in a week or two. Patients are usually followed by ourselves but also by their family doctor. Medical visits and blood tests are obtained every three months the first year and yearly thereafter.

Follow-up is crucial and difficult, and requires dedication. This is a new operation, unfamiliar to most health professionals. A certain reluctance of the medical profession towards surgical treatment of obesity renders the situation more difficult. Moreover, a tendency for these patients to underestimate the need for follow-up increases our obligation to be diligent.

The better results of BPD, in terms of weight loss, weight maintenance, and quality of life have never been challenged. It is its long-term metabolic consequences that have raised questions. We will now see what are the overall results of BPD with emphasis on the beneficial and detrimental impacts of this physiological change.

BENEFICIAL EFFECTS OF BILIOPANCREATIC DIVERSION
Weight Loss

Weight loss occured mainly during the first year and tapered off over another six months. This was followed by a mean weight gain of 1.4 kg/yr. In our most recent survey including all living patients (n = 569) a mean of 53 months (range 24–100 months) after duodenal switch, patients had lost 75% of their excess weight, 43% of their total weight, and the mean BMI had decreased from 48 to 31 kg/m^2. Ninety-two percent of these patients were no longer morbidly obese with a BMI <40 and 77% had a BMI <35. BMI <25 was present in 16% and <21, in 0.7% (Fig. 2) (26).

Quality of Life

Benefits on the quality of life were evident in all aspects of life, including self-confidence, acceptance by others, social activities, marital and sexual relations, daily routine activities, and professional work. Over 95% felt an improvement in each of these domains. On a scale of 5 between improvement and deterioration, mean scores were always above 4 in each domain.

Patients' own evaluations of their results were excellent. More than 85% were satisfied with their weight loss. Mean degree of overall satisfaction, taking into

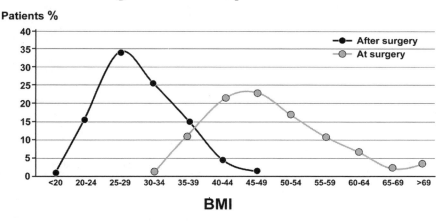

Change in BMI after biliopancreatic diversion

Figure 2 BMI distribution of 569 consecutive patients, a mean of 8 years after biliopancreatic diversion. BMI fell from 48 to 31. More than 90% of patients are no more morbidly obese with a BMI below 40 and 77% below 35.

account the side effects, was 4.4 on a scale of 5. Eating habits were normal in all without imposed restriction (26).

Comorbidities

The beneficial effect of BPD on comorbidity has been spectacular and has helped better understand the disease. It has dissipated many earlier concerns and paved the way for future obesity research. It has brought attention to the following: (1) the possible role of intestinal hormone in the process of diabetes, (2) the value of reducing, mainly, fat absorption in the prevention of arteriosclerosis, (3) the relationship between obesity and Syndrome X, (4) the relationship between obesity and liver disease, and (5) the detrimental effect of maternal obesity on newborn health.

1. *Impact on diabetes.* BPD is very efficient in curing diabetes. In our survey, 69 of 72 diabetic patients no longer required medical treatment. Among the three patients still requiring treatment, two were on oral medication instead of insulin. Furthermore, 35% of patients with fasting blood sugar above 6 mmol/L before surgery dropped to 3% after surgery.
   Procedures that include bypass of duodenum and proximal jejunum (gastric bypass or BPD) were found to be more efficient in curing diabetes (27–29) than pure restrictive procedures (30). At least one mechanism responsible for this improvement in glucose metabolism is the change in intestinal hormone release (27,29,31). BPD and gastric bypass cause a decrease in insulin response to a meal and an increase in insulin sensitivity. Bypassing the proximal intestine causes a decrease in hormones like enterogastrone and pancreatic polypeptide responsible for stimulating the secretion of insulin by the pancreas. On the other hand, entry of food directly into the distal intestine increases other hormones like enteroglucagon (GLPI) which decreases both glycogenolysis by the liver and the secretion

Table 1 Effect of Biliopancreatic Diversion on Lipid Metabolism

Serum levels	Before surgery	10 yrs after surgery
Serum triglycerides (mmol/L)	2.1 ± 1.3	0.7 ± 0.8[**]
Low-density lipoprotein (mmol/L)	3.3 ± 1.0	2.1 ± 1.2[**]
High-density lipoprotein (mmol/L)	1.1 ± 0.3	1.3 ± 0.4[*]
Total cholesterol (mmol/L)	5.2 ± 1.1	3.3 ± 0.8[**]
Chol/HDL ratio	5.3 ± 3.6	2.8 ± 1.0[**]

From a series of 689 consecutive patients submitted to a BPD. The improvement in lipid serum levels and in the artherosclerotic index persists 10 years after surgery.
[*]$p < 0.01$, [**]$p < 0.001$. *Abbreviations*: HDL, high-density lipoprotein; BPD, biliopancreatic diversion.

of glucagon from the pancreas. These hormonal changes decrease the post-prandial rise of blood glucose and the insulin response.

2. *The advantage of a selective decrease in fat absorption (Table 1)*. Efficient decrease of fat absorption after BPD represents an additional benefit and should reduce the risk of cardiovascular disease. It decreases triglycerides and low-density (32) lipoprotein cholesterol while increasing high-density lipoprotein cholesterol. These beneficial effects vary with the level of bile re-entry. The lower the re-entry, the greater the effect (33).

  It has also been shown (34) that after BPD, the decreased lipid absorption in itself further improves insulin sensitivity and glucose tolerance. This is an added favorable long-term factor for better health.

3. *Biliopancreatic diversion and Syndrome X (Table 2)*. BPD improves the metabolic disorder at its root even before clinical evidence of what is called "Syndrome X." Even patients with normal plasma levels of glucose and lipids and normal blood pressure before surgery were found to improve these parameters after surgery. Table 3 shows this improvement in a group of euglycemic, non-diabetic, normotensive patients or with normal plasma

Table 2 Effect of Biliopancreatic Diversion on Syndrome X Showing Lasting Improvement of Its Parameters

Parameters of Syndrome X	Before surgery (%)	10 yrs after surgery (%)
Diabetes	10	3
IGT (FBS > 6 g/L)	28	3
Hypertension	41	13
Systolic > 140 mmHg	30	10
Diastolic > 90 mmHg	18	1
Dyslipidemia	67	21
s-TG > 3	14	6
Chol/HDL > 5	46	10

From a series of 689 consecutive patients submitted to a biliopancreatic diversion. After surgery all components of Syndrome X were improved and remained so after 10 years of observation. *Abbreviations*: IGT, abnormal initial glucose tolerance; s-TG, serum triglyceride; HDL, high-density lipoprotein; FBS, fasting blood sugar.

Table 3 Effect of Biliopancreatic Diversion on Syndrome X Improvement of Its Parameters Even Within Normal Range

Parameters of Syndrome X	n	Before surgery	After surgery	p
Euglycemic, non-diabetic (FBS <6 g/L)	272	5.2	4.8	<0.003
Normal cholesterol (<6 mmol/L)	184	4.7	3.5	<0.001
Normal s-TG (<3 mmol/L)	251	1.8	1.3	<0.0001
Normal diastolic pressure (<90 mmHg)	25	73	68	<0.02

In a series of 689 consecutive patients submitted to a BPD. Before surgery there were 272 with normal FBS, 184 with normal cholesterol level, and 251 with normal s-TG level. In a subgroup of 110 patients with available both pre-and post operative blood pressure, 25 of them, before surgery, had normal blood pressure (<120/90). After surgery these parameters, characterizing Syndrome X, were all improved even when they were within the normal range before surgery as if BPD corrected hidden pathological situations. *Abbreviations*: FBS, fasting blood sugar; s-TG, serum triglycerides.

lipid concentrations. BPD improved glucose tolerance, decreased athero-sclerotic risk, and lowered diastolic blood pressure even if these were within the normal range before surgery. This emphasized how early and progressive is the damage from obesity and raises questions about the definition of what is considered normal.

4. *Biliopancreatic diversion and liver disease*. BPD can improve liver function and repair pre-existing liver damage caused by obesity. It decreases steatosis, fibrosis, and can even cure cirrhosis. In some, this beneficial effect is tempered by the adverse effects of the surgical stress and its complications of malnutrition and diarrhea.

Among 689 patients who had baseline wedge biopsies performed at the time of BPD, two or more follow-up liver biopsies were available for study in 104 patients. Mean steatosis evaluated on a scale of 0 to 3 decreased from 1.57 ± 0.98 to 0.52 ± 0.71 ($p < 0.0001$). It decreased in 80% of patients and increased in only 6%.

The effect of surgery on fibrosis was more complex. On a scale of 5, there was a slight increase from 1.34 ± 1.14 to 1.57 ± 1.17 ($p < 0.053$). It increased in some and decreased in others. There are two competing mechanisms influencing fibrosis. The surgery and its complications would be factors capable of increasing fibrosis, while on the other hand correction of the metabolic disorder would decrease it. It decreased in heavier patients, diabetics, patients with higher waist hip ratio, and patients with a higher initial grade of fibrosis with a greater initial metabolic disorder. On the other hand, it increased in patients without initial fibrosis or with diarrhea and malnutrition after surgery. Generally, fibrosis tended to decrease with time. Steatosis decreased even when fibrosis increased, but if steatosis increased, fibrosis also increased. Inflammation was present in 20% of patients initially. It disappeared in half but appeared in as many. There was no relationship between the change in steatosis or fibrosis and the change in inflammation. Glycogenated nuclei disappeared in 28 of 41 patients where they were present.

In our series (32), 14 patients were diagnosed as cirrhotic at the time of surgery, the liver being clearly nodular. BPD was done despite this unexpected finding. Twelve were still alive 101 months after surgery with normal liver function tests and in 10, two follow-up biopsies were available after a mean of 43 and 101 months, respectively. Fibrosis and inflammation continued to decrease over the years. In three, fibrous bridging disappeared and biopsy returned to normal. The beneficial effect of BPD on the liver is evident if malnutrition is avoided, even if cirrhosis is present before surgery.

5. *Biliopancreatic diversion, pregnancy, and the newborn.* There were concerns about the possible harmful effect of BPD on future pregnancies and newborns. Our study (35) showed that weight loss after BPD improved fertility and made pregnancies safer. In a comparison of birthweights of 379 children born before their mothers' surgery (n = 601; BMI = 47) with those of 80 children born after surgery (n = 77; BMI = 31), the percentage of children born with normal weight after surgery was found to be higher. Macrosomia decreased from 35% to 5% ($p < 0.0001$) while small infants have increased only from 5% to 17%. Without being statistically significant, stillbirth decreased from 9 to none after surgery. Longer follow-up of children born after surgery is needed to evaluate the expected benefit in terms of future obesity later in life. Our study is in progress and involves 150 such children born after BPD.

DETRIMENTAL EFFECT OF BILIOPANCREATIC DIVERSION

One cannot change the normal physiology without paying a price. After BPD there is a price to be paid. From the patient's perspective it seems an acceptable price for rendering an intolerable and untreatable disease into a tolerable and treatable one. In terms of improving quality of life, this is a most gratifying procedure for both patients and surgeons. Nevertheless BPD creates a "new disease" requiring clinical vigilance and continuous monitoring.

Prevalence of Side Effects

About 10% of patients have diarrhea requiring medical treatment. The number of stools increases to a mean of 2.6/day after surgery. Unpleasant and malodorous gas is present in a third of patients representing the most negative impact of BPD. This is relieved by avoidance of fat and certain foods, and often requires intermittent use of metronidazole. These side effects tend to subside with time (36) but may continue for years. They are probably due to undigested food in the colon.

Vitamin and Mineral Deficiencies

By decreasing fat absorption, BPD also compromises the absorption of fat soluble vitamins (A, D, E, and K). This is not a major issue, but requires lifelong surveillance. Supplements are relatively easily administered. Patients must take a commercial multivitamin plus added vitamin A (25,000 U) and vitamin D (50,000 U).

BPD also compromises the absorption of iron and calcium. Supplements of both must be taken permanently. Taking iron daily is not always easy. Compliance can be difficult. Yearly sampling reveals deficiency in iron (Fe < 10 mmol/L) in about 10% of patients and severe anemia in 6% (37). This is usually accompanied by fatigue. Anemia usually responds to an increase in the daily dose of iron from 300 to 900 mg. Over the years intramuscular administration had to be used for limited periods in 8% of patients because of intolerance to oral iron supplements.

Decreased calcium absorption after BPD has always been of concern. The simultaneous decrease in vitamin D worsened the risk of bone damage. Lifelong calcium supplementation is necessary and patients must take 500 mg of calcium daily. Compliance is not difficult. When serum calcium falls below 2.15 mg/L or parathyroid hormone increases above 100 ng/L, supplements must be increased.

In a prospective study (38) including bone histology, it was found that 10 years after BPD, bone loss was within normal limit in 85% of patients and that bone was relatively tolerant of this metabolic change. This is a notion that was well recognized years ago, when jejunoilial bypass was used. Provided close surveillance, use of appropriate supplements, and avoidance of malnutrition, the procedure will not be detrimental to the bones.

Risk of Protein Deficiencies

Mean serum albumin level remained stable after BPD. Nevertheless six months after surgery, hypoalbuminemia was present in 20% of patients followed by a return toward normal. Scopinaro et al. have shown that a BPD, constructed with a distal gastrectomy and a 50-cm common channel, decreased protein absorption by about 40%, and that for some reason intestinal endogenous protein loss was increased from the normal 6 g to 30 g a day (39). Consequently, daily requirements of protein must be increased from 40 g to 90 g. A normal American diet of 2000–2500 kcal contains 20% protein, that is 100 to 150 g of protein. With normal eating habits, protein requirements can be easily met, but if dietary stress or abnormal protein loss occur, such patients remain susceptible to protein deficiency. The re-hospitalization rate for this problem has been about 1% per year after duodenal switch. All hypoalbuminemia, albeit frequently asymptomatic, should be treated by diet adjustments and additional surveillance since serum albumin level remains a predictor of bone loss (38) and liver damage (data not yet reported).

Change in Intestinal Flora

After BPD, there is no "blind loop." Hence, bacterial overgrowth does not have the same impact as it did after JIB. Nevertheless BPD remains a procedure that favors bacterial overgrowth. Many factors contribute to changing bacterial status. Absence of bile and pancreatic juice (40), shortness of the gut (41), protein deficiency (42), and undigested food in the colon (43), have been shown to predispose to changes in intestinal flora. The relief of side effects with antibiotics (metronidazole) is testimony to a bacterial problem. The serious forms of bacterial overgrowth are rare but they may be life-threatening. There may be a link between bacterial overgrowth and increased endogenous protein loss, although this has not been sufficently studied. Bacterial overgrowth may be responsible for the occasional and apparently unexpected occurrences of protein deficiency in these patients that seem to respond to antibiotic treatments (31).

CONCLUSION

Bariatric surgery represents a major advancement in the treatment and indeed, in the comprehension of morbid obesity. It has brought great hope to these patients. It is a promising tool for research. Because these patients are incapable of normally disposing, day after day, extra calories taken above expenditure, they are faced with choosing between forceful restriction and changed intestinal absorption. In order to avoid the necessary lifelong, severe restriction hardly compatible with normal life, we favor changing intestinal absorption. Biliopancreatic diversion is the sole technique available for changing intestinal absorption. Not only does it give good results in terms of weight loss, maintenance of weight loss, and quality of life, but it also produces metabolic changes that are, in the long term, highly beneficial. In particular, biliopancreatic diversion increases glucose tolerance, improves the condition of the liver, and may decrease the risk of artherosclerosis. Biliopancreatic diversion also makes pregnancy safer and newborns healthier. Allowing normal free diet seems to be a contributing factor for easier psychological rehabilitation. The risks after BPD are nutritional deficiency and intestinal bacterial overgrowth. Both can be serious and even life-threatening, but these serious forms are infrequent, preventable, and curable. The key to success depends on appropriate follow-up that is clearly the surgeon's responsibility.

REFERENCES

1. Friedman JM. Obesity in the new millennium. Nature 2000; 404:632–634.
2. Lowell BB, Spiegelman BM. Towards a molecular understanding of adaptive thermogenesis. Nature 2000; 404:652–660.
3. Levine JA, Eberhardt NL, Jensen MD. Role of non exercice activity thermogenesis in resistance to fat gain in humans. Science 1999; 283:212–214.
4. Liebel RL, Rosenbaum M, Hirsch J. Change in energy expenditure resulting from altered body weight. N Engl J Med 1995; 332:621–628.
5. Brolin RE, Robertson LB, Kenler HA, Cody RP. Weight loss and dietary intake after vertical banded gastroplasty and Roux-en-y gastric bypass. Ann Surg 1994; 220:782–790.
6. Kenler HA, Brolin RE, Cody RP. Changes in eating behavior after horizontal gastroplasty and Roux-en Y gastric bypass. Am J Clin Nutr 1990; 52:87–92.
7. Andersen T, Hojlund Pedersen B, Henricksen JH, Uhrenholdt A. Food intake in relation to pouch volume, stoma diameter and pouch emptying after gastroplasty for morbid obesity. Scand J Gastroenterol 1988; 23:1057–1062.
8. Payne JH, DeWind LT. Surgical treatment of obesity. Am J Surg 1969; 118:141–147.
9. National Institutes of Health Consensus Development conference Statement. Am J Clin Nutr 1987; 41:904.
10. Gastrointestinal surgery for severe obesity: National Institutes of Health Consensus Development Conference Statement, March 91. Am J Clin Nutr 1992; 55:6155–6195.
11. Brolin RE. Update: NIH Consensus Conference. Gastrointestinal surgery for severe obesity. Nutrition 1996; 12:403–404.
12. Kral JG, Brolin RE, Buchwald H, Pories WJ, Sarr MG, Sugerman HJ, Wolfe BM. Research considerations in obesity surgery (Workshop summary). Obes Res 2001; 10:63.
13. Brolin RE, LaMorca LB, Cody RP, Piscataway NJ. Malabsorptive gastric bypass in patients with super obesity: a comparative study of Roux limb length. The Society for Surgery of the alimentary tract, 42nd Annual Meeting 2001: 65 (abstract 403).
14. Sugerman HJ, Starkey JV, Birkenhauer RA. A randomized prospective trial of gastric bypass versus vertical banded gastroplasty for morbid obesity and their effects on sweets versus non-sweets eaters. Ann Surg 1987; 205:613–624.

15. DeMaria EJ, Sugerman HJ, Meador JG, Doty JM, Kellum JM, Wolfe L, Szucs RA, Turner MA. High failure rate after laparoscopic adjustable silicone gastric banding for the treatment of morbid obesity. Ann Surg 2001; 233:809–818.

16. Thibault C, Marceau P, Biron S, Bourque RA, Béland L, Potvin M. The Angelchik antireflux prosthesis: long-term clinical and technical follow-up. Can J Surg 1994; 37:12–17.

17. Scopinaro N, Gianetta E, Civalleri D, Bonalumi V, Bachi V. Biliopancreatic bypass for obesity: 1. An experimental study in dogs. Br J Surg 1979; 66:613–617.

18. Scopinaro N, Gianetta E, Civalleri D, Bonalumi V, Bachi V. Biliopancreatic bypass for obesity. II. Initial experience in man. Br J Surg 1979; 66:618–620.

19. Scopinaro N, Gianetta E, Civarelli D, Bonalumi D, Bachi V. Two years of clinical experience with biliopancreatic bypass for obesity. Am J Clin Nutr 1980; 22:506–514.

20. Scopinaro N, Gianetta E, Friedman D, Adami GF, Traverso E, Bachi V. Evolution of biliopancreatic bypass. Clin Nutr 1986; 5(suppl):137–379.

21. Scopinaro N, Gianetta E, Friedman D, Traverso E, Adami GF, Vitale B, Marinari G, Cuneo S, Ballari F, Colombini M, Bachi V. Biliopancreatic diversion for obesity. Probl Gen Surg 1992; 9:362–379.

22. Clare MW. Equal biliopancreatic and alimentary limbs: an analysis of 106 cases over 5 years. Obes Surg 1993; 3:289–295.

23. Lemmens L. Biliopancreatic diversion: 170 patients in a 7 years follow-up. Obes Surg 1993; 3:179–180.

24. Marceau S, Biron S, Lagacé M, Hould FS, Potvin M, Bourque RA, Marceau P. Biliopancreatic diversion, with distal gastrectomy, 150 cm and 50 cm limbs: long term results. Obes Surg 1995; 5:302–307.

25. DeMeester TR, Fuchs KH, Ball CS, Albertrecci M, Smyrk TC, Marcus JN. Experimental and clinical results with proximal end-to-end duodenojejunostomy for pathologic duodenogastric reflux. Ann Surg 1987; 206:414–426.

26. Marceau P, Hould FS, Simard S, Lebel S, Bourque RA, Potvin M, Biron S. Biliopancreatic diversion with duodenal switch. World J Surg 1998; 22:947–954.

27. Sarson DL, Scopinaro N, Bloom SR. Gut hormone changes after jejunoileal (JIB) or biliopancreatic (BPD) bypass surgery for morbid obesity. Int J Obes 1981; 5:471–480.

28. Hickey MS, Pories WJ, MacDonald KG, Cory KA, Dohm GL, Swanson MS, Israel RG, Barakat HA, Considine RV, Caro JF, Houmard JA. A new paradigm for type 2 diabetes mellitus: could it be a disease of the foregut? Ann Surg 1998; 227:637–644

29. Sirinek RK, O'Dorisio Hill D, McFee A. Hyperinsulinism, glucose-dependent insulinotropic polypeptide, and the enteroinsular axis in morbidly obese patients before and after gastric bypass. Surgery 1986; 100:781–787.

30. Letiexhe MR, Scheen AJ, Gérard PL, Desaive C, Lefèbvre PJ. Postgastroplasty recovery of ideal body weight normalizes glucose and insulin mtabolism in obese women. Clin Endocrinol Metab 1995; 80:364–369.

31. Kellum JM, Kuenmerle JF, O'Dorisio TM, Rayford P, Martin D, Engle K, Wolf L, Sugerman HJ. Gastrointestinal hormone responses to meals before and after gastric bypass and vertical banded gastroplasty. Ann Surg 1998; 8:253–260.

32. Marceau P, Hould FS, Lebel S, Marceau S, Biron S. Malabsorptive obesity surgery. Surg Clin N Am 2001; 81:1113–1127.

33. Brolin Re, Bradley LJ, Wilson AC, Cody RP. Lipid risk profile and weight stability after gastric restrictive operations for morbid obesity. J Gastrointest Surg 2000; 4: 464–469.

34. Mingrove G, DeGaetano A, Greco AV, Capristo E, Benedetti G, Castagneto M, Gasbarrini G. Reversibility of insulin resistance in obese diabetic patients: role of plasma lipid. Diabetologia 1997; 40:599–605.

35. Marceau P, Biron S, Hould FS, Lebel S, Marceau S, Simard S, Kral JG. Outcome of pregnancies after obesity surgery. In: Guy-Grand B, Ailhaud G, eds. Progress in Obesity Research. John Libbey & Cie International Congress on Obesity 1999; 8:795–802.

36. Marceau S, Biron S, Lagacé M, Hould FS, Potvin M, Bourque RA, Marceau P. Bilio-pancreatic diversion, with distal gastrectomy, 250 cm and 50 cm limbs: long term results. Obes Surg 1995; 5:302–307.
37. Marceau P, Biron S, Hould FS, Lebel S, Marceau S. Malabsorption procedure in surgical treatment of morbid obesity. Probl Gen Surg 2000; 17:29–39.
38. Marceau P, Biron S, Lebel S, Marceau S, Hould FS, Simard S, Dumont M, Fitzpatrick LA. Does bone change after biliopancreatic diversion? J Gastroint Surg. 2002; 6: 690–698.
39. Scopinaro N, Adami GF, Marinari GM. Biliopancreatic diversion. World J Surg 1998; 22:936–946.
40. Slocum MM, Sittig KM, Specian RD, Deitch EA. Absence of intestinal bile promotes bacterial translocation. Am Surg 1992; 58:305–310.
41. Vanderhoof JA, Young RJ, Murray N, Kaufman SS. Treatment strategies for small bowel bacterial overgrowth in short bowel syndrome. J Pediatr Gastroenterology Nutr 1998; 27:155–160.
42. Li Ma, Specian RD, Rodney DB, Berg RD, Deitch EA. Effects of protein malnutrition and endotoxin on the intestinal mucosal barrier to the translocation of endogenous flora in mice. J Parenteral Nutr 1989; 13:572–578.
43. Sedman PC, Macfie J, Sagar P, Mitchell CJ, May J, Mancey-Jones B, Johnstone D. The prevalence of gut translocation in humans. Gastroenterology 1994; 107:643–649.

13

Laparoscopic Adjustable Silicone Gastric Banding

Jeff W. Allen
Department of Surgery and the Center for Advanced Surgical Technologies, University of Louisville School of Medicine, Louisville, Kentucky, U.S.A.

Christine J. Ren
New York University School of Medicine, New York, New York, U.S.A.

INTRODUCTION

The restrictive operation known as gastric banding has evolved from the open placement of a fixed piece of a woven mesh to its current state of laparoscopic positioning of an adjustable silicone ring just below the gastroesophageal junction. Adjustable gastric banding is a purely restrictive operation that relies on decreasing the consumption of food as the mechanism for weight loss. There is no malabsorptive component to this operation and therefore minimal risk of malnutrition. Adjustable gastric banding involves the surgical implantation of a silicone device circumferentially around the uppermost part of the stomach. The band creates a small proximal "pouch" that empties slowly, resulting in decreased appetite and early satiety.

The stoma created by the band can be made smaller or larger because of the inflatable balloon that is lining the inner lumen of the device. This balloon is, in turn, attached to a subcutaneous reservoir port via hollow tubing. Potential benefits of this particular bariatric operation include a high rate of laparoscopic completion, shortened hospital and off-work times, and a minimal risk of malnutrition (1). The novelty of the device, however, lies squarely on its adjustability. No previous bariatric operation of any variety has allowed the surgeon the ability to alter the patient's level of restriction post-operatively (and theoretically their weight loss). Injection of saline into the port results in inflation of the balloon and subsequent tightening of the band leading to a narrowed stoma. The band tightening or "adjustment" is performed on an individual basis according to the patients' weight loss and appetite. Although there are wide variations, a typical adjustment pattern would include tightening approximately five to six times in the first year and two to three times in the second year. Weight loss is gradual, averaging 1.02 lbs (0.45 to 0.90 kg) each week during the first two years after surgery. The only available device is the LapBand®, although the Swedish Adjustable Band is currently under investigation as an investigative device exemption prior to pre-market approval by the US Food and Drug Administration.

PATIENT SELECTION

The essential factors influencing the patient selection for silicone adjustable gastric band (LAGB) are no different than any other weight-loss operation (2). The guidelines set forth by the consensus conference of the National Institutes of Health in 1991 outline the basic recommendations for vertical banded gastroplasty (VBG) and gastric bypass and are summarized in Table 1 (3). While these have been broadly applied to bariatric surgery, in general, some specific issues related to the LAGB warrant further examination.

Because the LAGB is a purely restrictive operation, it is theorized that "sweet-eaters" will not sustain significant weight loss after this operation. The reasoning for this lies in the fact that LAGB patients attain weight loss solely by decreasing the amount of ingested calories, while gastric bypass patients also have some level of malabsorption. In addition, LAGB patients will not incur the "dumping syndrome" with carbohydrate meals as do some gastric bypass patients. Hudson et al. (4) compared the weight loss after LAGB between patients who scored highly on preoperative sweet-eating food surveys versus those who did not, and found no statistically significant difference in their weight loss. Based on this study, it does not appear reasonable to deny LAGB to a morbidly obese sweet-eater.

The NIH consensus conference did not make any recommendations about weight-loss surgery in children and adolescents. Operative therapy for obesity is emerging as a more-accepted treatment for these patients, however. The most common operation in America in this (and all) age groups is the gastric bypass. The long-term effects of gastric bypass performed on children or adolescents are not known. Vitamin deficiencies are more common with gastric bypass than with LAGB, and this patient population may be especially sensitive given their rapid growth phases. But the long-term effects of the LAGB in adolescents are also unknown. The effective duration of the integrity of the balloon over 30 to 60 or more years, the presumed life expectancy of these adolescents, is unknown nor is the risk of band erosion over this length of time known. At present, the Federal Drug Administration has set age guidelines on the only currently available LAGB, the LapBand System® (Inamed Health, Santa Barbara, California, U. S.). The minimum recommended age is 18 years, and while many surgeons have chosen to place the device in younger patients, this use is considered "off label."

One additional group continues to be controversial with respect to LAGB placement. Patients with a very high body mass index (BMI) (e.g., $> 60 \, \text{kg/m}^2$) are known by a variety of pseudonyms, including the "super-obese." Given the decreased average percent excess body weight loss associated with LAGB compared to gastric

Table 1 NIH Recommendations for Bariatric Surgery Patient Selection

Attempted non-operative methods of weight loss
Well-informed and motivated
Acceptable operative risk
BMI $> 40 \, \text{kg/m}^2$
BMI 35–40 kg/m^2 with high-risk co-morbid conditions and/or obesity-induced physical
  problems interfering with lifestyle

bypass, many surgeons believe that a band may not be appropriate for the super-obese patient. Others tend to recommend a staged procedure such as a gastric resection followed by a gastric bypass or duodenal switch (5). The benefit of LAGB in these patients is the possibility of a definitive, laparoscopic, clean case with the lowest risk. Fielding has reported good results in this population with an average reduction of BMI from $69 \, kg/m^2$ to $33 \, kg/m^2$ at three years (6). Additional, larger studies are needed to confirm the utility of LAGB in the super-obese.

Patients with connective tissue diseases, such as systemic lupus erythematosus, may be at a higher risk of the complication of band erosion. In addition, patients with the unusual allergic reaction to silicone should be identified. These potential operative candidates may be best advised to pursue gastric bypass.

OPERATIVE TECHNIQUE

Thromboembolic hose and sequential compression devices are generally used to prevent deep vein thrombosis. In addition, many patients receive an anticoagulant such as subcutaneous fractionated heparin. A first-generation cephalosporin is administered, and the patient is placed supine on the operating table; a minority of surgeons will prefer the lithotomy position and stand between the patient's legs. A standard surgical skin preparation is used. After establishing pneumoperitoneum, a brief exploration is undertaken, noting the size of the liver, location of adhesions, and any abnormality that may preclude the safe placement of the device.

Two slightly dissimilar methods for placement have evolved: the perigastric and pars flaccida techniques. The perigastric approach is the manner in which the early LAGBs were performed. It entails dividing the gastrohepatic ligament, identifying the right crus of the diaphragm, and then bluntly developing a generous retrogastric tunnel to the angle of His. After the tunnel is created, the LAGB is introduced into the abdominal cavity, pulled through behind the stomach, confirmed in place by an intragastric calibration tube, and locked into place. In most instances, the lesser sac is entered during the tunneling, and some surgeons advocate placing a mesh in the lesser sac to minimize mobility of the freed-up stomach. Gastric-to-gastric sutures (above and below the LAGB) to form a fundoplication are used to prevent migration of the stomach up through the device, a complication known as gastric prolapse. The tubing of the band is then exteriorized and attached to the adjustment port, which, in turn, is secured to the fascia of the anterior abdominal wall.

The pars flaccida approach is the more modern technique. Using this method, the peritoneal attachments overlying the angle of His are first freed up. Then, the gastrohepatic ligament is divided and the right crus of the diaphragm identified. The fatty tissue medial to the right crus is scored and a blunt grasping instrument is passed blindly behind the stomach to exit at the angle of His that was previously dissected. The band is then introduced and secured as mentioned above. This technique avoids the generous retrogastric tunnel.

The pars flaccida approach evolved because the perigastric technique was associated with high complication rates, most notably posterior gastric prolapse. In addition, the avoidance of the larger retrogastric tunnel eliminated the need for mesh, which carries an added risk of erosion and infection. In performing the pars flaccida technique, a significant amount of adipose tissue is occasionally included inside the band, a scenario that can lead to the problem of postoperative obstruction. To avoid this, the greater curve fat pad is excised, and occasionally, the fat along the lesser curve is incised. A "two-step" hybrid method of placement combines the peri-gastric and pars flaccida techniques and is occasionally used (7).

POSTOPERATIVE MANAGEMENT

Immediate

Postoperative care after LAGB is typically straightforward. Most patients are observed in a regular room. Patients with documented or suspected obstructive sleep apnea may require additional monitoring and/or continuous positive airway pressure device. Early ambulation is encouraged.

Early postoperative retching and vomiting by the patient should be avoided. Just as in anti-reflux surgery, vomiting immediately after surgery can result in suture failure. This will cause an acute gastric prolapse with "band slip." Aggressive anti-emetic therapy should be instituted in the operating room. Intraoperative intravenous administration of ondansetron/metoclopramide/ketorolac is one strategy. Additional intravenous anti-emetics are given liberally during the first 24 hours. Both patient and nursing staff are counseled on the importance of emesis prevention after surgery. Pain management involves subcutaneous injection of skin incisions with 0.25% bupivacaine, and intravenous ketorolac is administered as a standing order every six hours, with subcutaneous morphine for breakthrough pain.

Patients remain NPO (nothing per orum) until an upper gastrointestinal radiographic series (UGI) is performed the next morning, showing normal, rapid esophageal emptying, no extravasation of contrast, and adequate band placement with the patient lying in a 7-to-1 o'clock position. If the esophagram shows delayed emptying, the predicted normal clinical progression is increased swelling over 48 hours. It is advised that the patient remain NPO with intravenous hydration and anti-inflammatory medication (i.e., ketorolac).

Patients should be kept in the hospital if there is any evidence for delayed esophageal emptying, as stomal swelling usually maximizes 24 to 48 hours after band placement. This is particularly relevant when the pars flaccida technique is used. Incorporation of peri-gastric fat within the band can cause an external compression of the stomach and a greater likelihood of stomal narrowing. Communication with the radiologist is an important component to ensure that abnormal findings are reported. In 670 operations performed at New York University Medical Center, there have been no cases of perforation, five cases of stomal obstruction, and seven cases of delayed esophageal emptying. All obstructions were symptomatic at the time of esophagram. Those with delayed emptying were not symptomatic until 48 hours after surgery. In addition, it provides the surgeon with a baseline esophagram to document band positioning.

Patients are seen in the office at 10 to 14 days for their first follow-up visit to check their wounds and reiterate dietary guidelines. Due to the possible correlation between early vomiting and gastric prolapse (8,9), patients are placed on a diet that progresses from liquids to solids over the first six weeks after surgery. In weeks 1 and 2 clear liquids are introduced, weeks 3 and 4 pureed foods, and weeks 5 and 6 soft and flaky solid foods. This specifically excludes chicken, steak, and bread, which tend to form a large bolus that cannot transverse through the narrow band stoma. Tough, doughy, and dry foods are typically poorly tolerated for 6 to 12 months by the majority of patients after gastric banding. Patients are counseled not to eat and drink simultaneously in order to maximize the amount of time the gastric pouch is filled with food.

Nutritional deficiencies have not been widely reported after adjustable gastric banding. However, patients are encouraged to take a daily multivitamin. More importantly, patients should already have the nutritional knowledge and skills to make healthy food choices prior to any bariatric surgery, including gastric banding. Patients are counseled on avoiding high-calorie liquids and soft foods, such as chocolate and ice cream, since these items will be physically easy to eat, but will lead to weight regain or weight loss failure.

Long-Term: Band Adjustments

Adjustable gastric banding works on the basis of three mechanisms: (1) decreasing appetite, (2) creating satiety with a smaller amount of food, and (3) behavior modification. This is a direct function of a small gastric pouch (10–15 cc) and a narrow stomal opening that slows gastric emptying (12 mm). The gastric band acts in this capacity through external constriction of the stomach, which is gradually tightened in accordance with each individual. If no constriction is created, no restriction is experienced, and no weight is lost. Therefore, weight loss after gastric banding is contingent upon band adjustment. The band is useless if adjustments are not performed. Both patient and surgeon must understand this, otherwise loss will be suboptimal and the operation ineffective.

The band is left empty when initially placed. The first adjustment is performed six weeks postoperatively. This allows time for a capsule to form around the band, which secures its position around the stomach. Adjustments should be made while patients are eating solid food, so that the gastric pouch is properly stretched. An appropriately adjusted band probably also acts as an appetite suppressant. A sense of hunger, increased appetite, or increased snacking are signs that the band is not appropriately tightened. Individuals who do not eat as a response to hunger (i.e., emotional eaters) may continue to eat and fail to lose weight by grazing throughout the day or by eating soft, high-calorie foods and beverages. Soft and liquid foods empty faster than solids, and thus more can be ingested prior to the feeling of satiety. Thus, a band that is too tight will make solid-food ingestion difficult, but easy for creamy sugary liquids. This is an example of maladaptive behavior and may necessitate band loosening. The patient then requires additional dietary counseling to help correct this behavior.

Two general strategies to band adjustment exist: in-office adjustment using a clinical algorithm or radiographic adjustment under fluoroscopic guidance. In-office adjustments are quick and inexpensive, but require frequent visits due to inaccuracy of the adjustment. Radiographic adjustments are more cumbersome and expensive, but require fewer visits due to the more "accurate" adjustment visualized under fluoroscopy.

The maximum recommended amount of saline that a gastric band accommodates depends on the band type. The Lap-Band System recommends the maximum amount of saline in their 9.75- and 10-cm bands to be 4 cc and 9 cc in the 11-cm band.

Office-Based Adjustments

When performed in the office, the port is located by palpation. The band is adjusted by accessing the port percutaneously with a non-coring needle and subsequently injecting sterile saline, which tightens the band. Withdrawal of the saline results in band loosening with subsequent decreased restriction. The skin is cleansed with alcohol, and a non-coring needle on a 3-cc syringe filled with the desired amount of saline introduced through the skin into the access port. Successful port access is confirmed by feeling the needle hit the metal base of the access port and having free reflux of saline back into the syringe. Local anesthetic is unnecessary. This can be performed with the patients supine.

Radiographic or ultrasound assistance may be needed to help localize and mark the port, particularly in patients who have a thick wall of subcutaneous fat. The learning curve for port localization using palpation is surprisingly long and may take up to 100 cases. Our experience has shown that upon review of our first 200 consecutive Lap-Band patients (69% female, mean BMI 48.7), 660 adjustments were performed in the office (74% by NP, 26% by MD), and 98.2% were completed successfully. The nine patients (1.8%) who required fluoroscopy to localize the port were in the first 75 patients undergoing adjustments.

The amount of saline to inject for each adjustment is based on three variables: hunger, weight loss, and restriction. A properly adjusted band will induce the lack of hunger and appetite suppression. It should also induce a prolonged sense of satiety that lasts longer than two hours after a meal. Weight loss should be constant and gradual over the course of 18 to 36 months. The goal of weight loss is 1 to 2 lb/wk (0.45–0.90 kg/wk) or 6 to 10 lbs/mo (2.7–4.5 kg/mo). Lack of weight loss reflects a too large portion of intake and suboptimal restriction, indicating the band needs tightening. Lack of restriction to tough or doughy solid foods such as steak, chicken, or bread also signals the need for band adjustment. Initial adjustments measure approximately 1.0 cc but gradually decrease down to 0.2 cc, depending on appetite, weight loss, and food tolerance (10). For larger bands, such as Lap-Band V6, the initial injection is 3 cc. After each adjustment, the patient drinks a cup of water to ensure that he/she does not have outlet obstruction.

At New York University, the adjustments are performed in the office, and the patients are seen every 4 to 6 weeks for weight and appetite evaluation. The program is structured for patients to return for regular weigh-ins, progress evaluation, adjustments, nutritional reinforcement, and behavioral counseling. Frequent patient follow-up has a significant impact on percent excess weight loss (%EWL) achieved in just one year. Patients who return more than six times in the first year after gastric banding lose an average of 50% EWL, as compared to those who return six times or less who lose 42% EWL (10). The average number of adjustments in the first year was 4.5 and the second year was two times. The average amount of fluid present in the band after the first year was 1.9 cc.

Radiographic-Guided Adjustment

Real-time fluoroscopy allows for rapid localization of the port to assist in percutaneous access. The needle can be observed simultaneously as the skin is punctured and the port accessed. Free reflux of saline into the syringe confirms successful access. Fluoroscopy also allows for visualization of the esophagus, gastric pouch, band, diameter of outlet, and integrity of tubing/port system. The band is fully tightened, the patient drinks barium, and the fluid is either added or removed. Radiographic criteria for fluid removal include lack of esophageal emptying after five peristaltic waves, reflux, pouch dilatation with insufficient emptying, or obstruction (11). Radiographic criteria for fluid addition is an immediate passage of barium through the stoma or wide stomal outlet (approximately > 8 mm).

Fluoroscopy may show esophageal dilatation, gastric pouch dilation or prolapse, malfunctioning band or malpositioned band. These situations require immediate intervention such as the band to be loosened or surgical revision. This may be helpful, since not all of these abnormalities are necessarily reflected in clinical symptoms. Busetto et al. (12) found that in their 379 laparoscopic adjustable gastric banding (LAGB) patients, the average number of adjustments performed in the first year after surgery was 2.3 ± 1.7, and the mean maximum band filling after surgery was $2.8\,mL \pm 1.2\,mL$.

Although the number of follow-up visits and adjustments are much fewer with radiographic assistance, a greater investment in time, cost, and manpower is required. The surgeon must coordinate with a radiology facility for use of the fluoroscopy; this can be time- and cost-consuming. Unless the surgeon owns his/her own fluoroscopic C-arm, the average time to perform an adjustment is 15 to 30 minutes.

COMPLICATIONS

A morbidly obese patient undergoing abdominal surgery is generally at higher risk for surgical complications than a leaner individual. This is due, in part, to the disease processes associated with obesity, such as adult onset diabetes mellitus, hypertension, and sleep apnea. However, there are certain adverse clinical scenarios that are unique to gastric banding: prolapse, erosion, and pouch or gastroesophageal dilation. Despite these, LAGB is the safest bariatric operation available.

This procedure carries a 0.05% mortality rate (13), 5% 30-day morbidity rate, and delayed complication (gastric prolapse, erosion, port-tubing disconnection) rate of 12% (1,14–24) (Table 2). The Australian Safety and Efficacy Register of New Interventional Procedures-Surgical (ASERNIP-S), a subcommittee of the Royal Australasian College of Surgeons evaluated the LAGB against VBG and Roux-en-Y gastric bypass (RYGB), in terms of safety and efficacy. Their systematic review of the literature (121 studies) found LAGB to be safer than VBG and RYGB and to be effective up to four years after surgery. The median complication rate for LAGB was 11.3% (13) with very few studies having reported overall morbidity rates above 20%. The incidence of complications is inversely related to experience with the procedure.

Gastric Prolapse

Gastric prolapse is the most appropriate term for the situation that occurs when part of the stomach below the device herniates up through the band. This is also known as a "slipped band." The fundus is most commonly the involved portion of the stomach with prolapse. The herniated stomach will begin to preferentially receive ingested materials, and this causes engorgement and downward rotation of the band. As this process continues, a partial and sometimes complete gastric obstruction will result.

Table 2 Outcomes of Lap-Band System: Complications

Study	N	Mortality	Compli-cations (30 days) (%)	Gastric prolapse/ pouch dilatation (%)	Erosion (%)	Port/tubing problem (%)	Band removal
Dargent, 1999 (14)	500	0	2.2	5	0.6	1.0	–
Fielding, 1999 (15)	335	0	7.7	3.6	0	1.5	1.5
O'Brien, 2002 (16)	709	0	1.2	12.5	2.8	3.6	1.7
Vertruyen, 2002 (24)	543	0	1.2	4.6	1	3	0.6
Rubenstein, 2002 (1)	63	0	1.8	14.2	1.6	7.9	4.8
Favretti, 2002 (17)	830	0	3.9	2.1	0.5	11	1.6
Ren, 2002 (18)	115	0	13	2	0	7	2
Belachew, 2002 (19)	763	0.1	0.8	8	0.9	2.5	3.1
Angrisani, 2003 (20)	1893	0.53	10.2	4.8	1.1	4.1	–
Weiner, 2003 (21)	984	0	4.2	3.7	2.5	–	–
Ren, 2004 (22)	445	0.2	10.5	3.1	0.2	2.3	–
Sarker, 2004 (24)	154	1.2	–	3.2	0.6	4.5	–

–, not reported.

The three types of gastric prolapse are anterior, posterior, and concentric. The most common variety is the anterior prolapse, which is characterized by the greater curve being the lead point up through the band. The posterior gastric prolapse involves the lesser curvature of the stomach as the lead point. This uncommon variety is associated with devices placed using the perigastric technique. In the posterior prolapse, the herniated stomach comes to rest posterior to the band and the remaining stomach.

It is often difficult to distinguish the "concentric slip" from dilation of the pouch above the band. The latter may be due to non-compliance and overeating by the patient. A band that is over-inflated also can cause this scenario as can erroneous placement of the band too low. In addition, development of a hiatal hernia proximal to the band may promote pouch enlargement or slip.

Symptoms in a patient with a gastric prolapse include heartburn, nausea, food intolerance, vomiting, and occasionally back or abdominal pain. The symptoms are often indolent and may be confused for a band that is over-inflated. A patient with intense abdominal pain or signs of peritonitis should alert the surgeon to ischemia or perforation and requires urgent care.

Clinical suspicion and confirmatory radiographs are used in the diagnosis of gastric prolapse. A contrast esophagram is most commonly employed, but a plain film occasionally will suffice. The radiographic findings of gastric prolapse are listed in Table 3. The LAGB will appear to point at the patient's left hip instead at the left shoulder, which is the normal orientation. The presence of fundus or dilated stomach (especially an air-fluid level) above the band or a "wave sign" of herniated stomach overhanging the band are common. With gastric prolapse, a varying amount of obstruction is also seen. In some instances, it is difficult to distinguish a gastric prolapse from pouch dilation above the band. Hiatal hernia is inconsistently diagnosed by esophagram and endoscopy, with the only reliable diagnostic method being laparoscopy.

Table 3 Radiographic Features of Gastric Prolapse

Air fluid level above the band
Rotation of the band downward and to the patient's left
Wave sign
Partial to complete outlet obstruction
Increased amount of stomach above the band

The treatment of gastric prolapse is operative re-positioning of the LAGB. The severity of the gastric slip often correlates with the patient's symptoms. Intense pain may be indicative of ischemia and mandates emergent treatment. In some instances, especially where the patient has mild symptoms and non-diagnostic radiographic findings, removal of all fluid from the band and a period of observation would be appropriate.

The technical details of repairing a gastric prolapse include removal of all saline solution from the LAGB and placement of a decompressing nasogastric tube. After establishing pneumoperitoneum, the adhesions are incised, the device and prolapsed stomach identified, and the previous plicating sutures taken down. When possible, the herniated stomach above the band is simply reduced. Often this is not eminently achievable, and the band must be opened or removed and replaced. At this operation, assiduous gastric-to-gastric plicating sutures are especially important to prevent future prolapse. Simultaneous evaluation of the hiatus must be performed for the presence of a crural defect and hiatus hernia. Primary crural repair with non-absorbable suture is a necessary step to avoid recurrence of prolapse.

Erosion

Since the LAGB remotely resembles an Angelchik prosthesis, a common concern is that the device will undergo erosion into the gastric lumen at a high rate. Fortunately this has not often been the case, but when it occurs, an eroded band is a serious complication. A patient with an eroded band often is asymptomatic. Signs and symptoms include mild upper gastrointestinal discomfort, latent adjustment port site infection, heartburn, or a sudden change in the level of food restriction. Only rarely is the presentation that of an acute gastric perforation.

It is difficult to identify an eroded LAGB radiographically, except in extreme cases. The most useful diagnostic test is upper endoscopy to detect the device intraluminally. It is important to retroflex the endoscope to obtain good visualization just below the gastroesophageal junction, as there may be only a pinhole-sized erosion in this location. In addition, the LAGB should be deflated prior to endoscopic examination to allow unhindered passage of the endoscope through the banded stomach.

Since the eroded LAGB is an uncommon complication, there is limited data recommending treatment strategies. There is no current evidence to suggest that a small erosion will repair itself. As such, the treatment of choice is removal of the device. This, however, leaves the disease of obesity untreated and is nearly always poorly received by patients. With this in mind, the treatment options include replacement of the band at the same or a later operation or conversion to gastric bypass, again either simultaneously or in staged fashion. There may be a greater risk of band infection or another erosion should it be placed at the same time an eroded band is removed.

The technique associated with operating on an eroded LAGB is markedly different from treating gastric prolapse. Findings generally include a localized inflammatory reaction with dense adhesions and scar formation around the band. These often encase the band and tubing, making identification of the device difficult. Removal is accomplished by dissection along the tubing until the buckle is encountered, and then the band in this area is transected. The band that has migrated intraluminally will be discolored. A remnant gastrotomy defect may be difficult to demonstrate because of a "sealing effect," but when present should be closed.

Postoperative Obstruction

A small percentage of patients will develop severe dysphagia following LAGB placement. Usually this occurs early in the postoperative course during a confirmatory radiograph or when the patient first begins oral intake of fluids. Although the dysphagia is usually due to a mechanical problem, the spectrum of "postoperative obstruction" can include gastric ileus and gastroparesis. The technical factors contributing to postoperative obstruction include inadequate excision of perigastric fat, edema of the plicated stomach, hematoma at one of the sutures, or some degree of neuropraxia. An esophagram typically shows the band in good position and alignment, but with little or no flow of contrast material through the band.

Management of the obstruction includes continued hospitalization, intravenous fluids, bowel rest, and anti-inflammatory medications such as ketorolac. Postoperative obstruction will usually resolve with conservative management. Table 4 describes the outcome of 17 patients with this complication in our early experience of 386 patients (25). Upper endoscopy has been reassuring, but not necessarily therapeutic in our limited experience. However, obstruction for more than seven to 10 days may predispose to ischemia or future erosion, and an early return to the operating room for revision may be more prudent.

Emphasis should be placed on the prevention of postoperative obstruction. Strategies include minimizing the handling of the stomach during placement, decreasing the mass inside the device by excising the fat pad on the greater curve and/or incising a path in the fat along the lesser curve as needed (Fig. 1). With the recent availability and judicious use of larger gastric bands (e.g., LapBand® VG, Inamed Health, Santa Barbara California, U.S.) and using the techniques described above, the frequency of postoperative obstruction can be significantly decreased.

RESULTS

The LAGB has been available internationally for over 10 years, and American surgeons have relied upon the excellent results of foreign surgeons to justify the use of the device in America. These studies report weight loss occurring slower

Table 4 Immediate Management of Patients with Postoperative Obstruction

---

17 patients
15 resolved
  1 LAGB removed patient choice 11 days after placement
  1 LAGB removed fear of perforation 4 days after placement

---

and measuring slightly less than that of gastric bypass, but with good resolution of co-morbidities and low mortality rates (19,26–28). The LapBand System® has been in use outside of clinical trials in America for three years, and the current array of surgeons has benefited from several improvements in placement techniques and patient management strategies. The switch from the perigastric to pars flaccida placement technique has markedly decreased the rate of gastric prolapse, especially the posterior variety. In addition, the adherence to a more regimented adjustment protocol has improved weight-loss results and decreased problems such as gastroesophageal reflux and dilation.

At the University of Louisville, we recently reviewed our experience with the placement of 386 LAGB during the time period January 1, 2001, through December 31, 2003 (29). The average preoperative weight in our series was 302 lb (136 kg) corresponding to a BMI of 49 kg/m^2. Three patients required open conversion to laparotomy. There was one death, a sudden cardiac event in a patient with sleep apnea after an uncomplicated operation and with a negative autopsy. There have been 12 device explantations (4%). Reasons for LAGB removal are listed in Table 5. Twenty-one patients have two-year and 186 have one-year follow-up. They have lost an average of 53% and 42% of their excess body weight, respectively. Of the patients with at least two-year follow-up, four of seven diabetics are euglycemic while off all medications. Table 2 shows other surgeons results with Lap-Band.

Effect on Comorbidities

Dramatic improvement or resolution of serious medical comorbidities accompanies weight loss following LAGB. There are major improvements in Type II diabetes mellitus (1,30–32), dyslipidemia (33), obstructive sleep apnea (1,30,34), asthma (35), hypertension (1,33,36) and gastroesophageal reflux (37–39).

It is now well-recognized that Type II diabetes mellitus is the greatest health risk caused by obesity. Weight loss following LAGB surgery has a major impact on Type II diabetes mellitus, with resolution or remission of diabetes in 66% of patients and improved serum glucose in the remainder (30,31). Dolan et al. (32) found that in 88 LAGB patients with diabetes, there was a 51.1% EWL at two years and a BMI reduction of 11.7 kg/m^2. At a median of six months, 26 of 38 (68%) patients on oral hypoglycemic agents and six of 11 (55%) on insulin were off all medications. The only predictive factor for elimination of diabetes was 30% EWL. In

Table 5 Reasons for LAGB Removal

Subhepatic abscess 3 months after placement
Subhepatic abscess 3 weeks after placement
Subphrenic abscess 2 months after placement (open conversion)
Sepsis/obstruction 4 days after placement
Obstruction 11 days after placement
Dilation 7 months after placement
Gastric prolapse (patient request)
Erosion 18 months after placement
Erosion 9 months after placement
Excessive weight loss 17 months after placement
Excessive weight loss 24 months after placement
Development of AIDS (patient choice)

---

fact, weight loss after LAGB results in increased insulin sensitivity and increased pancreatic beta-cell function, particularly in those patients who were diabetic for less than seven years (31). Weight loss is the mechanism for diabetes resolution after LAGB, which may be different than after RYGB. Postulated hypotheses of gastrointestinal hormone changes after RYGB, in addition to weight loss, are still being investigated (40). For this reason, it will be interesting to see if conversion of a patient who fails control of their diabetes with a LAGB will get effective control after conversion to a gastric bypass. However, regardless of the operation, weight regain correlates with the return of Type II diabetes mellitus.

CONCLUSIONS

The LAGB is an effective weight loss operation. It is a less complicated operation than the more popular gastric bypass, with results that are nearly as good. The NIH guidelines for patient selection should be followed when evaluating a patient for LAGB. Surgeons who choose to place the gastric band need to be familiar with adjustment techniques as well as the unique complications associated with the LAGB, namely gastric prolapse, band erosion, and postoperative obstruction.

REFERENCES

1. Rubenstein RB. Laparoscopic adjustable gastric banding at a US center with up to 3-year follow-up. Obes Surg 2002; 12:380–384.
2. Dixon JB, O'Brien PE. Selecting the optimal patient for Lap-Band placement. Am J Surg 2002; 184(6B):17S–20S.
3. http://www.niddk.nih.gov/health/nutrit/pubs/gastric/gastricsurgery.htm
4. Hudson SM, Dixon JB, O'Brien PE. Sweet eating is not a predictor of outcome after Lap-Band placement. Can we finally bury the myth? Obese Surg 2003; 13:468–469.
5. Regan JP, Inabnet WB, Gagner M, Pomp A. Early experience with two-stage laparoscopic Roux-en-Y gastric bypass as an alternative in the super-super obese patient. Obes Surg 2003; 13(6):861–864.
6. Fielding GA. Laparoscopic adjustable gastric banding for massive superobesity (>60 body mass index kg/m^2). Surg Endosc 2003; 17:1541–1545.
7. Rubin M, Spivak H. Prospective study of 250 patients undergoing laparoscopic gastric banding using the two-step technique: a technique to prevent postoperative slippage. Surg Endosc 2003; 17:857–860.
8. Fielding GA. Reduction in incidence of gastric herniation with Lap-Band: experience in 620 cases (abstr). Obes Surg 2000; 10:136.
9. Dargent J. Pouch dilation and slippage after adjustable gastric banding: is it still and issue? Obes Surg 2003; 13:111–115
10. Shen R, Dugay G, Rajaram K, Cabrera I, Siegel N, Ren CJ. Impact of patient follow-up on weight loss after bariatric surgery. Obes Surg 2004; 14:514–519.
11. Favretti F, O'Brien PE, Dixon JB. Patient management after Lap-Band placement. Am J Surg 2002; 184:38S–41S.
12. Busetto L, Segato G, De Marchi F, Foletto M, De Luca M, Favretti F, Enzi G. Postoperative management of laparoscopic gastric banding. Obes Surg 2003; 13:121–127.
13. Chapman AE, Kiroff G, Game P, Foster B, O'Brien P, Ham J, Maddern GJ. Laparoscopic adjustable gastric banding in the treatment of obesity: a systematic literature review. Surgery 2004; 135:326–351.

14. Dargent J. Laparoscopic adjustable gastric banding: lessons from the first 500 patients in a single institution. Obes Surg 1999; 9:446–452.

15. Fielding GA, Rhodes M, Nathanson LK. Laparoscopic gastric banding for morbid obesity. Surg Endosc 1999; 13:550–554.

16. O'Brien PE, Dixon JB, Brown W, et al. The laparoscopic adjustable gastric band (Lap-Band): a prospective study of medium-term effects on weight, health and quality of life. Obes Surg 2002; 12:652–660.

17. Favretti F, Cadiere GB, Segato G, et al. Laparoscopic banding: selection and technique in 830 patients. Obes Surg 2002; 12:385–390.

18. Ren CJ, Horgan S, Ponce J. U.S. experience with the Lap-Band system. Am J Surg 2002; 184:46S–51S.

19. Belachew M, Belva PH, Desaive C. Long-term results of laparoscopic adjustable gastric banding for the treatment of morbid obesity. Obes Surg 2002; 12:564–568.

20. Angrisani L, Furbetta F, Doldi SB, et al. Lap-Band adjustable gastric banding system: the Italian experience with 1863 patients operated on 6 years. Surg Endosc 2003; 17: 409–413.

21. Weiner R, Blanco-Engert R, Weiner S, Matkowitz R, Schaefer L, Pomhoff I. Outcome after laparoscopic adjustable gastric banding—8 years experience. Obes Surg 2003; 13:427–434.

22. Ren CJ, Weiner M, Allen JW. Favorable early results of gastric banding for morbid obesity: the American experience. Surg Endosc 2004; 18:543–546.

23. Sarker S, Herold K, Creech S, Shayani V. Early and late complications following laparoscopic adjustable gastric banding. Am Surg 2004; 70:146–149.

24. Vertruyen M. Experience with Lap-Band system up to 7 years. Obes Surg 2002; 12: 569–572.

25. Shen R, Ren CJ. Removal of peri-gastric fat prevents acute obstruction after Lap-Band® surgery. Obes Surg 2004; 14:224–229.

26. Dixon JB, O'Brien P. Changes in comorbidities and improvements in quality of life after Lap-Band placement. Am J Surg 2002; 184(6B):51S–54S.

27. Allen JW, Coleman MG, Fielding GA. Lessons learned from laparoscopic gastric banding for morbid obesity. Am J Surg 2001; 182:10–14.

28. Dargent J. Adjustable gastric banding: lessons from the first 500 patients in a single institution. Obes Surg 1999; 9:446–452.

29. Allen JW. Three-year follow-up of patients undergoing laparoscopic adjustable gastric banding. Annual Meeting of the Society of Laparoscopic Surgeons, Sept 30, 2004.

30. Abu-Abeid S, Keidar A, Szold A. Resolution of chronic medical conditions after laparoscopic adjustable silicone gastric banding for the treatment of morbid obesity in the elderly. Surg Endosc 2001; 15:132–134.

31. Dixon J, O'Brien P. Improvement in insulin sensitivity and cell function (HOMA) with weight loss in the severely obese. Diab Med 2003; 20:127–134.

32. Dolan K, Bryant R, Fielding G. Treating diabetes in the morbidly obese by laparoscopic gastric banding. Obes Surg 2003; 13:439–443.

33. Bacci V, Basso MS, Greco F, et al. Modifications of metabolic and cardiovascular risk factor after weight loss induced by laparoscopic gastric banding. Obes Surg 2002; 12:77–82.

34. Dixon JB, Schachter LM, O'Brien PE. Sleep disturbance and obesity; changes following surgically induced weight loss. Arch Intern Med 2001; 161:102–106.

35. Dixon JB, Chapman L, O'Brien P. Marked improvement in asthma after Lap-Band surgery for morbid obesity. Obes Surg 1999; 9:385–389.

36. Dixon JB, O'Brien PE. Changes in co-morbidities and improvements in quality of life after Lap-Band placement. Am J Surg 2002; 184:51S–54S.

37. Dixon JB, O'Brien PE. Gastroesophageal reflux in obesity: the effect of Lap-Band placement. Obes Surg 1999; 9:527–531.

38. Iovino P, Angrisani L, Tremolaterra F, et al. Abnormal esophageal acid exposure is common in morbidly obese patients and improves after a successful Lap-band system implantation. Surg Endosc 2002; 16:1631–1635.

39. Dolan K, Finch R, Fielding G. Laparoscopic gastric banding and crural repair in the obese patient with a hiatal hernia. Obes Surg 2003; 13:772–775.

40. Clements RH, Gonzalez QH, Long CI, Wittert G, Laws HL. Hormonal changes after Roux-enY gastric bypass for morbid obesity and the control of Type-II diabetes mellitus. Am Surg 2004; 70:1–4.

14

Outcomes of Laparoscopic Adjustable Gastric Banding

Paul E. O'Brien
*The Centre for Obesity Research and Education (CORE), Monash University,
Melbourne, Victoria, Australia*

INTRODUCTION

The Benefits of Weight Loss

Obesity is a major and increasing health problem across all areas of the world with a prevalence of more than 50% among the adult population in all Western communities and 64% of those in the United States (1). The increasing prevalence is associated with a parallel increase of obesity-related diseases, in particular, type 2 diabetes and the diseases of the metabolic syndrome. The final solution to this epidemic for the community can only be by prevention, but the increasing prevalence indicates that the preventive strategies have not begun to take effect.

Bariatric Surgery Provides the Only Effective Option

For the individual with the problem, the options are limited. Medical therapies of improved eating practices, increased exercise and activity, supplemented by behavioral modification programs and pharmocotherapy, generally achieve only a modest and transient effect. Numerous observational studies of bariatric surgical therapies have shown them to be effective in achieving good weight loss and major improvements in health and quality of life. However, the use of surgical treatment for severe obesity is infrequent. On the basis that there are 23 million people in the United States with severe obesity (BMI > 35) and that approximately 100,000 bariatric procedures were performed in 2003, it can be estimated that, each year, less than one in 200 of the severely obese are treated by a bariatric surgical procedure.

What Is the Best Surgical Option?

In this review we present an argument for the relative effectiveness and safety of the two dominant surgical options used globally today. We hope the data presented will assist the surgeon and the patient in selecting a preference. However, it must be stressed that both options are safe and effective when applied correctly, and are many times more powerful than any alternative options from the range of medical therapies and endoscopic procedures. The message regarding the benefits of bariatric surgery overall can be lost if there is too much debate between surgeons and too much concentration on the differences between different operations, leaving the critical differences between the "medical" options and bariatric surgery poorly communicated. Currently, with less than one in 200 who suffer the problem of severe obesity seeking bariatric surgical treatment, the surgical option is irrelevant as a solution at a community level. A greater focus on stressing the overall benefits of bariatric surgery and identifying and incorporating what the community regards as the characteristics of the ideal bariatric procedure is important in changing this relevance.

Characteristics of the Ideal Surgical Procedure

Table 1 lists the characteristics which should be present if surgical treatment is likely to become broadly acceptable.

- Bariatric procedures need to be performed laparoscopically. The patient will require it, not wanting the pain and the scars and the long recuperation. The surgeon will not be able to justify the higher perioperative complication rates.
- They need to be safe, very safe. There cannot be mortality. Even the 0.5% to 1.0% that is the norm for Roux-en-Y gastric bypass (RYGB) should be regarded as unacceptable.
- They must be effective, not only in achieving weight loss but also in improving the comorbidities of obesity and quality of life (QOL).
- The effects must be durable. They need to be shown to last for years—5, 10, 15 years—if they are to be considered worthwhile.
- There should not be even a low need for revisional surgery. There is no broadly accepted incidence that could be acceptable, but possibly a revisional surgery rate of less than 5% during the first 10 years would be a reasonable target.
- There must be minimal side effects. Particularly worrying are the late nutritional side effects of RYGB and BPD. Why exchange one problem for another?
- With up to 20% of the adult population needing help, an operative procedure has to be able to be done by the broad general surgical group. It must be relatively straightforward, or death or complications will ensue.

Table 1 Attributes of an Ideal Bariatric Operation

Minimally invasive
Safe
Effective—weight loss, comorbidities, QOL
Durable—effective over time
Low reoperation rate
Minimal side effects
Technically feasible broadly
Reversible
Controllable / adjustable

- Whatever we do today is unlikely to be the best treatment in 20 years time; so the procedure should be easily and totally reversible so that future options are not excluded.
- It needs to be controllable. If the day of the operation is the last chance we have for setting the parameters, it is likely that, with time, the settings of the procedure will be sub-optimal. This does not allow for a durable outcome. The recidivism of the RYGB is a powerful demonstration of this issue.

LAPAROSCOPIC ADJUSTABLE GASTRIC BANDING

Introduction

Laparoscopic adjustable gastric banding (LAGB) was introduced in the early 1990s as an approach with the potential for a safe, controllable, and reversible method for achieving significant weight loss. The first procedure was performed by Cadiere in 1992 (2) using the device developed for open placement by Kuzmak in the 1980s (3). The first device designed for laparoscopic placement was the BioEnterics® Lap-Band® system (LAGB®) which was introduced into surgical practice in 1993 (4). Since then more than 130,000 Lap-Bands have been placed and there are more than 100 full papers on its use. Additional devices have subsequently become available, but only for the Swedish adjustable gastric band (SAGB®) are there any published data available on the outcomes.

Key Attributes of LAGB

Adjustability. This is the most important single factor in achieving good weight loss without hurting people. Figure 1 shows the 10 cm Lap-Band and the recently released Vanguard (Lap-Band VG), of approximately 11 cm circumference, without fluid and with saline added. The decrease in the area leads to an increase in the sense of satiety and a more rapid sense of fullness after eating.

The volume of fluid added is titrated against the weight loss and against the sense of satiety, and the sense of restriction achieved. A gentle progression of weight loss over time is the result. With the gastric stapling procedures, such as gastric bypass and gastroplasty, there is no control of the settings of tightness from the day of operation. Weight loss occurs rapidly, possibly at the expense of QOL. After 12 to 24 months, no further weight loss occurs and a progressive increase in weight is usual (5). With the option of adjustability, the LAGB is able to induce a less severe rate of weight loss over a period of two to three years followed by maintenance of that weight loss which has now been measured out to six years and more (Fig. 3).

Laparoscopic placement. The LAGB can be placed laparoscopically in almost all patients who have not had previous gastric surgery, regardless of the size of the patient (6). The procedure can be readily done in less than one hour with less than one-day length of stay, and is associated with only modest discomfort and enables a rapid return to normal activities. The procedure has proved to be remarkably safe, no doubt partly due to the minimally invasive approach.

Reversibility. It should be hoped and expected that whatever treatments for obesity are available today, they will be replaced by better treatment in the next 20 years. It is an asset of the LAGB that it can be removed easily and the stomach allowed to return to normal configuration. An 18-year-old patient will be less than

Lap Band 10 cm – No added fluid   Lap Band VG – No added fluid

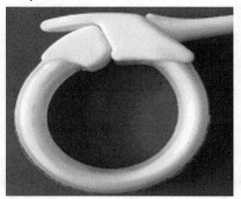 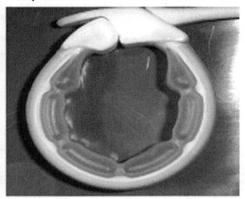

Lap Band 10 cm – 2 ml saline added   Lap Band VG – 5ml saline added

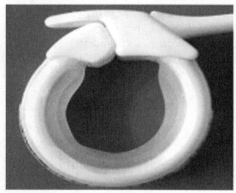 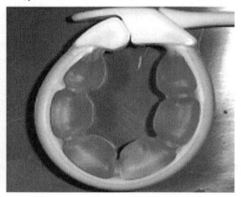

Figure 1 The two commonly used forms of LAGB with no added fluid and with saline added. Note the decrease in area within the band.

40 in 20 years time and thus retains the option of moving to improved treatments if and when appropriate.

Sources of Data

There are three major sources of outcome data for this review.

1. Data have been derived from the published reports by our group during the last three years. These reports have been based on a prospective collection of data on all patients we have treated since 1994 and includes data on perioperative complications, weight changes, and changes in health and QOL.
2. Outcome data have been taken from a formal systematic review of the outcomes after LAGB performed by the Australian Safety and Efficacy Review of New Interventional Procedures—Surgical (ASERNIP-S) (7). This group is funded by the Australian government to evaluate the safety and efficacy of new procedures, strictly using the methodology of evidence-based medicine.

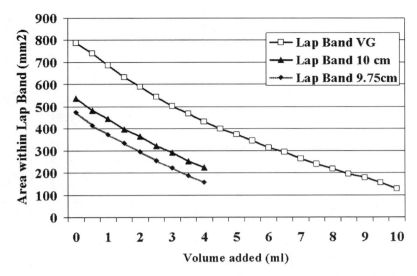

Figure 2 Graphs of the reducing area within the Lap-Band for added volumes of saline. Note that the 10-cm band without saline has an area equivalent to the Lap-Band VG with 2.5 mL added.

3. The systematic review included reports available up to September 2001. Those reports on LAGB or RYGB that have been published after closure of the ASERNIP-S search and which include at least 50 patients and at least three years of follow-up have been included.

Outcomes

Safety

Lap-Band placement has proved to be a safe procedure. The Systematic Review of all the published literature on safety and efficacy of LAGB (7) showed a mortality rate of 0.05%. When compared with the gastric stapling procedures, the mortality rate was 10 times greater for RYGB (0.5%) and six times greater for vertical banded gastroplasty (8). The morbidity rates were also reported by ASERNIP-S to be lower with an incidence of 10.7% of patients having early or late complications after LAGB compared with 27.4% after RYGB and 23.6% after VBG.

In our group of five surgeons and more than 2000 patients having Lap-Band placement, there have been no deaths. Early complication rate for the patients having laparoscopic placement was 1.8% (9). The commonest problem has been infection at the site of the subcutaneous access port, a problem which necessitates removal of the port and subsequent replacement.

The incidence of complications is inversely related to the experience with the procedure. Figure 3, adapted from the data in the ASERNIP-S review, shows the relationship between the number of patients in the series and the incidence of complications. It serves to emphasize the "learning curve" associated with this procedure.

Efficacy

The efficacy of any bariatric procedure must be measured in terms of the problem for which the procedure was done, and thus must include not only weight loss but also

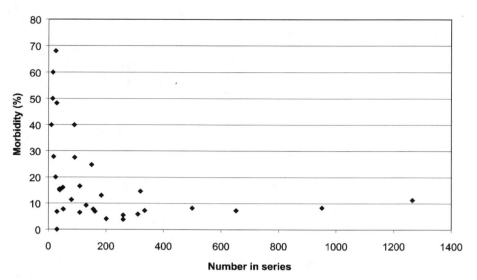

Figure 3 The "learning curve" for LAGB. There is a significant negative relationship ($r = -0.62$, $p < 0.001$) between series size and morbidity in series reporting the outcomes of LAGB surgery. Few studies containing less than 50 patients have been able to achieve acceptable outcomes. The morbidity figure contains both early and late complications. Derived from ASERNIP-S systematic review of LAGB (8).

measures of the effects on comorbidities and QOL. As the intention of bariatric surgery is to achieve a lifelong benefit, efficacy measures should be taken at a minimum of four to five years after the operation. In this section we provide a summary of published results and our own outcomes of weight loss, change in a selection of major comorbidities, and changes in QOL.

   Weight loss. Figure 4 contains a summary of all reports of weight loss expressed as percentage of excess weight lost (%EWL) available to us on

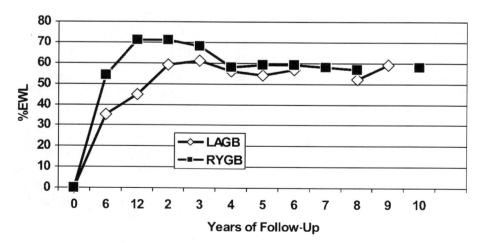

Figure 4 A comparison of the %EWL after LAGB and RYGB. Data include all published series with an initial recruitment of at least 50 patients reporting data at three years or more following surgery. There were eight RYGB studies and seven LAGB studies.

1 February 2004. The median %EWL at three, four and five years is 61%, 56%, and 54%, respectively. For comparison, the median %EWL for RYGB at these time intervals, as reported from the systematic review, was 69%, 58%, and 59%. The differences between the effects of the two operations on weight loss at five years is not significant. Sadly, after more than 20 years experience with RYGB, we have only patches of follow-up data beyond five years.

There is an important difference in the pattern of weight loss. Maximal weight lost after RYGB generally occurs at 12 to 18 months after the operation, followed by a steady decline in the effects. In contrast, as shown in Figure 4, the Lap-Band generates a slower, but continuing, weight loss during the first two to three years, followed by stability of weight over the first six years (9). This more gentle initial weight loss followed by a more durable maintenance is attributable to the adjustability of the band and represents one its most valuable features.

Changes in the comorbidities of obesity. Obesity generates a wide range of illnesses, to the point where it could now reasonably be regarded as the worst pathogen in the Western communities. The following are a summary of the changes in a selection of these comorbidities to illustrate the major health benefits that can be achieved by Lap-Band placement. These effects have been achieved through weight loss per se, or the mechanical effect of the band by its position, or the immediate reduction of food intake after placement. Some effects are therefore seen quite early after the procedure whereas others are most apparent after maximal weight loss at two to three years.

Type 2 diabetes mellitus is the paradigm of an obesity-related illness. Fifty patients were followed for one year after Lap-Band placement (10). There was a significant improvement in all measures of glucose metabolism with complete remission of diabetes in 32 patients (64%), improvement of control in 13 (26%), and five (10%) were relatively unchanged. Importantly, duration of time with diabetes was a predictor of outcome, indicating that early treatment of obesity is indicated in the newly diagnosed diabetic.

Insulin resistance is the central feature of the metabolic syndrome in association with hypertension, dyslipidemia, and visceral obesity. The condition is strongly associated with non-alcoholic steatohepatitis, polycystic ovary syndrome and increased risk of cardiovascular events. The serum insulin and fasting blood glucose showed a marked fall in association with weight loss after Lap-Band placement and the levels remained down over a four-year period. No patient with insulin resistance before operation has become diabetic subsequently. Insulin sensitivity, as measured by HOMA%S, improved from 37.5% to 62% in 254 patients during the first year after Lap-Band placement. Pancreatic beta cell function, as measured by HOMA%B, also significantly improved (11). Thus the basic mechanisms for the appearance and progression of type 2 diabetes are halted.

Gastroesophageal reflux disease (GERD) is more than twice as prevalent in the morbidly obese (12). Eighty-seven patients who had moderate or severe GERD have been followed for at least 12 months after Lap-Band placement. seventy-three (89%) have had total resolution of the problem, as defined by the absence of symptoms without treatment for the previous month. Preoperative and postoperative pH study and manometry have been performed on 12 of these patients who had severe symptoms preoperatively. The mean DeMeester score was 38 ± 15 preoperatively and 7.9 ± 8 at follow-up ($p < 0.001$). In all but one of these patients symptoms had resolved completely. Others also have demonstrated that a correctly placed band reduces gastroesophageal reflux (13,14). Furthermore, in my own series of

1500 patients, followed closely for up to eight years by clinical assessment, numerous barium studies, endoscopies, a number of 24-hour pH studies, and esophageal manometry measurements, there has been no significant evidence of an evolving pattern of esophageal dysfunction.

Obstructive sleep apnea and other sleep disturbances have been studied in 313 patients prior to Lap-Band placment and repeated at one year after operation in 123 of the patients (15). There was a high prevalence of significantly disturbed sleep in both men (59%) and women (45%). Observed sleep apnea was decreased from 33% to 2%, habitual snoring from 82% to 14%, abnormal daytime sleepiness from 39% to 4%, and poor sleep quality from 39% to 2%.

Depression is common in the morbidly obese. Does the presence of obesity cause the person to be depressed or does depression cause the person to eat too much? We have investigated the effect of weight loss induced by Lap-Band placment on depression as measured by the Beck Depression Inventory (BDI) (16). Preoperative BDI on 487 consecutive patients was a mean of 17.7 ± 9.5, a level within the range for moderate depression. Weight loss was associated with a significant and sustained fall in BDI scores with a mean score of 7.8 ± 6.5 ($N = 373$) at one year after surgery. By four years after surgery, the 134 patients studied had lost 54% of excess weight and had a BDI of 9.6 ± 7.7. Although a small number remained in the major depressive illness category, the shift of the majority to normal values for BDI strongly indicates that most of the depression of obesity is reactive to the problem of obesity rather than a cause of obesity and is resolved by weight loss.

Changes in QOL. The physical and psychosocial limitations of obesity add considerably to the morbidity of the disease, and improvement in QOL is one of the most gratifying outcomes of bariatric surgery. A number of studies clearly demonstrate major QOL improvements following Lap-Band placement (17,18). We reported a large prospective study of QOL after the Lap-Band placement, based on the Medical Outcomes Trust Short Form-36 (SF-36). The SF-36 is a reliable, broadly used instrument that has been validated in obese people. In our study, 459 severely obese subjects had lower scores compared with community normal values for all the eight aspects of QOL measured, especially the physical health scores. Lap-Band placement provided a dramatic and sustained improvement in all measures of the SF-36. Improvement was greater in those with more preoperative disability, and the extent of weight loss was not a good predictor of improved QOL. Mean scores returned to those of community normal values by one year after surgery, and remained in the normal range throughout the four years of the study. It is significant that patients who required revisional surgery during the follow-up period achieved the same improvement in measures of QOL. Similar improvements in QOL have been demonstrated in patients having Lap-Band placement for previously failed gastric stapling (19).

DISCUSSION

Lap-Band placement is proving to be a safe, effective, and gentle procedure which enables major and durable weight loss in association with improvement or resolution of a broad range of serious health problems. Its characteristics of adjustability and reversibility are unique and important. We have studied the predictors of effectiveness (20–22) and have not identified any subgroups that do not achieve a worthwhile effect from the procedure. It appears, in our data, to be equally effective in the superobese and the obese, in the sweet-eaters and the non–sweet-eaters, and in those with psychiatric disease or failed gastric stapling (19,20,22). As we believe it requires an active partnership between the patient and the surgeon, we have not used the procedure in the mentally defective and those with malignant hyperphagia such as Prader-Willi syndrome. Treatment of this group of patients is controversial but may be helped by a malabsorptive procedure (23,24).

CONCLUSIONS

Lap-Band placement is proving to be safe and effective. In view of the attributes of adjustability, safe laparoscopic placement and reversibility, it should be considered the optimal initial approach for the control of obesity and its comorbities.

REFERENCES

1. Flegal KM, Carroll MD, Ogden CL, Johnson CL. Prevalence and trends in obesity among US adults, 1999–2000. JAMA 2002; 288:1723–1727.
2. Cadiere GB, Bruyns J, Himpens J, Favretti F. Laparoscopic gastroplasty for morbid obesity. Br J Surg 1994; 81:1524.
3. Kuzmak LI. A review of seven years' experience with silicone gastric banding. Obes Surg 1991; 1:403–408.
4. Belachew M, Legrand MJ, Defechereux TH, Burtheret MP, Jacquet N. Laparoscopic adjustable silicone gastric banding in the treatment of morbid obesity. A preliminary report. Surg Endosc 1994; 8:1354–1356.
5. Hall JC, Watts JM, O'Brien PE, Dunstan RE, Walsh JF, Slavotinek AH, Elmslie RG. Gastric surgery for morbid obesity. The Adelaide Study. Ann Surg 1990; 211:419–427.
6. Fielding GA. Laparoscopic adjustable gastric banding for massive superobesity (>60 body mass index kg/m^2). Surg Endosc 2003; 17:1541–1545.
7. Chapman AE, Kiroff G, Game P, Foster B, O'Brien P, Ham J, Maddern GJ. Laparoscopic adjustable gastric banding in the treatment of obesity: a systematic literature review. Surgery 2004; 135:326–351.
8. Chapman A, Kiroff G, Game P, Foster B, O'Brien P, Ham J, Maddern G. Systematic review of laparoscopic adjustable gastric banding in the treatment of obesity. ASERNIP-S Report No. 31, Adelaide, South Australia, 2002.
9. O'Brien PE, Dixon JB, Brown W, Schachter LM, Chapman L, Burn AJ, Dixon ME, Scheinkestel C, Halket C, Sutherland LJ, Korin A, Baquie P. The laparoscopic adjustable gastric band (Lap-Band): a prospective study of medium-term effects on weight, health and quality of life. Obes Surg 2002; 12:652–660.
10. Dixon JB, O'Brien P. Health outcomes of severely obese type 2 diabetic subjects 1 year after laparoscopic adjustable gastric banding. Diabetes Care 2002; 25:358–363.
11. Dixon JB, Dixon AF, O'Brien PE. Improvements in insulin sensitivity and beta-cell function (HOMA) with weight loss in the severely obese. Diabetes Med 2003; 20:127–134.
12. Dixon JB, O'Brien PE. Gastroesophageal reflux in obesity: the effect of lap-band placement. Obes Surg 1999; 9:527–531.
13. Angrisani L, Iovino P, Lorenzo M, Santoro T, Sabbatini F, Claar E, Nicodemi O, Persico G, Tesauro B. Treatment of morbid obesity and gastroesophageal reflux with hiatal hernia by Lap-Band. Obes Surg 1999; 9:396–398.
14. Weiss HG, Nehoda H, Labeck B, Peer-Kuhberger MD, Klingler P, Gadenstatter M, Aigner F, Wetscher GJ. Treatment of morbid obesity with laparoscopic adjustable gastric banding affects esophageal motility. Am J Surg 2000; 180:479–482.

15. Dixon JB, Schachter LM, O'Brien PE. Sleep disturbance and obesity: changes following surgically induced weight loss. Arch Intern Med 2001; 161:102–106.
16. Dixon JB, Dixon ME, O'Brien PE. Depression in association with severe obesity: changes with weight loss. Arch Intern Med 2003; 163:2058–2065.
17. Horchner R, Tuinebreijer MW, Kelder PH. Quality-of-life assessment of morbidly obese patients who have undergone a Lap-Band operation: 2-year follow-up study. Is the MOS SF-36 a useful instrument to measure quality of life in morbidly obese patients? Obes Surg 2001; 11:212–218, discussion 219.
18. Weiner R, Datz M, Wagner D, Bockhorn H. Quality-of-life outcome after laparoscopic adjustable gastric banding for morbid obesity. Obes Surg 1999; 9:539–545.
19. O'Brien P, Brown W, Dixon J. Revisional surgery for morbid obesity—conversion to the lap-band system. Obes Surg 2000; 10:557–563.
20. Dixon JB, Dixon ME, O'Brien PE. Preoperative predictors of weight loss at 1-year after Lap-Band surgery. Obes Surg 2001; 11:200–207.
21. O'Brien P, Brown W, Dixon J. Revisional surgery for morbid obesity—conversion to the Lap-Band system. Obes Surg 2000; 10:557–563.
22. Hudson SM, Dixon JB, O'Brien PE. Sweet eating is not a predictor of outcome after Lap-Band placement. Can we finally bury the myth?. Obes Surg 2002; 12:789–794.
23. Soper RT, Mason EE, Printen KJ, Zellweger H. Gastric bypass for morbid obesity in children and adolescents. J Pediatr Surg 1975; 10:51–58.
24. Grugni G, Guzzaloni G, Morabito F. Failure of biliopancreatic diversion in Prader-Willi syndrome. Obes Surg 2000; 10:179–181, discussion 182.

15

Part II of Debate: Laparoscopic Roux-en-Y Gastric Bypass

Eric J. DeMaria

Department of Surgery, Duke University, Durham, North Carolina, U.S.A.

INTRODUCTION

The history of abdominal surgery for the treatment of obesity is replete with novel procedures introduced by clinicians who substitute enthusiasm for data in their quest for the "holy grail" of a cure for obesity. The result is an unfortunate history of human experimentation upon a population of patients so desperate for life-saving weight loss, that they put their blind trust in surgeons offering a cure in the absence of convincing long-term outcome data to prove benefit that is worth the risk. The sacrifices of a previous generation of desperate patients combined with the scientific diligence of a small cadre of surgeons committed to bringing scientific sanity to the new speciality of bariatric surgery have made it no longer necessary for patients to choose unproven surgical procedures. The ideal characteristics of a bariatric surgical procedure are suggested in Table 1.

ROUX-EN-Y GASTRIC BYPASS

Historical Perspective Comparisons with Restriction

Introduced by Mason in the 1960s, the Roux-en-Y gastric bypass (RYGB) is the "gold standard" of weight-loss surgery to which all other procedures must be compared. At the National Institutes of Health Consensus Conference in 1991 (1), a panel of experts performed a careful review of the available literature on the subject of weight-loss surgery and determined that the RYGB and the vertical banded gastroplasty (VBG) were the two weight-loss operations demonstrating favorable outcomes with low morbidity which justified a consensus that they were effective for the treatment of morbidly obese patients. The RYGB clearly resulted in a greater magnitude of weight-loss than the VBG. The consensus panel stated, "The success rate for weight-loss is higher with the Roux-en-Y gastric bypass. This higher success must be balanced with the higher complication rate of the RYGB." This statement has proven to be true to the present time when comparing restrictive procedures like the laparoscopic adjustable gastric banding (LAGB) to RYGB. Over time, the NIH

Table 1 Proposed Characteristics of the Ideal Bariatric Procedure

---

•Laparoscopic access for bariatric procedures offers significant benefit to obese patients, particularly a decrease in wound-related morbidity and quicker postoperative recovery time with decreased incisional pain. Laparoscopic procedures are ideally developed based upon concepts from traditional "open" surgery which have been proven to be effective in the long-term
•The greatest value of a bariatric procedure is in reducing or eliminating the serious co-morbid complications of obesity. Although some degree of risk is inherent in any invasive procedure in severely obese patients, risk–benefit analysis must demonstrate a uniformly high degree of benefit to justify risk
•The procedure must be permanent as experience has taught that procedure reversal invariably leads to recurrent obesity in the long-term. If patients have "control" of the outcome of the surgery they may sabotage the ultimate result over time. The effects must be durable. They need to be shown to last for years—at least 10 years and preferably lifelong—if they are to be considered worthwhile
•There should be a low need for revisional surgery
•Side effects, particularly nutritional, are an inevitable risk with dramatic and rapid reductions in body weight. Their prevention and reversal must be straightforward and successful
•Failed weight loss must be a minimal risk. If morbidly obese patients are to accept any degree of surgical risk, they must have the promise of dramatic and lasting weight loss that allows a confidence that co-morbid conditions will resolve. Wide adoption of relatively ineffective procedures will compromise this confidence as well as acceptance

---

consensus led most American surgeons performing weight-loss surgery to predominately perform the RYGB or gastric restriction procedures (VBG, gastric banding) in their patients. The controversy over whether the higher risk of RYGB is worth the greater potential for weight loss and its resultant health benefits continues today.

A review of the medical literature on the subject of weight-loss surgery reveals multiple prospective randomized controlled studies comparing RYGB to other procedures, particularly the restrictive procedure, VBG (2–7). Two prospective randomized studies in the early 1980s established the superiority of RYGB by comparing it to gastric partitioning (3,4). In both of these studies, patients undergoing gastric bypass achieved superior weight loss without significant late consequences when compared to those undergoing partitioning alone.

In 1989, after a randomized study found a greater weight-loss efficacy with the RYGB than with VBG, a prospective study compared the VBG with RYGB and looked at a selective assignment of the technique based on a patient's dietary habits (5) to provide some insight into why RYGB might provide superior weight loss to restrictive procedures. This study demonstrated that patients who crave high caloric density sweets experienced significantly less weight loss after VBG than patients without sweets-eating behavior on dietary screening. Postoperative dumping symptoms in response to oral sugar intake, which is common after RYGB and does not usually occur after gastric restriction, is the likely mechanism of the superior weight loss (EWL) found after RYGB in sweets-addicted patients. Superior long-term excess weight loss was found after RYGB when compared to VBG ($71\pm21\%$ vs. $55\pm19\%$, respectively), but with a higher risk of complications following RYGB, including a slightly higher rate of postoperative morbidity and more micronutrient and metabolic derangements (notably anemia, iron deficiency, and low vitamin B_{12} levels). Most of these were easily correctable with vitamin supplementation.

Over the years, many authors have supported the concept that a surgical procedure should provide at least a 50% reduction in calculated excess weight to be considered effective, particularly in terms of providing significant resolution of obesity co-morbidities. Two studies have examined this outcome parameter in RYGB as compared to VBG (6,7). In the Adelaide study (6), only 48% of patients undergoing VBG lost more than 50% of their excess weight, whereas 67% of those undergoing RYGB lost more than 50%. No difference in perioperative morbidity was seen between the groups. In a study from Canada (7), similar results were reported where 58% of RYGB achieved a loss of more than 50% of their excess weight compared to only 39% of those undergoing VBG.

It is fair to say that every prospective randomized trial comparing the gastric restrictive procedure VBG to the RYGB procedure has demonstrated superior weight loss after RYGB. As the RYGB has demonstrated superior weight loss results compared to the VBG, many surgeons have abandoned the VBG. However, it is important to note that proponents of VBG have claimed weight loss results comparable to RYGB in the surgical literature. Buchwald (8) cited a compilation of studies in which the average reduction of excess weight was nearly the same as gastric bypass in one-year follow-up. Clearly proponents of the VBG, including its originator Dr. Mason (University of Iowa), became convinced that it was a superior procedure in terms of complications and provided equivalent weight loss to RYGB. However, over time most American surgeons have turned to performing the RYGB procedure for most patients because of its higher degree of reliability for weight loss. This trend includes the recent obesity surgery practice at the VBG originator's institution, the University of Iowa (James W. Maher, personal communication, 2004). Furthermore, long-term data on the effectiveness of VBG have raised concerns that it is not a durable weight loss procedure. One study from the Mayo clinic (9) demonstrated that only 25% of patients maintained a durable weight loss of greater than 50% of excess at 10-year follow-up.

A compilation of series presented by Buchwald (8) demonstrated a remarkably reproducible reduction in excess weight in multiple published studies of RYGB (Table 2). A subsequent meta-analysis of 136 fully extracted studies in the medical literature (10) examined various bariatric procedures and revealed a difference in post-procedure mortality of 0.5% for RYGB versus 0.1% for banding. Although associated with lower mortality, banding provided less weight loss and lower resolution of co-morbid conditions. Reduction of excess weight was 47% after banding compared to 62% after gastric bypass.

Unlike the newer adjustable gastric banding operation, long-term outcome data are available for RYGB. Pories et al. (11) have reported follow-up to 14 years with maintenance of an average of 50% reduction (100 lbs) in excess weight after RYGB. Sugerman et al. (12), in a study of adolescents undergoing RYGB, demonstrated an overall average reduction in excess weight of 56% at 10 years and 33% at 14 years postoperatively. However, further scrutiny of the data clarified that a minority of patients regained significant amounts of weight which skewed the means. Removal of five of 18 patients from the 10-year analysis improved the EWL to 75% and removal of a single patient at 14 years improved the overall mean to 61% of excess weight. Thus the conclusion is more accurately presented as a minority of patients re-gain the lost weight in the long term, while the majority do quite well more than a decade after surgery. It is likely that long-term failure results from failed adherence to behavioral modification concepts including dietary indiscretions and a lack of physical activity.

Table 2 Outcomes of Gastric Bypass Surgery According to a Review of Compiled Studies by Buchwald

Author	n	1 yr%EWL
Wittgrove	500	77
Buchwald	92	57
Jones	312	78
Schauer	275	69
Higa	850	69
Kalfarentzos	38	64
Oh	194	69
Freeman	40	60
Pories	608	69
Howard	20	78
Sugerman	20	66
Total	2949 pts	69% EWL

Source: From Ref. 8.

Laparoscopic RYGB

Laparoscopic access for RYGB, pioneered by Wittgrove and Clark in the early 1990s (13), is a much newer concept than the "open" RYGB, but the scientific literature includes a growing number of large cohort series which documents the safety of this access technique and demonstrates that the weight loss realized is what one would expect based upon the history of the open approach (14–16). Three prospective randomized controlled studies have compared laparoscopic to open gastric bypass (17–19). Nguyen et al. randomized 155 patients to undergo either an open or a laparoscopic gastric bypass (17). The laparoscopic approach resulted in longer operative time, less blood loss, shorter hospital stay, earlier return to normal activity, higher incidence of anastomotic strictures, and greater overall cost. One-year weight loss was comparable between groups. In another study from Sweden, 51 patients were randomized to either laparoscopic or open RYGB ($n = 30$ laparoscopic, $n = 21$ open) (18). In this study, 23% of the patients were converted to an open operation. Also, 26% of the remaining patients in the laparoscopic group underwent further surgery due to bowel obstruction at the retro-colic window for the Roux limb. While not specifically addressed in this paper, this rate of conversion and the subsequent re-operation is higher than what has been reported in other cohort studies or the above detailed prospective study, suggesting some technical issues or early learning-curve impact on these outcomes. With this in mind, this study found significant differences with the laparoscopic group requiring lower amounts of post-operative narcotic analgesia and shorter hospital stay. Weight loss was comparable at one year postoperatively.

LAPAROSCOPIC ADJUSTABLE GASTRIC BANDING (LAGB)

LAGB shares a similar mechanism of action to the VBG and other forms of gastric partitioning surgery. Its mechanism of action is via gastric restriction with no malabsorptive component to the procedure. In this section, a review of the available literature on this procedure is provided.

International Studies

Angrisani et al. reported their experience with 1265 patients undergoing LAGB (20). These included 258 male and 1007 female patients with a mean body mass index (BMI) of 44.1 kg/m^2. Follow-up was obtained up to 48 months and the mean BMI decreased to 31.5 kg/m^2 at that point. The percentage of patients seen in follow-up was only in the range of 60%. No intra-operative or complication-related mortality was reported. Postoperative mortality was 0.55% ($n = 7$), higher than the usually cited procedure-related mortality of 0.1%. LAGB-related complications occurred in 11.3% ($n = 143$) with pouch dilatation diagnosed in 65 (5.2%), band erosion in 24 (1.9%), and port or connecting tube-port complications in 54 patients (4.2%). A number of these complications required re-operation or revision.

Weiner et al. reported the German experience with the LAGB in 984 consecutive patients over an eight-year period (21). In this series, the initial BMI was 46.8 kg/m^2. Median follow-up was 55 months and there were no conversions or mortalities. Mean EWL was 59% after eight years and the BMI decreased from 46.8 to 32.3 kg/m^2. Five of the first 100 patients ultimately underwent band removal with conversion to laparoscopic RYGB. Fourteen patients underwent a "banded" RYGBP conversion for failed weight loss. The best weight loss was achieved during the first two years after LAGB, in contrast to other claims that weight loss progresses over the long term with this procedure. Complications included gastric perforation and band slippage, and 17 patients required repeat surgical interventions during the following years.

In a series of 1250 patients, O'Brien et al. reported LAGB to be a very safe procedure with a low mortality rate (22). Although the early complication rate was very low, late complications of prolapse or erosions were frequent, particularly during their early experience. Weight loss was maximal during the first two to three years after surgery and averaged 56% of excess at five years. Major improvements in co-morbid conditions were reported in association with weight loss after LAGB, particularly for the resolution of type 2 diabetes. Gastroesophageal reflux disease, obstructive sleep apnea, and depression were other major co-morbid conditions that showed improvement.

Favretti et al. demonstrated similar results in a series of 830 patients (23). The initial mean BMI was 46 kg/m^2. The reported conversion rate was 2.7% without a mortality although major complications requiring re-operation developed in 3.9% ($n=36$). These included one gastric perforation (requiring band removal) and one gastric slippage (requiring repositioning). Late complications included 17 gastric slippages (treated by band repositioning in 12 and band removal in five), nine malpositionings (all treated by band repositioning), four gastric erosions (all treated by band removal), three psychological intolerance (requiring band removal), and one HIV sero-conversion (band removed). Reservoir leakage was described as a minor complication although it required re-operation in 91 patients (11%). Regarding weight loss, a high incidence of failure in the long term was noted. An error in the manuscript suggested 20% of patients failed to lose at least 30% of excess weight, but the actual calculation from the authors' table of three-year results revealed this failure incidence to be nearly 30% (Table 3). The authors suggest failure arose in most cases from patients losing "compliance with dietetic, psychological and surgical advice" which, of course, represents an opinion rather than something proven by their analysis. Changes in eating behavior towards liquid and semi-solid sweets intake in patients following restrictive operations do occur, as patients try to ingest substances that pass the band without causing obstruction and is the likely source of

Table 3 Table of Percent Excess Weight (%EWL) Modified from Figure 3 of Favretti et al. (23) Reporting Weight Loss in 479 Patients Undergoing LAGB with at Least Three-Year Follow-Up Data

Range of %EWL	Number of patients	Total population (%)
0–10	30	6.3
11–20	42	8.8
21–30	70	14.6 Failures =29.67
31–40	82	17.1
41–50	89	18.6
51–60	64	13.4
61–70	42	8.8
71–80	26	5.4
81–90	25	5.2
91–100	9	1.8
	Sum =479 patients	=100%

Although the manuscript claims 20% of patients failed the procedure with loss of 30% or less of excess weight, one can see that this represents an error as nearly 30% of patients failed the procedure by this definition (n=30+42+70=142 of 479 total patients = 29.6% of total population).

most non-compliance. It should be remembered that recidivism is a well-known characteristic of clinically severe obesity and, while surgeons often blame their patients for their failures, a more "ideal" bariatric procedure would perform independently of patient compliance to minimize poor long-term weight loss outcomes. The overall reduction in the BMI in this study was significant—from the initial 46.4 to 37.3 at one year, 36.4 at year two years, 36.8 at three years, and 36.4 kg/m^2 at five years. Clearly some patients did well in the five-year term while many did not.

In the series of 400 patients undergoing LAGB reported by Chevallier (24), mean BMI fell from 43.8 to 32.7 kg/m^2 with a mean EWL of 53% at two years follow-up. There were no mortalities reported. There were 12 conversions (3%) with complications requiring an abdominal re-operation in 10% of the patients. These included gastric perforation ($n = 2$), gastric necrosis ($n = 1$), slippage ($n = 31$), incisional hernia ($n = 2$), and a need to reconnect the tubing ($n = 4$).

Szold et al. reported preliminary results of their experience with the LAGB in 715 patients followed up prospectively for the management of peri-operative and long-term complications (25). The mean age of the patients was 34 years with a mean BMI of 43.1 kg/m^2. Their mean operative time was 78 minutes with a postoperative hospitalization time of 1.2 days. There were six intra-operative complications (0.8%), eight early postoperative complications (1.1%), and no deaths. Late complications included band slippage or pouch dilation in 53 patients (7.4%), band erosion in three patients, and port complications in 18 patients. In 57 patients (7.9%), 69 major re-operations were performed. Six patients (0.84%) underwent re-operation during the first three postoperative days: one for a bleeding trocar site, and five for band repositioning because of band malposition and outlet obstruction. All early repositioning procedures were performed through a laparotomy. Band dislodgment or pouch dilation occurred in 53 patients (7.4%). All these patients had radiographic studies to prove band dislodgment, and all underwent laparoscopic surgery for band repositioning or band removal. The reasons for band removal were patient request or patient refusal of regular follow-up evaluation in 20 patients, band erosion in three patients, and previous band repositioning in nine patients. In addition, 18 procedures were performed on the ports, most with the patient under local anesthesia. The data for 181 patients with a follow-up period longer than two years were studied to obtain long-term follow-up information. A total of 121 patients (67%) were available for a mean follow-up period of 30 months with a drop in BMI from 43.3 to 32.1 kg/m^2.

Only a few authors have reported data on resolution of major co-morbidities after LAGB placement. In a series of 295 patients with a mean BMI of 45 kg/m^2 undergoing the LAGB, reduction in co-morbidity was scaled relative to the preoperative co-morbidity level as having been cured, improved, unchanged, or worsened (25). The preoperative frequencies of co-morbidities in this study were typical of most obesity surgery series and included hypertension 52%, diabetes 20%, dyspnea 85%, peripheral edema 63%, sleep apnea 36%, arthralgia 89%, gastroesophageal reflux 57%, reduced self-esteem 95%, reduced general physical performance 96%, hyperlipidemia 39%, hyperuricemia 36%, and menstrual problems 22%. EWL was 40% after one year, 46% after two years, 47% after three years, and 54% after four years follow-up. After four years, the rate of cure of the co-morbidities were hypertension 58%, diabetes 75%, dyspnea 85%, arthralgia 52%, reflux 79%, self-esteem 45%, and general physical performance 58%. Improvement was also found in stress incontinence, sleep apnea, peripheral edema, and regulation of menstruation. Greater weight loss was associated with a greater reduction in dyspnea and arthralgia and improved self-esteem and physical performance, whereas the authors claimed hypertension, diabetes, reflux, and edema improved independent of the amount of weight loss. In essence, major co-morbidities were cured in 50% to 80% and improved, but not cured in 10% to 40% of all patients undergoing the LAGB in this series.

Another device, the so-called Swedish Adjustable Gastric Band (SAGB) has been compared with other laparoscopic bariatric procedures including the gastric bypass, LAGB and VBG (26). In a series of 454 patients undergoing laparoscopic SAGB, the average weight lost was 35.5 kg after one year, reaching an average of 54 kg after three years. The mean EWL was 72% after three years, and the BMI decreased from 46.7 to 28.1 kg/m^2. Marked improvement in co-morbidities was also reported in patients undergoing the SAGB. Complications requiring re-operation occurred in 8% and no mortality was reported in this series. In a series of 824 patients undergoing laparoscopic SAGB over a five-year period (28), EWL of >50% was achieved in 83% of the patients after the initial treatment. At the end of the follow-up period, mean EWL was 30, 41, 49, 55, and 57% after one, two, three, four and five years, respectively. There were no intra- or post-operative deaths reported in the series. Intra-operative conversion rate was 5% with a peri-operative complication rate of 1.2%. Long-term complications occurred in 191 patients (23%) related primarily to the band (16%) or to the access-port or tubing (7%).

American Experience

LAGB is the most commonly performed bariatric procedure in Europe and Australia, and has been shown to result in significant long-term weight loss and resolution of co-morbidities. A common theme in international studies appears to be a lower degree of obesity, as measured by BMI, than is seen in many U.S. obesity surgery centers. Initial clinical trials undertaken under the supervision of the US Food and Drug Administration (FDA) with the LAGB have not reproduced the results of studies performed elsewhere in the world. Newer American studies are more encouraging, although subject to less rigorous controls and scrutiny than the strict FDA protocols.

The first FDA-monitored clinical trial to evaluate the LAGB in morbidly obese patients began in April 1995 and was called the A-trial. This trial included eight centers and 299 patients who were followed for 36 months. Eighty-nine percent ($n=259$) had the band placed laparoscopically using the peri-gastric technique, whereas 11% ($n=33$) had the band implanted by laparotomy. The average %EWL was 26.5 at six months, 34.5 at 12 months, 38 at 24 months, and 36 at 36 months.

Our group reported our clinical experience with the Lap-Band at one of the eight original U.S. centers performing LAGB as part of the FDA monitored A-trial (29). Thirty-seven patients were enrolled and underwent laparoscopic placement of the device with successful placement in 36 patients. One patient required an open conversion to a gastric bypass following an intra-operative gastric perforation. Patients were followed up for up to four years after surgery for weight loss and resolution of co-morbidities. Five patients were lost after (14%) a mean follow-up of two years, but at the last available follow-up had achieved only 18% EWL. The LAGB devices were ultimately removed in more than half ($n=19$) of the patients between 10 days and more than four years after surgery. Most patients undergoing device removal were converted to a gastric bypass. The most common reason for removal was inadequate weight loss in the presence of a functioning band. The primary reasons for removal in others were infection, leakage from the inflatable silicone ring causing inadequate weight loss, and band slippage. Bands were also removed in two others as a result of symptoms related to esophageal dilatation. Significant radiograpic evidence of esophageal dilatation developed in 18 of 25 patients (71%) who underwent preoperative and long-term postoperative contrast evaluation. Of these, 13 (72%) patients had prominent dysphagia, vomiting, or reflux symptoms. Of the remaining patients with bands in situ, eight desired band removal and conversion to a gastric bypass for inadequate weight loss. Six of the remaining patients had persistent morbid obesity two years after surgery, but refused to undergo further surgery. Overall, only four patients achieved a BMI of less than 35 and/or at least a 50% reduction in excess weight. Based on these results, the LAGB was not felt to be an effective and durable surgical modality for the treatment of morbid obesity. Inadequate weight loss was more prominent in the African-American cohort for unknown reasons but consistent with general observations about racial differences in weight loss outcomes after bariatric procedures.

The second FDA-monitored clinical trial, called the B-trial, began in 1999 and also followed patients for up to 36 months (30). The single published report from the B-trial involved 63 patients who underwent LAGB between March 1999 and June 2001 at a single center. All of these patients underwent laparoscopic placement of the Lap Band with placement done via the classic high peri-gastric dissection above the lesser sac. The operative time decreased from a mean of 197 minutes for the first 10 patients to 120 minutes for the last group with an average hospital stay of 1.4 days. The average %EWL was 27.2 at 6 months, 38.3 at 12 months, 46.6 at 24 months, and 53.6 at 36 months. Before surgery, 46 of 63 patients (73%) suffered from a serious co-morbidity. Following LAGB, all showed marked improvement.

More complications occurred in trial-A as compared to the published 63 patients in trial-B. When compared to trial-B, nausea or vomiting occurred in 51% of patients in trial A versus 23%, gastroesophageal reflux in 34% versus 2%, gastric prolapse (band slippage)/pouch dilatation in 24% versus 5%, stoma obstruction in 14% versus 0%, esophageal dilatation in 10% versus 6%, port problems in

15% versus 8%, and erosions in 1% in both groups. Peri-operative complications in trial-B included one intra-operative gastric perforation which was closed and did not prevent band placement. Two deaths occurred during the course of trial-A: one due to "mixed drug intoxication" a week after explantation of the device and the other due to multiple pulmonary emboli a day after explantation of the Lap Band and conversion to an RYGB. No deaths were reported among the 63 trial-B patients.

Doherty et al. reported their experience with the adjustable gastric banding (ASGB) procedure in a prospective study of 62 patients over an eight-year period (31). Patients were characterized by a mean body weight of 145 kg and a mean BMI of 49 kg/m^2. In the ASGB cohort, the BMI decreased from 50 to 36 kg/m^2 over a three-year period and then increased to 44 kg/m^2 at eight years after operation. In the Lap-Band cohort, the BMI decreased from 47 to 40 kg/m^2 at one year and then increased to 43 kg/m^2 at six years after operation. There were no operative mortalities. Thirty abdominal re-operations were necessary to correct complications related to the implanted device. The adverse events included infected band (1.6%), obstructive aneurysmal deformity of the inflatable bladder component of the band (3.2%, $n=2$; ASGB), enlarged pouch with obstructive angulation of the outlet channel (17.7%, $n=11$; seven ASGB, four Lap-Bands), herniation of the distal stomach through the band into the posterior lesser sac causing obstruction (23%, $n=14$; 11 ASGB, three Lap-Bands). Seven subjects voluntarily withdrew from the study because of minimal or no weight loss. Twenty-seven implantable devices (18 ASGB, nine Lap-Bands) were removed by the time of publication. After 116 months, only 26 subjects (42% of participants) remained. Their conclusions suggested that adjustable gastric banding was neither effective nor durable for the surgical treatment of morbid obesity.

As centers persisting with LAGB treatment have gained experience with larger numbers of patients, more favorable data have begun to emerge from the U.S. centers. An initial clinical series reported by Ren et al. provided short-term data on nearly 500 patients undergoing the LAGB at four U.S. medical centers (32). Of these, 115 patients were followed for at least nine months and 43 for at least 12 months. The reported %EWL was 35.6 at nine months and 41.6 at 12 months. The average BMI decreased from 47.5 kg/m^2 to 37.3 kg/m^2 in 12 months. Conversion to an open procedure was necessary in one patient (1%). Acute peri-operative complications occurred in four patients (3%) and included two stoma obstructions, one hemorrhage, and one case of pneumonia. The acute stoma obstructions, secondary to edema, were treated conservatively with intravenous hydration and resolved spontaneously. Wound infection occurred in five patients (4%). These were conservatively managed with oral antibiotics and resolved in all but one patient, in whom a port abscess developed that required port removal three weeks postoperatively and a subsequent port replacement six months postoperatively. There were no device-related mortalities, but 12 patients developed complications requiring operative management (13%). These included eight port displacements or tubing breaks (7%), two elective explantations (2%), two gastric prolapse (2%), and one gastric pouch dilatation (1%).

Another series authored by Ren et al. described favorable early results of LAGB at two American academic centers (33). In this series of 445 patients, the mean BMI was 49.6 kg/m^2 with a mean total body weight of 299 lbs. Only one case required conversion to a laparotomy (bleeding). Mean length of stay was 1.1 days and there was one death. Additional complications included band slippage in 14 patients (3.1%), gastric obstruction without slip in 12 (2.7%), port migration in two (0.4%), tubing disconnections in three (0.7%), and port infection in five (1.1%). Two bands (0.4%) were removed due to intra-abdominal abscess two months after placement. There was one band erosion (0.2%). Ninety-nine patients with one-year follow-up lost an average of 44% of excess body weight. Although no data were provided on resolution of co-morbidities, this series suggested comparable weight loss to European studies.

Grade A Evidence

There are no randomized controlled studies to date which compare RYGB to LAGB; thus randomized comparison data do not definitively answer the question of superiority between the two procedures. In the absence of such direct comparison data, one must ask if it is reasonable to view the LAGB and VBG procedures as equivalent procedures, since they share the common mechanism of gastric restriction. Conceptually, VBG and LAGB are similar procedures in which a banded outlet is utilized to create a small proximal gastric pouch. The primary difference is in the area of adjustability of the band diameter. A further incentive to analyze whether or not LAGB and VBG can be considered comparable procedures is that there are many studies in the literature which directly compare RYGB and VBG, and the outcomes of these studies are relevant to the discussion if a reasonable argument can be made that VBG and LAGB are comparable procedures.

In fact, LAGB and VBG have been directly compared in a single randomized trial (34) in which VBG was demonstrated to result in superior weight loss to LAGB. This result provides a strong counter-argument to the concept that the adjustability of the LAGB device promotes superior weight loss to other restrictive procedures by virtue of its adjustability which allows the band diameter to be repeatedly narrowed to enhance the device's impact on oral intake. While this adjustability component of the LAGB has been touted to enhance weight loss, its primary value may alternatively be in the reduction of postoperative vomiting which occurred following VBG in 5% to 9% of the patients (34).

Adjustability is touted to produce "gentle progressive weight loss" over a long-term follow-up up to seven years following LAGB (22). Scientific scrutiny of the weight loss following LAGB refutes this claim. Table 4 demonstrates weight loss data used to make this claim about weight loss progression including the standard deviations for each mean value reported. The large variance in each mean reported for each postoperative time point makes it highly unlikely that one value differs from the others beyond the two-year time point. The authors have not reported that statistics prove this claim of ongoing weight loss beyond two years, and the small difference between means in the presence of such large variance almost certainly reflects merely "noise" in the measurements. In fact, to the best of this author's knowledge, no surgical procedure for weight loss has been demonstrated to provide ongoing weight loss more than 18 months to two years after the procedure. The additional claim that weight loss is "gentle" for LAGB is furthermore easily explained by the need to market the device to the public in a way that is more palatable to the consumer / prospective patient. It is regrettable that such terms have been allowed to emerge in the scientific literature. Another justifiable term to describe the weight loss curve after LAGB is "slower" which clearly fails to provide the same degree of marketability as "gentle." Most studies clearly confirm that the slower weight loss of LAGB provides an overall less weight loss than gastric bypass (20–25,36,37).

A non-randomized "best-practice" comparative study of LAGB with RYGB was reported by Biertho et al. (36). In this analysis, 456 patients undergoing the

Table 4 Modified Presentation of Data from O'Brien et al. (22) Demonstrating Annual Percentage of Excess Weight Lost (%EWL) Following LAGB (mean $\pm$ SD)

Months	n	%EWL
12	492	47 ± 16
24	336	53 ± 18
36	273	53 ± 22
48	112	52 ± 23
60	32	54 ± 23

Note: The wide variance in means for each annual time point making progression of weight loss over the five-year term unlikely by any statistical methodology.

laparoscopic RYGB at a U.S. center were compared to 805 LAGB performed in the European institutions. The BMIs, complication rates, mortality, and EWL up to 18 months were reported. The 805 patients underwent the laparoscopic Swedish Adjustable Gastric Banding (SAGB, Obtech) performed as the initial surgical treatment of their obesity. Patients with a BMI above $50 \, kg/m^2$ were usually considered for gastric bypass. Preoperative BMI was higher at $49.4 \, kg/m^2$ in the RYGB group versus $42.2 \, kg/m^2$ in the LAGB group. Peri-operative major complication rates were 2.0% after RYGB versus 1.3% after SAGB, and the early postoperative major complication rates were 4.2% versus 1.7%, respectively. Mortality rate was 0.4% in the RYGB group versus 0% in the SAGB group. The global EWL was 36.3% for RYGB versus 14.7% for LAGB at three months, 52% versus 22% at six months, 67% versus 33% at 12 months, and 75% versus 40% at 18 months, respectively. Long-term follow-up for the LAGB group showed an EWL of 47% at two years, 56% at three years, and 58% at four years.

Band Adjustment

A critique of the LAGB procedure must also include the observation that good weight loss outcomes do not automatically follow once the procedure is completed. Although there are failures in the long term after RYGB, often such patients develop weight re-gain due to habitual dietary indiscretion years after a successful procedure. With the LAGB procedure, adjustment of the device appears to be critical in reaching weight loss goals, yet there is very little in the scientific literature to guide strategies for band adjustment. It has become clear that frequent adjustments during the postoperative period enhance weight-loss results in a program dedicated to an intensive follow-up of the patients undergoing this procedure (38). It is not clear that wide application of this simpler procedure, which can be done by general laparoscopic surgeons lacking a commitment to obesity treatment, will ever provide similar results to those reported by the dedicated bariatric surgery pioneers of LAGB in the scientific literature. Will surgeons who are technically capable of performing this "easier" laparoscopic procedure be motivated to follow their patients closely with frequent band adjustments to "fine tune" the result over time for each patient? Already cited above are worrisome data from one of the recognized European pioneers of LAGB (21) in which 30% of patients experienced failed weight loss in seven-year follow-up. That an internationally acclaimed pioneer in LAGB would identify such a high failure rate does not bode well for the broader application of this procedure by surgeons who are less dedicated to understanding the procedure as its application becomes more widespread.

LAGB Conversion

Favorable outcomes have led some to suggest that LAGB should be the preferred initial procedure for all morbidly obese patients, with more complex revisional gastrointestinal procedures reserved for weight-loss failure. In fact, many bariatric surgeons in the United States today are allowing patients to choose their own surgical procedure. This provides an insight into the relative lack of clear data demonstrating how to successfully tailor the choice of operation to the individual patient in this rapidly growing new speciality. A flaw in this line of thinking also rests in the assessment of surgical risk for revisional versus primary procedures. Revision to proximal gastric bypass from a failed primary gastroplasty procedure carries a higher risk of complications, particularly anastomotic leak, than does a primary gastric bypass operation. A similar increase in the risk of postoperative complications has been demonstrated after a failed LAGB. Regarding conversion of LAGB to gastric bypass (39), our group found conversions were technically difficult to perform and fraught with serious complications—three patients developed intra-operative gastrojejunal leaks requiring intra-operative repair, whereas another developed postoperative bleeding requiring re-exploration. One patient who was converted to RYGB laparoscopically developed a gastrojejunal anastomotic leak postoperatively that healed with three weeks of outpatient intravenous nutrition. Three of five patients requiring open conversion developed ventral hernias necessitating repair.

Finally, one could question the logic of performing a procedure on all candidates that has been shown to carry a 20% to 30% outright failure rate (23,29), when it would make more sense to analyze subgroups of morbidly obese patients to determine predictors which signal that successful long-term weight loss is more likely with a given procedure. Proponents of LAGB claim that it is a technically less-challenging surgical procedure than the gastric bypass and that most re-operations for complications can be performed laparoscopically with low morbidity and short hospitalizations.

Comorbidity Resolution

Turning to co-morbid conditions, the LAGB has provided inferior resolution of these to parallel its inferior weight-loss results. Studies of weight-loss surgery have reliably shown that resolution of co-morbid conditions parallels the amount of weight loss and reaches a high degree after RYGB in nearly every study published to date. Pories' work provides an excellent example regarding the high rate of cure of type 2 diabetes after RYGB (40). Similar results were shown by Sugerman et al. (41) who found that diabetes resolved completely in 83% of the diabetic cohort among 1025 surgical patients treated with gastric bypass between 1981 and 2000. Patients who resolved their diabetes or hypertension had greater EWL than those who did not. Given that the LAGB procedure demonstrates weight loss in the lower range of the above categories, one would anticipate a lower resolution of diabetes following this procedure. The literature confirms this observation. Furthermore, it is quite likely that bypass of the stomach, duodenum, and upper jejunum may provide an independent mechanism for the control of diabetes in addition to the effects of weight loss (41,43).

Buchwald et al.'s meta-analysis (10) reveals significant benefit for sufferers of serious co-morbidities after RYGB as compared to gastric banding, correlating with the superior weight loss outcome described previously in this review. Co-morbidity resolution data included improvement in diabetes in 48% of patients after banding compared to improvement in 84% of patients after gastric bypass. Hypertension was cured in 43% of patients after banding compared to the cure in 68% of patients after gastric bypass. One can postulate that given the superior resolution of co-morbidity found after RYGB, make it the procedure of choice for patients suffering from these conditions as a complication of obesity.

CONCLUSION

In summary, the RYGB is the only weight-loss operation that has been shown through prospective randomized studies to be superior in terms of weight loss to either the jejunoileal bypass, gastric partitioning alone, or VBG. Laparoscopic access for RYGB is feasible and demonstrates comparable outcomes to the well-studied open procedure. There are no high-grade evidence studies from which to draw any conclusions about the role of adjustable gastric banding procedures as compared to the gastric bypass. On the favorable side, LAGB appears to be a simpler laparoscopic procedure with lower operative risk than RYGB, but this decreased risk is realized at the cost of inferior weight loss, a higher outright failure risk in the range of 20% to 30% of all patients, and an inferior resolution of co-morbid conditions.

Patients with lower BMI, similar to those typically operated upon in international centers, may do better with weight loss after LAGB than heavier patients, while African-Americans and patients with severe co-morbid conditions such as diabetes are likely to be less satisfactory candidates. It remains unclear if a broader application of the LAGB treatment for obesity around the world will replicate the published results by surgical pioneers of the device as the outcome appears to be dependent on rigorous follow-up and compliance. Concerns about esophageal dilatation, band erosions, and the potential for device failure cannot be adequately addressed by long-term data with this relatively new procedure.

RYGB remains the gold standard procedure to treat morbid obesity by virtue of its well-documented long-term reliability for producing substantial weight loss and resolution of co-morbid conditions.

REFERENCES

1. Gastrointestinal surgery for severe obesity: National Institutes of Health Consensus Development Conference Statement. Am J Surg 1992; 55:615S–619S.
2. Griffen WO Jr, Young L, Stevenson CC. A prospective comparison of gastric and jejunoileal bypass procedures for morbid obesity. Ann Surg 1977; 186(4):500–509.
3. Laws HL, Piantadosi S. Superior gastric reduction procedure for morbid obesity. A prospective, randomized trial. Ann Surg 1981; 193(3):334–340.
4. Pories WJ, Flickinger EG, Meelheim D, et al. The effectiveness of gastric bypass over gastric partition in morbid obesity. Consequence of distal gastric and duodenal exclusion. Ann Surg 1982; 194(4):389–399.

5. Sugerman HJ, Londrey GL, Kellum JM, et al. Weight loss with vertical banded gastroplasty and Roux-Y bypass for morbid obesity with selective versus random assignment. Am J Surg 1989; 157(1):93–102.

6. Hall JC, Watts JM, O'Brien PE, et al. Gastric surgery for morbid obesity. The Adelaide study. Ann Surg 1990; 211(4):419–427.

7. Mclean LD, Rhode BM, Forse RA, Nohr CW. Surgery for obesity—an update of a randomized trial. Obes Surg 1995; 5(2):145–150.

8. Buchwald, H. Overview of bariatric surgery. J Am Coll Surg 2002; 194(3):367–375.

9. Balsiger BM, Poggio JL, Mai J, Kelly KA, Sarr MG. Ten and more years after vertical banded gastroplasty as primary operation for morbid obesity. J Gastrointest Surg 2000; 4(6):598–605.

10. Buchwald H, Avidor Y, Braunwald E, et al. Bariatric surgery: a systematic review and meta-analysis. JAMA 2004; 292(14):1724–1737.

11. Pories WJ, Swanson MS, Macdonald KG, et al. Who would have thought it? An operation proves to be the most effective therapy for adult-onset diabetes mellitus. Ann Surg 1995; 222(3):339–350.

12. Sugerman HJ, Sugerman EL, DeMaria EJ, et al. Bariatric surgery for severely obese adolescents. J Gastrointest Surg 2003; 7(1):102–107.

13. Wittgrove AC, Clark GW, Tremblay LJ. Laparoscopic gastric bypass, Roux-en-Y: preliminary report of five cases. Obes Surg 1994; 4(4):353–357.

14. Wittgrove AC, Clark GW. Laparoscopic gastric bypass Roux-en-Y in 500 patients: technique and results, with 3–60 months follow-up. Obes Surg 2000; 10(3):233–239.

15. Schauer PR, Ikramuddin S, Gourash W, et al. Outcomes after laparoscopic Roux-en-Y gastric bypass for morbid obesity. Ann Surg. 2000; 232(4):515–529.

16. DeMaria EJ, Sugerman HJ, Kellum JM, et al. Results of 281 consecutive total laparoscopic Roux-en-Y gastric bypasses to treat morbid obesity. Ann Surg 2002; 235(5): 640–647.

17. Nguyen NT, Goldman C, Rosenquist CJ, et al. Laparoscopic versus open gastric bypass: a randomized study of outcomes, quality of life, and costs. Ann Surg 2001; 234(3): 279–289.

18. Westling A, Gustavsson S. Laparoscopic vs. open Roux-en-Y gastric bypass: a prospective, randomized trial. Obes Surg 2001; 11(3):284–292.

19. Lujan JA, Frutos MD, Hernandez Q, et al. Laparoscopic versus open gastric bypass in the treatment of morbid obesity: a randomized prospective study. Ann Surg 2004; 239(4): 433–437.

20. Angrisani L, Furbetta F, Doldi SB. Results of the Italian multicenter study on 239 superobese patients treated by adjustable gastric banding. Obes Surg 2002; 12(6):846–850.

21. Weiner R, Blanco-Engert R, Weiner S. Outcome after laparoscopic adjustable gastric banding—8 years experience. Obes Surg 2003; 13(3):427–434.

22. O'Brien PE, Dixon JB. Lap-band: outcomes and results. J Laparoendosc Adv Surg Tech 2003; 13(4):265–270.

23. Favretti F, Cadiere G, Segato G, et al. Laparoscopic banding: selection and technique in 830 patients. Obes Surg 2002; 12(3):385–390.

24. Chevallier JM, Zinzindohoue F, Elian N. Adjustable gastric banding in a public university hospital: prospective analysis of 400 patients. Obes Surg 2002; 12(1):93–99.

25. Szold A, Abu-Abeid S. Laparoscopic adjustable silicone gastric banding for morbid obesity: results and complications in 715 patients. Surg Endosc 2002; 16(2):230–233.

26. Mittermair RP, Weiss H, Nehoda H. Laparoscopic Swedish adjustable gastric banding: 6-year follow-up and comparison to other laparoscopic bariatric procedures. Obes Surg 2003; 13(3):412–417.

27. Frigg A, Peterli R, Peters T. Reduction in co-morbidities 4 years after laparoscopic adjustable gastric banding. Obes Surg 2004; 14(2):216–223.

28. Steffen R, Biertho L, Ricklin T. Laparoscopic Swedish adjustable gastric banding: a five-year prospective study. Obes Surg 2003; 13(3):404–411.

29. DeMaria EJ, Sugerman HJ, Meador JG, et al. High failure rate after laparoscopic adjustable silicone gastric banding for treatment of morbid obesity. Ann Surg 2001; 233(6):809–818.

30. Rubenstein RB. Laparoscopic adjustable gastric banding at a U.S. center with up to 3-year follow-up. Obes Surg 2002; 12(3):380–384.

31. Doherty C, Maher JW, Heitshusen DS. Long-term data indicate a progressive loss in efficacy of adjustable silicone gastric banding for the surgical treatment of morbid obesity. Surgery 2002; 132(4):724–728.

32. Ren CJ, Horgan S, Ponce J. US experience with the Lap-Band system. Am J Surg 2002; 184(6B):46S–50S.

33. Ren CJ, Weiner M, Allen JW. Favorable early results of gastric banding for morbid obesity: the American experience. Surg Endosc 2004 18(3):543–546.

34. Ashy AR, Merdad AA. A prospective study comparing vertical banded gastroplasty versus laparoscopic adjustable gastric banding in the treatment of morbid and superobesity. Int Surg 1998; 83(2):108–110.

35. Papakonstantinou A, Alfaras P, Komessidou V, et al. Gastrointestinal complications after vertical banded gastroplasty. Obes Surg 1998; 8(2):215–217.

36. Biertho L, Steffen R, Ricklin T. Laparoscopic gastric bypass versus laparoscopic adjustable gastric banding: a comparative study of 1,200 cases. J Am Coll Surg 2003; 197: 536–547.

37. Weber M, Muller MK, Bucher T, et al. Laparoscopic gastric bypass is superior to laparoscopic banding for treatment of morbid obesity. Ann Surg 2004; 240(6):975–982.

38. Fox SR, Fox KM, Srikanth MS, et al. The Lap-Band system in a North American population. Obes Surg 2003; 13(2):275–280.

39. Kothari SN, DeMaria EJ, Sugerman HJ, et al. Lap-band failures: conversion to gastric bypass and their preliminary outcomes. Surgery 2002:131(6); 625–629.

40. Pories WJ, Albrecht RJ. Etiology of type II diabetes mellitus: role of the foregut. World J Surg 2001; 25(4):527–531.

41. Sugerman HJ, Wolfe LG, Sica DA, et al. Diabetes and hypertension in severe obesity and effects of gastric bypass-induced weight loss. Ann Surg 2003; 237(6):741–748.

42. Hickey MS, Pories WJ, MacDonald KG Jr, et al. A new paradigm for type 2 diabetes mellitus: could it be a disease of the foregut? Ann Surg 1998; 227(5):637–644.

16

Complications of Laparoscopic Bariatric Surgery

Daniel M. Herron
Section of Bariatric Surgery, Department of Surgery, Mount Sinai School of Medicine, New York, New York, U.S.A.

INTRODUCTION

The growth of morbid obesity in the United States has now reached epidemic proportions. Recent estimates suggest that 365,000 deaths per year in the United States may be attributed to poor diet and physical inactivity (1). This epidemic has resulted in the geometric growth of bariatric surgery nationwide. Prior to 1996, American surgeons performed a total of 16,000 to 20,000 bariatric operations each year (2). The American Society for Bariatric Surgery (ASBS) estimates that over 100,000 such procedures were performed in the United States in 2003. Of these operations, more than half were laparoscopic.

Patients undergoing bariatric surgery are considered to be at high risk for surgical complications regardless of whether their surgery is open or laparoscopic. First, the obese abdomen presents substantial technical challenges with regards to exposure, retraction, and bowel manipulation. Second, the severely obese patient may suffer from numerous comorbidities such as hypertension, sleep apnea, venous stasis, restrictive lung disease, and diabetes—just to name a few—any one of which may increase the risk of perioperative complications. Finally, all bariatric surgery is elective, thus decreasing both the patient's and the surgeon's tolerance for complications.

It is self-evident that any bariatric surgeon must be intimately familiar with the diagnosis and management of bariatric surgical complications. With the recent surge in bariatric procedures, however, it is becoming increasingly necessary for any general surgeon who may be called upon to treat surgical emergencies in the emergency department to be knowledgeable of the evaluation and management of such complications. While entire volumes have been written on the management of perioperative complications, this chapter is intended to serve as a brief overview of the most common problems that may occur in the perioperative period after laparoscopic or open bariatric procedures, specifically those involving stapled pouch formation and multiple gastrointestinal anastomoses, such as Roux-en-Y gastric bypass (RYGB) or biliopancreatic diversion with duodenal switch.

LEAKS

Enteric leaks—whether from the stomach, intestine, or one of the anastomoses—are amongst the most feared complications of bariatric surgery. In the RYGB operation, leaks may occur at a number of different locations.

- Gastric pouch staple line
- Gastric remnant staple line
- Terminal (stapled) end of Roux limb
- Proximal anastomosis (gastrojejunostomy)
- Distal anastomosis (jejunojejunostomy)
- Gastric wall (transmural perforation)
- Intestinal wall (transmural perforation)

Enteric leaks typically present in the immediate postoperative period, usually during the initial hospitalization. Unlike the normal-weight patient, the obese one may not complain of any abdominal pain or tenderness even in the presence of florid peritonitis. Fever or tachycardia may be the only presenting signs.

The incidence of enteric leaks varies considerably in different studies. In their first 99 cases, Wittgrove and Clark reported four leaks at the circular-stapled gastro-jejunostomy, giving a leak rate of 4% (3). This rate decreased as the authors gained additional experience. In a subsequent report of their first 500 patients, the authors reported 11 leaks (2.2%) (4).

In contrast to Wittgrove, Higa's group utilized a two-layer hand-sewn gastro-jejunostomy. In reviewing his group's first 400 laparoscopic RYGBs, Higa did not identify any leaks from the proximal anastomosis (5). However, six patients suffered from disruption of the staple line along the gastric pouch, one patient suffered an early gastric pouch perforation, and one patient suffered from disruption of the staple line on the gastric remnant due to obstruction of the distal anastomosis.

The gastric pouch and the proximal anastomosis can be assessed intraopera-tively for leakage using a number of techniques. An orogastric tube can be inserted into the pouch or proximal Roux limb and used to instill air or methylene blue to reveal leaks. Some surgeons routinely perform intraoperative upper endoscopy to visually inspect the pouch and proximal anastomosis, and insufflate under direct vision (6). Air leakage may be identified by submerging the pouch and proximal anastomosis under saline irrigation. Methylene blue leakage is usually immediately apparent, or may be detected by placing a clean surgical sponge adjacent to the staple line or anastomosis and carefully inspecting it after it is withdrawn. Some authors, including Higa, do not feel that any type of leak test is necessary (5).

Postoperatively, the bariatric patient with an enteric leak may or may not complain of excessive abdominal pain. Their physical examination may or may not reveal peritoneal irritation. Interestingly, bariatric patients frequently remain afebrile in the presence of a leak (7).

The most reliable clinical finding suggesting leakage is the presence of tachy-cardia. A review of nine patients with enteric leakage after laparoscopic RYGB revealed that eight were tachycardic above 120 beats/min while the remaining one was tachycardic to 110 beats/min (7). Only 16% of controls were tachycardic to more than 120 beats/min.

Respiratory distress is another sensitive indicator of enteric leakage. Indeed, many bariatric surgeons feel that the onset of respiratory distress after gastric bypass represents enteric leakage until proven otherwise. In Hamilton et al.'s study, six of the nine patients with leaks (67%) demonstrated respiratory distress, while only 10% of controls did (7).

The presence of a leak may be confirmed with imaging. Either a water-soluble contrast swallow or a CT of the abdomen and pelvis may be used. Interestingly, imaging may have extremely poor sensitivity. In Hamilton et al.'s study, all patients had a water-soluble upper GI study performed on postoperative day 1. Only two of the nine patients with leaks demonstrated leakage on imaging studies (7). Upper GI contrast studies are extremely poor at identifying leaks at the distal anastomosis; CT may be more useful if this diagnosis is clinically suspected (8). The most reliable diagnostic modality remains laparoscopic or open re-exploration.

The treatment of leaks depends upon the severity of the clinical presentation. A small, contained leak in a minimally symptomatic, stable patient may be managed with antibiotics and observation alone. Most leaks, however, mandate immediate return to the operating room for abscess drainage, peritoneal washout and drain placement. The perforation may also be patched with omentum, similar to a Graham patch repair. It is essential to place enteric feeding access if there is concern about postoperative nutrition. In the gastric bypass patient, the best location for enteral access is the gastric remnant, as it allows bolus feedings without the risk of reflux. If a gastrostomy is technically unfeasible, a feeding jejunostomy placed in the mid-biliopancreatic limb is acceptable.

INTESTINAL OBSTRUCTION FROM INTERNAL HERNIA

Intestinal obstruction from internal herniation has been reported as an extremely rare event in the open bariatric surgery literature (9). One of the frequently mentioned advantages of laparoscopic surgery is the decrease in the formation of intra-abdominal adhesions. This "advantage" may paradoxically contribute to a higher incidence of internal hernia formation in laparoscopic procedures.

Internal hernias may form at one of three sites:

- Distal anastomosis mesenteric defect.
- Petersen hernia space.
- Mesocolic tunnel.

The potential hernia space at the mesenteric defect of the distal anastomosis exists in all gastric bypasses regardless of the Roux position. Similarly, the Petersen space—the area behind the Roux limb—is present in both antecolic and retrocolic bypasses, although the space is substantially larger in the former approach. The potential hernia space at the mesocolic tunnel only exists if the Roux limb is brought up through a retrocolic approach.

Symptoms of internal herniation span a broad range of severity, from mild intermittent abdominal pain to bowel necrosis, gastric perforation, and death (10). In a typical case, the patient may complain of intermittent epigastric pain, sometimes postprandial, sometimes radiating to the back that may vary in intensity from mild cramping to incapacitating pain.

Several authors have reviewed the incidence of internal hernia formation after laparoscopic gastric bypass. Higa retrospectively reviewed his group's experience with 2000 patients between 1998 and 2001 (11). Sixty-six internal hernias occurred in 63 patients, for an overall internal hernia formation rate of 3.1%. The majority of the patients (52%) in his series presented with acute bowel obstruction, while a slightly smaller number (41%) presented with abdominal pain. Only 5% of patients were asymptomatic, with their hernias identified incidentally on a subsequent surgery. Of note, 67% of the patients herniated at the mesocolic tunnel—Higa's group uses the retrocolic Roux limb exclusively. Distal anastomosis mesenteric hernias comprised 21% of the cases, while Petersen's space was the least common location, present in only 7%.

Several other authors have identified the mesocolic tunnel as a substantial source of internal herniation with resultant small bowel obstruction. Felsher et al. identified two patients with small bowel obstruction secondary to mesocolic herniation in a series of 115 laparoscopic RYGBs (12). Filip et al. found a 5% incidence of mesocolic herniation in a series of 100 laparoscopic RYGBs, despite the fact that his group sutured the bowel to the mesentery at this site (13). Champion and Williams found six internal hernias occurring in their series of 711 laparoscopic RYGBs—four at the mesocolic tunnel, one at Petersen's space and one at the distal anastomosis mesenteric defect (14). Partway through their series, Champion and Williams changed their surgical technique from a retrocolic to an antecolic approach, and in doing so noted a decrease in the incidence of small bowel obstruction from 4.5% to 0.4%. For this reason, they advocate placing the Roux limb in the antecolic position in order to reduce or eliminate the possibility of mesocolic tunnel herniation.

It is of interest to note that imaging studies are of limited use in the diagnosis of internal hernias. In Higa's study, 71% of patients underwent a preoperative CT scan or contrast swallow. Fully 20% of these patients demonstrated no pathologic radiologic findings (11).

Treatment of internal herniation is usually straightforward, requiring reduction of the herniated bowel and suture closure of the hernia space. If bowel has herniated through the mesocolic tunnel, it may either be reduced and aggressively resutured or divided from the gastric pouch and re-anastomosed in an antecolic position. If herniation has irreversibly compromised the vascular supply of a segment of bowel, the necrotic area must be resected, with reconstruction of the alimentary channel utilizing a segment of the biliopancreatic limb if necessary.

BLEEDING

Intra-abdominal and gastrointestinal bleeding after gastric bypass is not uncommon. In a review of 275 laparoscopic gastric bypass patients from the University of Pittsburgh, postoperative bleeding was identified in nine patients (3%) (15). The majority of these patients required packed red blood cell transfusion.

Gastrointestinal bleeding accounted for three of the nine cases of postoperative bleeding identified in the Pittsburgh study (15). Intraluminal gastrointestinal bleeding may occur along a staple line in the gastric pouch or gastric remnant, or along the proximal or distal anastomosis. The majority of intraluminal bleeding will resolve spontaneously. Proximal anastomotic bleeding in the immediate postoperative period may be diagnosed and treated with upper endoscopy and injection of vasoconstrictors. While this may be safely accomplished in the endoscopy suite, some surgeons feel it is safer to perform such endoscopy in the operating room with the anastomosis under direct laparoscopic visualization. Bleeding at the distal anastomosis is typically beyond the reach of the endoscope; if persistent, it may require reoperation with revision or oversewing of the anastomosis.

Intra-abdominal bleeding was more common than GI bleeding in the Pittsburgh series, accounting for two-thirds of the bleeding complications. Only one patient required reoperation, and this was accomplished by laparoscopy. Intra-abdominal bleeding may occur along the stomach, at the short gastric vessels, from the spleen, along a divided edge of omentum or mesentery, or elsewhere. The bleeding source may be difficult or impossible to localize; in the only patient reoperated for such bleeding in the Pittsburgh series, no bleeding site was found (15).

STRICTURE FORMATION

Stricture formation is one of the most common complications after both open and laparoscopic RYGB, with an incidence ranging from 0.6% to 20% (16,17). The gastrojejunostomy is the most common location for stricture formation, but strictures may form at the mesocolic tunnel or at the distal anastomosis as well.

While the cause of strictures has not been identified, it may be due to a relative ischemia or tension at the site of the anastomosis. This explanation is plausible for the gastrojejunostomy site, but does not explain why strictures may also form at the mesocolic tunnel or at the jejunojejunostomy. Some feel that stricture formation is analogous to keloid formation in a skin wound.

Gastrojejunal strictures typically present within two months after surgery. The diagnosis of gastrojejunal stenosis is made primarily by history. The patient may report rapidly worsening nausea, dysphagia, or food intolerance starting six to eight weeks after the operation. It is usually unnecessary to perform a contrast study; the diagnosis is confirmed with upper endoscopy and simultaneously treated with endoscopic balloon dilatation. A balloon of 12 to 18 mm diameter may be used. Typically, the balloon is inflated to three or four atmospheres of pressure and held for 30 to 60 seconds (18). A significant subset of patients may require two or more dilatations to achieve a durable result.

In Nguyen et al.'s review of 185 laparoscopic RYGB patients, 29 (15.7%) suffered from stricture formation at the gastrojejunostomy (18). The rate was substantially higher in patients where the 21-mm circular stapler was used compared to the 25-mm circular stapler (27% vs. 9%, $p < 0.01$). Of the patients with strictures, 24 (83%) had complete symptomatic resolution after a single endoscopic treatment. Four patients (14%) required a second dilation and one patient (3%) required a third. There was no significant difference in excess weight loss at one year between patients with strictures and those without.

The University of Pittsburgh group measured a 3.1% incidence of gastrojejunal narrowing in their series of 450 patients who underwent laparoscopic RYGB (19). This group presented an average of 2.7 months after the surgery. Of these 14 patients, nine (64%) responded to a single endoscopic dilatation, while five (36%) required two or more. Interestingly, one patient required six endoscopies for persistent vomiting, although the anastomosis remained patent after the third dilatation procedure.

DeMaria et al. compared 33 laparoscopic RYGB patients to 73 patients undergoing an open operation during the same time period (20). He found no difference in the rate of stenosis formation between the two groups (24% vs. 20%, $p = $ NS). These data are in disagreement with Nguyen's 2001 prospective randomized trial comparing laparoscopic ($n = 79$) and open ($n = 76$) RYGB operations. Strictures formed in 2.6% of the open surgery patients versus 11.4% of the laparoscopic patients (21).

If the Roux limb is placed retrocolic, stenosis of the mesocolic tunnel may occur. In one of the largest published series of laparoscopic gastric bypasses ($n = 1500$), Higa reports a mesocolic stenosis rate of 0.7% (22). In this situation endoscopic balloon dilatation is ineffective; surgical lysis of the mesocolic scar is required.

PULMONARY EMBOLISM

Deep vein thrombosis (DVT) with pulmonary embolism is one of the most common causes of mortality following bariatric surgery. Every patient undergoing a bariatric procedure possesses at least three risk factors for DVT: morbid obesity, limited ambulation, and postoperative status. Most additionally suffer from some degree of venous stasis. In Higa's series of 1040 patients undergoing laparoscopic gastric bypass, the greatest source of operative mortality was pulmonary embolism. One death occurred perioperatively, while two others occurred more than one month postoperatively (5). No nonfatal pulmonary emboli were identified. Thus, the overall incidence of pulmonary embolism in this series was 3/1040 (0.3%). While this data is similar to that of Schauer's series of 275 patients and Shepherd's study of 700 gastric bypass patients, a 1997 study from Sweden revealed a substantially higher incidence of pulmonary embolism (2.4%) (15,23,24).

Most bariatric surgeons agree that early ambulation is a key element of DVT prophylaxis. Additionally, there is a consensus that sequential compression devices may contribute to a reduced DVT risk. The use of pre- and post-operative heparin, however, is more controversial. A survey of members of the American Society for Bariatric Surgery revealed that 50% adhere to a fixed-dose protocol of unfractionated heparin—typically 5000 units given subcutaneously every eight to twelve hours (25). Some data suggest that a weight-based regimen—giving substantially higher doses of non-fractionated heparin (15,000 units or more)—may provide better DVT prophylaxis with minimal increase in bleeding complications (23). Other authors favor low-molecular weight heparin as standard prophylaxis (26). To date, there is no high-quality data strongly favoring one approach.

CHOLELITHIASIS

Both obesity and rapid weight loss have been implicated as risk factors for gallstone formation. Thus, many surgeons feel that the diagnosis and treatment of gallstones must be actively pursued in the bariatric patient. The most aggressive approach, advocated by Fobi et al., is the routine performance of cholecystectomy during bariatric operations (27). Other authors prefer a selective approach, performing concomitant cholecystectomy only if gallstones are identified during preoperative workup (28). A third approach is to treat bariatric patients the same as the general population, evaluating and treating for gallstones only if symptoms are present (29).

O'Brien and Dixon advocate the latter, most conservative approach for their patients undergoing placement of an adjustable gastric band. In their 2003 study of 1000 patients, only those with a preoperative history of symptomatic cholelithiasis underwent preoperative imaging, with concomitant cholecystectomy performed if the imaging was positive (29). Of those patients with intact gallbladders after their bariatric surgery, 6.8% subsequently went on to have cholecystectomy during a median follow-up period of 42 months. They concluded that treatment of only symptomatic gallstones was the most rational approach to cholelithiasis.

However, patients undergoing gastric bypass or duodenal switch operations present a substantially different scenario from those undergoing banding. First, they typically lose weight at a faster rate than band patients. Second, their duodenum is excluded from the alimentary path, eliminating the option of endoscopic retrograde cholangiopancreatography (ERCP) should choledocholithiasis develop. For these reasons, Sugerman et al. recommended routine intraoperative ultrasound of the gallbladder in his 1995 study of open gastric bypass patients, with cholecystectomy if either stones or sludge were detected (30). In his study he randomized patients with an intact gallbladder to receive placebo or one of three different doses of ursodiol. In the group receiving placebo, 32% were noted to develop gallstones at six months. Of the 124 patients receiving 600 mg of ursodiol or more per day, only 2% to 6% developed cholelithiasis. While Sugerman's group concluded that selective cholecystectomy/postoperative ursodiol treatment was an effective treatment paradigm, he did not demonstrate any poor outcomes due to cholecystitis or choledocholithiasis in the placebo group. To date, the best approach to treating asymptomatic gallstones in the gastric bypass patient has not been further clarified.

MARGINAL ULCER

Marginal ulcers are those that occur at, or just distal to, the gastrojejunostomy. Their occurrence has been tied to larger amounts of acid in the gastric pouch and breakdown of the staple line separating the gastric pouch from the gastric remnant (31). Nonsteroidal anti-inflammatory drugs may also lead to marginal ulcer formation, although this has not been clinically proven. Some surgeons routinely check for *Helicobacter pylori* preoperatively and treat a positive result in hopes of reducing the incidence of marginal ulcer, but the efficacy of this approach remains unknown.

MacLean et al. demonstrated a substantially lower rate of ulcer formation in gastric bypass patients when the pouch was divided from the gastric remnant, rather than stapled in continuity (3% vs. 16%) (31). Some data suggest that the formation of a very small pouch at the cardia of the stomach may further reduce this incidence to less than 1% (15,32).

Patients with marginal ulcer may complain of a burning sensation or discomfort in the epigastric region. Nausea or vomiting may occur due to inflammation and edema near the gastrojejunostomy. Upper GI bleeding is a rare presentation of marginal ulcer. Patients whose ulcer is due to spontaneous reconnection of the stomach pouch and remnant may present with weight regain. Finally, some patients with marginal ulcer may remain asymptomatic.

The diagnosis of marginal ulcer may be easily confirmed with upper endoscopy. Treatment usually includes medical therapy with H2 blockers or proton pump inhibitors (32). Conservative treatment with H2 blockade and sucralfate will result in healing of 95% of marginal ulcers (33). Surgical intervention may be required if the ulceration is a result of gastro-gastric fistula or if the ulcer does not respond to medical therapy.

INCISIONAL HERNIA

One of the clear advantages of the laparoscopic approach to bariatric surgery is its substantially reduced risk of incisional hernia. In Nguyen et al.'s prospective randomized trial comparing laparoscopic and open gastric bypass, six of 76 patients (8%) undergoing open gastric bypass developed a ventral incisional hernia, while none of the laparoscopic patients did (21). Studies with longer follow-up, such as Sugerman et al.'s 1996 review of 968 patients undergoing open gastric bypass, suggest that the true incidence of ventral hernia may be higher, up to 20% or more (34).

In laparoscopic procedures, most surgeons feel that port sites 10 mm or larger in diameter should be closed with sutures, particularly those at the level of the umbilicus or below. While this can be accomplished using standard open suturing technique, the use of a transfascial suture passer may facilitate this maneuver substantially. Other authors feel that fascial closure is unnecessary—Higa et al. reported an acceptably low incisional hernia rate (0.3%) in his review of 1040 patients undergoing laparoscopic gastric bypass without fascial closure (35).

When hernias do occur, they may be repaired using either laparoscopic or open surgical technique. Waiting until the patient's weight has stabilized will reduce the intra-abdominal pressure on the repair, and may reduce the risk of recurrence. However, the benefits of waiting until 12 to 18 months after the original procedure need to be weighed against the risk of incarceration or strangulation during that time.

PRESSURE-RELATED COMPLICATIONS: RHABDOMYOLYSIS AND COMPARTMENT SYNDROME

Careful positioning of the patient is a critical component of a safe bariatric operation. Whether the patient is placed in the supine or the split-leg position, it is critical to avoid any pressure points to the trunk or extremities. Cases of rhabdomyolysis after both open and laparoscopic gastric bypass have been reported (36,37). Compartment syndrome is also a risk, particularly if surgery is performed in the lithotomy position or if operative times are excessive (38). Use of an operative table that allows the legs to be separated without being elevated or flexed will confer all of the positioning advantages of lithotomy positioning, while minimizing the potential for compartment syndrome or lower-extremity nerve compression injuries.

LAPAROSCOPIC VS. OPEN BARIATRIC SURGERY

Substantial controversy exists at present regarding whether the laparoscopic or open approach to bariatric surgery offers a lower incidence of complications. The largest published series of laparoscopic gastric bypasses to date demonstrates a remarkably low complication rate with results comparable to or better than any open series (22). However, the results of one group's performance cannot be generalized to the entire cohort of bariatric surgeons in the United States.

At the time of submission of this article, a PubMed search on the keywords "randomized, prospective, gastric bypass" returned only three randomized prospective trials comparing laparoscopic to open RYGB (21,39,40). Only two of these studies included more than 100 patients (21,40). These two studies support the hypothesis that the incidence of most major complications (death, anastomotic leak, etc.) is similar in the laparoscopic and open groups. However, several important differences were identified. Lujan et al.'s 2004 study noted two significant differences: a lower incidence of abdominal wall hernias and a shorter hospital stay in the laparoscopic group (40). Nguyen et al.'s 2001 study similarly noted a lower incidence of wound-related complications (infection and hernia) and a shorter length of stay in the laparoscopic group. Both studies confirmed that intermediate-term weight loss (12–24 months) is similar for both groups. Interestingly, a higher percentage of the laparoscopic group in Nguyen et al.'s study demonstrated a "good or better" BAROS outcome at six months after surgery (97% vs. 82%) (21).

CONCLUSION

In order to optimize the conditions under which bariatric surgery is performed and to minimize the risk of complications, the American College of Surgeons has published "Recommendations for Facilities Performing Bariatric Surgery" (41). Published in 2000, these recommendations include the following points:

- Bariatric surgery should be performed by a team of experienced surgeons, anesthesiologists, nurses, and nutritionists. Recovery room and nursing staff should be trained in the management of the severely obese.
- Operating rooms used for bariatric surgery should be designed to accommodate the unique needs of the severely obese patient.
- Hospital facilities, such as intensive care units, radiology departments, and rehabilitation facilities should be appropriately equipped to care for bariatric patients (41,42).

In order to specifically address the issues associated with laparoscopic bariatric surgery, the Society of American Gastrointestinal Endoscopic Surgeons (SAGES) has published "Guidelines for the clinical application of laparoscopic bariatric surgery" (43). These guidelines reinforce the Consensus Statement published by the NIH in 1991 and outline the appropriate integration of laparoscopic techniques into a bariatric surgery practice (44).

It is well established that there is a substantial learning curve involved in starting a bariatric practice, whether it be laparoscopic or open. Estimates of the laparoscopic learning curve range from 75 to 100 cases (45–47). To address this issue, the American Society for Bariatric Surgery has published "Guidelines for granting privileges in bariatric surgery" (48). In addition, SAGES published "Guidelines for institutions granting bariatric privileges utilizing laparoscopic techniques" (49). These documents set forth minimum standards for the credentialing of both open and laparoscopic bariatric surgeons. Several different pathways are described, depending upon whether the surgeon has received formal residency or fellowship training in laparoscopic and bariatric procedures.

With the geometric growth of bariatric surgery over the past five years, the field has come under intense scrutiny by the media, insurance companies, and zealous plaintiff's attorneys. It may not be unreasonable to suggest that the survival of bariatric surgery in the United States will depend upon minimizing complications and poor outcomes to the fullest extent possible. This goal will be facilitated by strict adherence to the nationally recognized guidelines described here. In addition, patient selection must be performed very carefully, with the choice of bariatric procedure carefully tailored to each patient's physiologic and lifestyle issues. Surgical and nutritional follow-up must be lifelong. If these recommendations are followed, it is the author's hope that complications will be kept to a minimum, and that bariatric surgery will continue to provide an effective treatment alternative in the fight against the obesity epidemic (42).

REFERENCES

1. Mokdad AH, Marks JS, Stroup DF, Gerberding JL. Actual causes of death in the United States, 2000. JAMA 2004; 291(10):1238–1245.
2. Steinbrook R. Surgery for severe obesity. NEJM 2004; 350:1075–1079.
3. Wittgrove AC, Clark GW, Schubert KR. Laparoscopic gastric bypass, Roux-en-Y: technique and results in 75 patients with 3–30 months follow-up. Obes Surg 1996; 6:500–504.
4. Wittgrove AC, Clark GW. Laparoscopic gastric bypass, Roux-en-Y—500 patients: technique and results, with 3–60 month follow-up. Obes Surg 2000; 10:233–239.
5. Higa KD, Boone KB, Ho T, Davies OG. Laparoscopic Roux-en-Y gastric bypass for morbid obesity: technique and preliminary results of our first 400 patients. Arch Surg 2000; 135:1029–1034.
6. Wittgrove AC, Clark GW, Tremblay LJ. Laparoscopic gastric bypass, Roux-en-Y: Preliminary report of 5 cases. Obes Surg 1994; 4:353–357.
7. Hamilton EC, Sims TL, Hamilton TT, Mullican MA, Jones DB, Provost DA. Clinical predictors of leak after laparoscopic Roux-en-Y gastric bypass for morbid obesity. Surg Endosc 2003; 17:674–684.
8. Blachar A, Federle MP, Pealer KM, Ikramuddin S, Schauer PR. Gastrointestinal complications of laparoscopic Roux-en-Y gastric bypass surgery: clinical and imaging findings. Radiology 2002; 223(3):625–632.
9. Jones KB. Biliopancreatic limb obstruction in gastric bypass at or proximal to the jejunojejunostomy: a potentially deadly, catastrophic event. Obes Surg 1996; 6:485–493.
10. Serra C, Baltasar A, Bou R, Miro J, Cipagauta LA. Internal hernias and gastric perforation alter a laparoscopic gastric bypass. Obes Surg 1999; 9:546–549.
11. Higa KD, Ho TC, Boone KB. Internal hernias after laparoscopic Roux-en-Y gastric bypass: incidence, treatment and prevention. Obes Surg 2003; 13:350–354.
12. Felsher J, Brodsky J, Brody F. Small bowel obstruction after laparoscopic Roux-en-Y gastric bypass. Surgery 2003; 134(3):501–505.
13. Filip JE, Mattar SG, Bowers SP, Smith CD. Internal hernia formation after laparoscopic Roux-en-Y gastric bypass for morbid obesity. Am Surg 2002; 69(7):640–643.
14. Champion JK, Williams M. Small bowel obstruction and internal hernias after laparoscopic Roux-en-Y gastric bypass. Obes Surg 2003; 13:596–600.
15. Schauer PR, Ikramuddin S, Gourash W, Ramanathan R, Luketich J. Outcomes after laparoscopic Roux-en-Y gastric bypass for morbid obesity. Ann Surg 2000; 232:515–529.
16. Fobi MAL, Lee H, Holness R, Cabinda D. Gastric bypass operation for obesity. World J Surg 1989; 22:925–935.
17. Abdel-Galil E, Sabry AA. Laparoscopic Roux-en-Y gastric bypass—evaluation of 3 different techniques. Obes Surg 2002; 12:639–642.
18. Nguyen NT, Stevens CM, Wolfe BM. Incidence and outcome of anastomotic stricture after laparoscopic gastric bypass. J Gastrointest Surg 2003; 7(8):997–1003.
19. Ahmad J, Martin J, Ikramuddin S, Schauer P, Slivka A. Endoscopic balloon dilatation of gastroenteric anastomotic stricture after laparoscopic gastric bypass. Endoscopy 2003; 35(9):725–728.
20. DeMaria EJ, Schweitzer M, Kellum JM, Sugerman HJ. Prospective comparison of open versus laparoscopic Roux-en-Y gastric bypass for morbid obesity [abstr]. Obes Surg 2000; 10:131.

21. Nguyen NT, Goldman C, Rosenquist CJ, Arango A, Cole CJ, Lee SJ, Wolfe BM. Laparoscopic versus open gastric bypass: a randomized study of outcomes, quality of life, and costs. Ann Surg 2001; 234(3):279–291.
22. Higa KD, Ho T, Boone KB. Laparoscopic Roux-en-Y gastric bypass: technique and 3-year follow-up. J Laparoendosc Adv Surg Tech 2001; 11(6):377–382.
23. Shepherd MF, Rosborough TK, Schwartz ML. Heparin thromboprophylaxis in gastric bypass surgery. Obes Surg 2003; 13:249–253.
24. Eriksson S, Backman L, Ljungstrom K. The incidence of clinical postoperative thrombosis after gastric surgery for obesity during 16 years. Obes Surg 1997; 7:332–335.
25. Wu EC, Barba CA. Current practices in the prophylaxis of venous thromboembolism in bariatric surgery. Obes Surg 2000; 10:7–13.
26. Kalfarentzos F, Stavropoulou F, Yarmenitis S, Kehagias I, Karamesini M, Dimitrako-poulos A, Maniati A. Prophylaxis of venous thromboembolism using two different doses of low-molecular-weight heparin in bariatric surgery: a prospective randomized trial. Obes Surg 2001; 11:670–676.
27. Fobi M, Lee H, Igwe D, Felahy B, James E, Stanczyk M, Fobi N. Prophylactic cholecystectomy with gastric bypass operation: incidence of gallbladder disease. Obes Surg 2002; 12:350–353.
28. Hamad GG, Ikramuddin S, Gourash WF, Schauer PR. Elective cholecystectomy during laparoscopic Roux-en-Y gastric bypass: is it worth the wait? Obes Surg 2002; 13: 76–81.
29. O'Brien PE, Dixon JB. A rational approach to cholelithiasis in bariatric surgery: its application to the laparoscopically placed adjustable gastric band. Arch Surg 2003; 138:908–912.
30. Sugerman HJ, Brewer WH, Shiffman ML, Brolin RE, Fobi MA, Linner JH, MacDonald KG, MacGregor AM, Martin LF, Oram-Smith JC. A multicenter, placebo-controlled, randomized, double-blind, prospective trial of prophylactic ursodiol for the prevention of gallstone formation following gastric bypass-induced rapid weight loss. Am J Surg 1995; 169:91–97.
31. MacLean LD, Rhode BM, Nohr C, Katz S, McLean AP. Stomal ulcer after gastric bypass. J Am Coll Surg 1997; 185(1):1–6.
32. Sapala JA, Wood MH, Schuhknecht MP, Sapala MA. Marginal ulcer after gastric bypass: a prospective 3-year study of 173 patients. Obes Surg 1998; 8:505–516.
33. Sanyal AJ, Sugerman HJ, Kellum JM, Engle KM, Wolfe L. Stomal complications of gastric bypass: incidence and outcome of therapy. Am J Gastroenterol 1992; 87: 1165–1169.
34. Sugerman HJ, Kellum JM Jr, Reines HD, DeMaria EJ, Newsome HH, Lowry JW. Greater risk of incisional hernia with morbidly obese than steroid-dependent patients and low recurrence with prefascial mesh. Am J Surg 1996; 171:80–84.
35. Higa KD, Boone KB, Ho T. Complications of the laparoscopic Roux-en-Y gastric bypass: 1040 patients—what have we learned? Obes Surg 2000; 10:509–513.
36. Wiltshire JP, Custer T. Lumbar muscle rhabdomyolysis as a cause of acute renal failure after Roux-en-Y gastric bypass. Obes Surg 2003; 13:306–313.
37. Torres-Villalobos G, Kimura E, Mosqueda JL, Garcia-Garcia E, Dominguez-Cherit G, Herrera MF. Pressure-induced rhabdomyolysis alter bariatric surgery. Obes Surg 2003; 13:297–301.
38. Gorecki PJ, Cottam D, Ger R. Lower extremity compartment syndrome following a laparoscopic Roux-en-Y gastric bypass. Obes Surg 2002; 12:289–291.
39. Westling A, Gustavsson S. Laparoscopic vs. open Roux-en-Y gastric bypass: a prospective, randomized trial. Obes Surg 2001; 11(3):284–292.
40. Lujan JA, Frutos MD, Hernandez Q, Liron R, Cuenca JR, Valero G, Parrilla P. Laparoscopic versus open gastric bypass in the treatment of morbid obesity: a randomized prospective study. Ann Surg 2004; 239(4):433–437.

41. Committee on Emerging Surgical Technology and Education, American College of Surgeons. Recommendations for facilities performing bariatric surgery. Bull Am Coll Surg 2000; 85(9):20–23.
42. Herron DM. The surgical management of severe obesity. Mt Sinai J Med 2004; 71(1): 63–71.
43. Guidelines for the clinical application of laparoscopic bariatric surgery. SAGES Website, 2003 July. http://www.sages.org/sg_pub30.html.
44. Gastrointestinal surgery for severe obesity. NIH Consensus Statement Online, Mar 25–27 1991; 9(1):1–20. http://odp.od.nih.gov/consensus/cons/084/084_statement.htm.
45. Oliak D, Ballantyne GH, Weber P, Wasielewski A, Davies RJ, Schmidt HJ. Laparoscopic Roux-en-Y gastric bypass: defining the learning curve. Surg Endosc, publ. online 29 October, 2002.
46. Schauer P, Ikramuddin S, Hamad G, Gourash W. The learning curve for laparoscopic Roux-en-Y gastric bypass is 100 cases. Surg Endosc 2003; 17:212–215.
47. Nguyen NT, Rivers R, Wolfe BM. Factors associated with operative outcomes in laparoscopic gastric bypass. J Am Coll Surg 2003; 197(4):548–555.
48. Guidelines for granting privileges in bariatric surgery. ASBS Website, 2003. http://www.asbs.org/html/guidelines.html.
49. Guidelines for institutions granting bariatric privileges utilizing laparoscopic techniques. SAGES Website, 2003 May. http://www.sages.org/sg_pub31.html.

17

Postoperative Follow-Up and Nutritional Management

Scott A. Shikora and Margaret M. Furtado
Obesity Consult Center, Center for Minimally Invasive Obesity Surgery,
Tufts-New England Medical Center, Boston, Massachusetts, U.S.A.

INTRODUCTION

As a field of surgery, bariatric procedures have never been safer or more effective for achieving meaningful and sustainable weight loss. However, all of the currently performed operations result in dramatic changes in gastrointestinal anatomy, physiology, and/or dietary habits. Unfortunately, a good surgical result does not ensure a successful outcome. Even after excellent weight loss, patients must still be carefully followed long term to guard against the development of nutritional or gastrointestinal complications (Table 1).

The long-term consequences of bariatric surgery will vary according to the procedure performed. Some are common to all procedures while others may be specific to one operative procedure. For the nutritional derangements, the etiology may be multifactorial, i.e., secondary to the dramatic reduction of macronutrient and micronutrient intake, altered dietary choices, and/or nutrient malabsorption. The degree of the deficiencies will be determined not only by the specific operative procedure, but also by the dietary habits of the individual patient. Some deficiencies may develop quickly, while others, slowly and in an insidious manner. In regard to gastrointestinal consequences, the presenting signs and symptoms may be unique for the specific procedure or those seen commonly after any gastrointestinal surgery. With both nutritional and gastrointestinal complications, misdiagnosis, inability to diagnose, or delay in diagnosis, may all have severe consequences. Therefore, a solid knowledge of these issues and an understanding of the treatments are necessary to minimize their impact and achieve the best outcomes.

COMMONLY PERFORMED BARIATRIC PROCEDURES

To understand the potential long-term consequences of bariatric surgery, it is important to first understand the more commonly performed procedures. Each is described at length elsewhere in the book. In this chapter, only the laparoscopic adjustable

Table 1 Long-Term Considerations of Bariatric Surgery

Nutritional issues
  Malnutrition
  Vitamin and mineral deficiencies
  Weight loss failure
  Dehydration
  Anemia
  Dumping syndrome
Gastrointestinal issues
  Nausea
  Constipation
  Abdominal pain
  Marginal ulcers
  Incisional hernias
  Vomiting
  Diarrhea
  Gallstones
  Gastritis
  Intestinal obstructions

---

gastric band (LAGB), the short limb Roux-en-Y gastric bypass (RYGB), and the biliopancreatic diversion with or without duodenal switch (BPD+/−DS) will be considered. These procedures are all effective for weight loss, but all achieve it by different mechanisms. The LAGB is a procedure where an inflatable silicone band is placed around the uppermost stomach. A small gastric pouch of 15 to 30 cc is created in the process, which is partially obstructed by the narrow band. Weight loss is due exclusively to the restriction of nutrient intake created by the small gastric pouch reservoir and the narrow outlet. The RYGB also relies on a small gastric pouch reservoir of 15 to 30 cc which is created by surgical stapling devices. The pouch drains through a narrow anastomosis to a Roux limb of the jejunum. Weight loss is due predominantly to nutrient restriction. However, the bypass of the fundus, duodenum, and proximal jejunum may contribute to the weight loss by influencing gut hormones. The BPD +/−DS is a predominantly malabsoptive procedure. A partial gastrectomy is preformed resulting in a large gastric pouch (200 cc) which mildly reduces the gastric reservoir volume. An anastomosis is created between the distal ileum to the stomach pouch or duodenum. Nutrients bypass the majority of the small bowel. Weight loss is mainly due to the limited intestinal absorptive capacity in the terminal ileum.

THE SIGNIFICANCE OF LONG-TERM FOLLOW-UP

For all of the bariatric procedures, long-term follow-up is critical for success and patient well-being. During the first year, patient monitoring is most critical. Weight loss is analyzed and patients are evaluated for overall heath, medication titration, activity level, dietary habits, bowel function, and hydrational status. After the first postoperative year, patients are seen less frequently. However, at these visits, patients should be assessed for nutritional deficiencies, appropriateness of their diet, weight maintenance, the presence of symptoms, and for overall health and well-being.

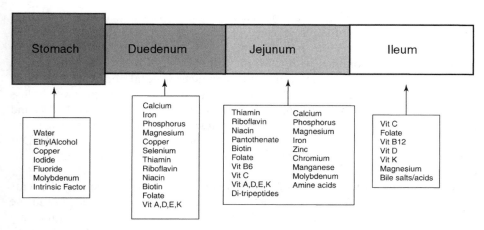

Figure 1 Sites of nutrient absorption in the GI tract.

NUTRITIONAL DEFICIENCIES

To understand the potential deficiencies that can develop after surgery, it is also important to know where along the gastrointestinal tract the macro- and micro-nutrients are absorbed (Fig. 1). Some nutrients are preferentially absorbed more proximally in the GI tract and others more distally. In addition, certain nutrients require specialized mixing for maximal absorption. For example, iron represents both. It is preferentially absorbed in the proximal small intestine and is best absorbed after contact with an acid environment. Procedures that re-route the nutrient stream away from the gastric acid and/or the proximal small intestine can be assumed to put patients at risk for an iron deficiency. Therefore, the type and severity of nutrient deficiency will vary according to the operative procedure performed (Table 2).

PROTEIN-CALORIE MALNUTRITION

The gastric restrictive procedures including the RYGB rarely cause protein-calorie malnutrition. The weight loss seen is predominantly from fat with only minimal changes in lean body tissue (1,2). However, protein malnutrition can occur in patients with dysfunctional eating habits such as anorexia or the avoidance of protein food sources, and is seen in patients with protracted vomiting. For the

Table 2 The Likelihood of Vitamin/Mineral Deficiencies After Various Bariatric Procedures

Procedure	Iron	Folate	Vitamin B$_{12}$	Calcium	Vitamin D	Thiamine
LapBand/ VBG	**	**	*	*	*	*
GBP	**	**	***	**	**	*
BPD	***	**	***	**	**	*

*Not very likely.
**Somewhat likely.
***Highly likely.

malabsorptive procedures, such as the distal gastric bypass and the BPD+/−DS, malnutrition is not uncommon as ingested protein may be poorly absorbed and lost in the stool. The incidence has been reported to be approximately 7% to 21% (3). Hypoalbuminemia is common within six months after surgery, but gradually returns to preoperative levels. Tacchino et al. studied changes in total and segmental body composition at 2,6,12, and 24 months post-op BPD, and discovered that weight loss with BPD was achieved with an appropriate decline of lean body mass (LBM) and with all parameters reaching, at stable weight, values similar to weight-matched controls (4). However, the yearly hospitalization rate for protein deficiency after BPD is 1%. Persistent hypoalbuminemia leads to revisional surgery in 1% to 2% of patients after BPD with duodenal switch (5).

Unfortunately, the diagnosis of protein malnutrition may not be easy. Patients are expected to rapidly lose weight, and serum protein levels will often stay in the normal range until late (6–8). Therefore, for all bariatric patients, dietary monitoring is important during weight loss and in the long term. Clinical signs of protein malnutrition can be seen even in overweight patients. We recommend that gastric bypass patients take in approximately 60 to 80 g of protein daily. Higher intake may be necessary for the malabsorptive procedures, and should be guided by serum protein levels as well as diet and bowel habit activity.

Severe calorie deficiency (cachexia) is also unusual after bariatric surgery but may be seen in patients with protracted vomiting, diarrhea, or anorexia. Treatment includes nutritional supplementation (even involuntary if necessary), correction of any underlying anatomical abnormalities (i.e., stricture, obstruction), and/or psychologic intervention as indicated. For the most extreme or intractable cases, common channel limb lengthening or even reversal may be necessary.

DEHYDRATION

Mild dehydration is commonly seen in the early postoperative period for all of the bariatric procedures and is mainly due to decreased intake. For the gastric restrictive procedures, patients have difficulty drinking the necessary fluid volumes as they adapt to very small gastric capacities. With the malabsorptive procedures, the frequent watery stools are a source of significant fluid loss. With any of these operations, vomiting or diarrhea may exacerbate fluid losses. Dehydration typically occurs in the first few months following surgery, during the summer months, and after gastrointestinal illnesses. On the basis of body weight, obese patients require a greater amount of fluid per day than their lean counterparts to maintain normal fluid balance. This volume is obtained directly from the liquid drunk and indirectly from the water constituent of the food eaten. Once dehydrated, these patients have great difficulty "catching up" because they cannot drink fluid quickly. Standard fluid recommendations are impossible given the heterogeneity of the patients. In addition, there are no mathematical equations that accurately estimate fluid needs in the obese. Patients are instructed to use thirst and urine concentration as a guide for fluid intake. For patients not vomiting, fluid status can be managed by encouraging patients to travel with a fluid source (e.g., sports bottle) and drink continuously throughout the day one swallow at a time until the symptoms of dehydration are relieved. For those patients with vomiting, intravenous fluid may be necessary to restore the lost intravascular volume.

It is therefore critical that patients drink enough fluid postoperatively to prevent dehydration. Dehydration may also increase the likelihood of nausea, which may exacerbate intolerance to the diet or fluids. Some patients may even require more than the recommended 64 ounces of fluid per day, especially if they are physically active or live in a warm climate. Patients should be instructed to monitor their hydration status via awareness of potential signs of dehydration, such as dizziness and dry skin, and concentrated urine. Patients should be reminded that meeting their fluid goal takes precedence over food, including even protein intake. Whenever possible, postoperative patients suffering from dehydration who are unable to ingest adequate protein from solid foods alone should include high-protein, low-carbohydrate liquid supplements in their diet to better meet fluid and protein needs. In order to minimize the risk of dumping syndrome, patients are often advised to select those supplements with approximately 13 g (or less) of "sugars" per serving.

NAUSEA AND VOMITING

Nausea and vomiting are common after gastric restrictive surgery. In most cases, nausea and vomiting are caused by dysfunctional eating habits, such as overeating, eating too fast, or not chewing food well. However, other causes must be ruled out including dumping syndrome, medication intolerance, anastomotic strictures, and marginal ulcers. A thorough history may help differentiate causes. For example, a patient who develops a solid food intolerance approximately four to six weeks after surgery, which necessitates a change in diet to only liquids, may have an anastomotic stricture. On the other hand, a patient who gets nauseated or vomits only on occasion without any obvious pattern, is most likely to be eating incorrectly (e.g., too quickly, excessive volume of food).

VITAMIN DEFICIENCIES

Vitamin and/or mineral deficiencies are prevalent after all bariatric procedures and in particular, after GBP and BPD (8–25). After surgery, all patients may be at risk for an array of dietary vitamin and/or mineral deficiencies and therefore should comply with lifelong supplementation. It should be noted that micronutrient deficiencies may develop slowly and may not become evident until years after surgery (Table 3). Therefore, patients need to be followed yearly.

Table 3 Nutritional Deficiencies Can Be Seen Months After Gastric Bypass Surgery

	% Abnormal	Mean abnormal value	Month first observed
Potassium	56 (7)	3.2 ± 0.1 mEq/L	6 ± 10
Magnesium	34 (4)	1.3 ± 0.1 mEq/L	15 ± 16
Albumin	0 (5)	–	–
Vitamin A	10 (5)	11 ± 6 ug/dL	31 ± 22
Vitamin B_{12}	64 (3)	166 ± 27 pg/mL	28 ± 18
Folate	38 (11)	1.8 ± 0.6 ng/mL	15 ± 11
Iron	49 (4)	43 ± 11 ug/dL	27 ± 12

% Abnormal pre-op. *Source*: Adapted from Ref. 8.

The gastric restrictive procedures generally cause few micronutritional deficiencies (11). This is presumably because nutrients are not diverted from the duodenum and gastric mixing is essentially normal. However, deficiencies may develop in those patients with intractable vomiting or among those with suboptimal nutrient intake. Intake may be inadequate since the meal size is dramatically reduced, and because many patients change their dietary choices. For example, many of these patients do not tolerate red meat, so they may avoid it altogether. Gastric bypass patients will be at risk for deficiencies for the same reasons as the restrictive procedure patients are, but will be at an additional risk due to the fact that the nutrient stream bypasses the fundus, duodenum, and proximal jejunum causing malabsorption of iron, folate, calcium, and vitamin B_{12}. The malabsorptive procedures such as the BPD+/–DS place patients at even greater risk for deficiencies of the above vitamins and calcium, as well as for the fat-soluble vitamins (A, D, E, K), electrolytes such as sodium, potassium, chloride, phosphorus, magnesium, and possibly even zinc (15,22). For all bariatric patients, serum levels need to be aggressively followed yearly, and supplementation should be prescribed judiciously. Since many bariatric programs rely on different supplementation protocols, there is no consensus as to what represents the optimal regimen. However, there is general agreement concerning the importance of lifelong surveillance of patients' vitamin/mineral status. Table 4 presents the

Table 4 Vitamin/Mineral Supplementation Protocols for Treating Deficiencies (Obesity Consult Center, Tufts-NEMC, Boston, Massachusetts)

All patients postoperatively
  Complete MVI with iron P.O. qd
  Calcium with vitamin D 1200–1500 mg P.O. qd
  Patients should be advised against taking a calcium supplement that does not include vitamin D
Specific vitamin/mineral
  Iron
    Fe sat $< 10\%$ and Ferritin < 10 ng/mL or Fe sat $< 7\%$ (regardless of ferritin)
      Supplement with $FeSO_4$ 325 mg plus 250 mg vitamin C P.O. qd.
      Increase to TID as tolerated. Patient is instructed to take with orange juice
  Folate
    If RBC folate level is low:
      First replete vitamin B_{12} if it is low
      1 mg of folate P.O. qd × 3 months
  Vitamin B_{12}
    If neurologic symptoms (regardless of level) or if level is < 100 mcg/dL:
      Vitamin B_{12} 1000 mcg IM q week × 4 weeks, then 1000 mcg IM q month × 4 months and recheck
    If level is 100–150 pg/dL:
      Vitamin B_{12} 1000 mcg IM q month, and recheck in 3–4 months
    If level is 150–250 pg/dL:
      Vitamin B_{12} 1000 mcg P.O. qd, and recheck in 3–4 months
      Vitamin B_{12} can also be administered sublingual or by nasal spray
  Vitamin D
   If low serum vitamin D level:
      Vitamin D 50,000 IU P.O. q week for 6–8 weeks; recheck level in 3–6 months
      If vitamin D level in 3–6 months is normal, go back to baseline post-op supplements, and recheck in 3 months
      Ensure that the patient is taking 1200–1500 mg elemental calcium per day

---

specific vitamin and mineral supplementation protocol of the Obesity Consult Center at Tufts-New England Medical Center in Boston.

Iron

Iron deficiency is commonly found in bariatric patients, and in particular, in pre-menopausal women (13,16,21,24,25). It manifests as a microcytic anemia. The etiology for iron deficiency is multifactorial. It is partly due to the nutrient restriction that limits the intake of dietary iron. In addition, after GBP and the BPD, malabsorption of iron also occurs. Iron absorption is facilitated by gastric acid. After GBP, gastric acid production is dramatically reduced in the small gastric pouch (12). In addition, iron is predominantly absorbed in the duodenum and proximal jejunum. Both GBP and BPD re-route the nutrient stream from the upper stomach "pouch" directly into the jejunum or ileum thereby avoiding the duodenum altogether. Therefore, patients are unlikely to maintain normal serum levels of iron or iron saturation after these procedures. The BPD+/−DS keeps the duodenum in the nutrient circuit but bypasses all of the jejunum. Lastly, patients who do not tolerate or avoid meat in their diet are more likely to be iron-deficient (7). However, for all patients found to be deficient, it is recommended that they be supplemented with 325 mg of $FeSO_4$ orally one to three times daily. Patients prescribed supplementation should be monitored for possible side effects of oral iron, such as constipation. If repletion is unsuccessful orally, parenteral iron infusions may be required.

Folic Acid

Folic acid deficiency is also a potential complication following bariatric surgery. It can manifest as macrocytic anemia, leukopenia, thrombocytopenia, glossitis, or megaloblastic marrow. For the most part, folate deficiency is thought to be predominantly due to decreased intake and not to malabsorption, and is easily corrected by oral vitamin supplementation (9). It has also been shown to be less likely in meat eaters than meat avoiders (7). Vitamin B_{12} is also necessary for the conversion of methyltetrahydrofolic acid to tetrahydrofolic acid, therefore, a B_{12} deficiency may result in a folate deficiency. Unfortunately, serum folate levels are more indicative of acute dietary insufficiency of folate than more chronic tissue levels (8). Red blood cell folate levels change more gradually and are thought to be more predictive of tissue levels. However, the significance of lower red blood cell folate levels is questioned since few patients actually develop megaloblastic anemia. The usual recommendation for supplementation is 1 mg of folate daily.

Vitamin B_{12}

Deficiencies of vitamin B_{12} have been reported to commonly occur following GBP (13,17,21,24). Some reports describe the incidence of low serum B_{12} levels as occuring in 26% to 70% of GBP patients. Significant deficiencies can lead to macrocytic anemia, megaloblastosis of the bone marrow, leukopenia, thrombocytopenia, glossitis, or neurologic derangements. However, despite the high incidence of low serum levels, few patients develop these sequelae. The normal absorption of vitamin B_{12} is a complex process. The vitamin must first be freed from the food source, particularly meat protein. This is facilitated by gastric acid. The free B_{12} is then bound to R-protein in the stomach. Within the duodenum, R-protein is cleaved from the vitamin, which then binds to intrinsic factor (IF). The B_{12}–IF complex then travels intact through the intestinal tract and is absorbed into the circulation in the distal ileum.

As with iron and folate, B_{12} intake is diminished after bariatric surgery. Absorption of available B_{12} may also be deranged. The gastric pouch produces little acid, thereby preventing the normal cleavage of B_{12} from its food source (12). Several studies have reported that oral crystalline B_{12} can be absorbed and normal serum levels maintained in GBP patients (10,12). Some researchers have suggested that a significant etiology for the B_{12} deficiency after GBP is the decrease in IF (26,27). Marcuard et al. demonstrated low IF levels in 53% of GBP patients with B_{12} deficiency (28). However, some of these patients had low levels of B_{12} and IF prior to surgery. In addition, other studies have reported normal Schillings tests on GBP patients suggesting that the IF mixing is adequate despite the bypass of the duodenum.

There is a general consensus that few GBP patients can adequately maintain normal serum B_{12} levels from diet alone (9,10). Interestingly, Avinoah et al. found better B_{12} (as well as iron and folate) levels in patients who were able to tolerate meat compared to those who could not (7). In many patients, acceptable vitamin B_{12} serum levels can be obtained if the vitamin is taken orally. Several of the studies recommend 500 to 600 mcg daily. If a mild or moderate deficiency is identified, our practice is to orally supplement with 1000 mcg daily. If oral supplementation does not replete the deficiency, or if it is severe, intramuscular injections (1000 mcg) can be administered monthly.

Vitamin B_{12} deficiency should be much less likely after LAGB procedures where the nutrient stream is not diverted and after BPD+/−DS where gastric acid production is less altered than after GBP and the terminal ileum is kept intact. If a deficiency is identified, poor dietary choices, suboptimal intake, and/or non-adherence with vitamin supplementation may be implicated.

Other vitamin and mineral deficiencies may occur and include vitamin A noted in 10% of patients, hypokalemia in 56%, and hypomagnesemia in 34% of GBP patients (8). However, these were not considered significant, as no patient experienced night blindness, and low potassium and magnesium levels were easily corrected with oral supplementation. There is a risk of deficiency of fat soluble vitamins (A, D, E, K) after the malabsorptive procedures (15,22).

Thiamine deficiency is generally uncommon after bariatric surgery. However, it must always be considered for any patient who presents with intractable vomiting and dehydration. Rehydration with a glucose-based intravenous fluid without the supplementation of thiamine can result in Wernicke–Korsakoff syndrome (29–31).

GASTROINTESTINAL ISSUES

Abdominal Pain

Abdominal pain can be encountered anytime after surgery and can be due to causes both related and unrelated to the operation. Generally speaking, the workup would be the same as for any patient presenting with abdominal pain after any abdominal procedure. The evaluation should always begin with a thorough history and physical exam. In most cases, this will eliminate many potential causes of pain. The history should ascertain the location, quality, timing, and pattern of any pain complaint. The exam should be particularly focused on localizing any tenderness and evaluating the surgical wound for evidence of herniation. Incisional hernias can be found in up to 25% of patients after open surgery and should be strongly considered in patients who have had postoperative wound infections (32). In addition to incisional hernias, other potential causes include marginal ulceration and gallstones. Other causes of pain will include dumping syndrome, fatty food intolerance, overeating, internal hernia, adhesions, and constipation. There are also other causes of abdominal pain that can occur independent of surgery, and include duodenal ulcer (very uncommon in this population), renal stones, musculoskeletal strains, diverticulitis, etc.

Gallbladder Disease

Gallstone formation results from a derangement of the normal concentrations of biliary cholesterol, lecithin, and bile salts. Conditions that increase the likelihood of gallstone formation include obesity (33), rapid weight loss, both medically and surgically induced (34,35), and even bariatric surgery itself (36). Therefore, a significant number of patients will have gallstones at the time of their bariatric surgery or will develop gallstones during the first year or so after bariatric surgery. For example, in our program, approximately 25% of patients had undergone cholecystectomy sometime in their past. Another 25% were found to have stones during their pre-operative evaluation. All of these patients had cholecystectomy at the time of GBP. Approximately 30% of the remaining patients have gone on to develop symptomatic gallstones after GBP. This is consistent with published series that report the likelihood of post-bariatric surgery gallstone formation to be between 10% and 42% (35–37). The great discrepancy in incidence may reflect the difference between routine postoperative gallbladder evaluation and evaluation only for symptoms. Given the relative inability to utilize ERCP after GBP, gallstone disease can become a significant problem in these patients. Complications are well known. Therefore, a rational approach for management is necessary.

There is little controversy concerning the operative management of the patient found preoperatively to have gallstones. Few bariatric surgeons would dispute the need to perform concomitant cholecystectomy. However, the management of the "normal" gallbladder is not conclusive. Some centers strongly advocate concomitant cholecystectomy, as it avoids the potential complications of gallbladder disease and also a second surgery (38). Another argument for concomitant cholecystectomy is that pre-operative assessment of the gallbladder is limited by body habitus and even overlying bowel gas. Further, both ultrasound and operative palpation can miss extremely small stones, bile crystals, sludge, and cholesterolosis. Laparoscopic surgery eliminates the ability to palpate the gallbladder.

Other centers, such as ours, will not typically remove a normal gallbladder at time of obesity surgery. It adds to operative time, blood loss, and has inherent risks such as bleeding, bile leak, bile duct injury, etc. For many of the extremely obese patients, it may adversely affect the ability to do the bariatric operation through a mini-laparotomy approach. For laparosopic procedures, the trocar sites are not best suited to address the gallbladder. The introduction of laparoscopic surgery has made cholecystectomy after bariatric surgery (and even common bile duct exploration) minimally invasive and of low risk (39). Although it does require a second operative procedure, the patient's subsequent weight loss and improvement in overall health may somewhat offset the risks of the second operative procedure and anesthesia. In addition, ERCP can be performed safely through the excluded fundus which can be accessed laparoscopically.

Currently there are no prospective randomized trials to determine which of the above approaches is superior. Either seems acceptable. A recent survey of American

Society of Bariatric Surgery found that 32.5% of surgeons performed concomitant cholecystectomy (40). Additionally, the likelihood increased with the complexity of the procedure, only 7% for gastric restrictive procedures and 100% for BPD+/−DS and distal GBP procedures.

A third approach involves the postoperative administration of ursodiol. This medication decreases the likelihood of gallstone formation. A randomized prospective trial by Sugerman et al. demonstrated a dramatic reduction in stone formation in post-GBP patients taking 600 mg of ursodiol given daily for 6 months (41). Gallstone formation was reduced from 32% to 2% ($p < 0.001$). However, patient compliance, possible medication side effects, and cost ($600.00 yearly), may influence the effectiveness of this option.

Intestinal Obstruction

As with any abdominal surgery, intestinal obstruction can occur after bariatric surgery. Not surprisingly, it would be less common after a procedure such as the LAGB and more likely after GBP or BPD+/−DS. Although a bowel obstruction might be a consequence of postoperative adhesion formation, intestinal obstruction can also be due to internal herniation. Internal herniation is a condition where intestine migrates into an intra-abdominal space and obstructs. These spaces are created during the surgical procedure but can be enlarged by the subsequent weight loss. There are three distinct areas for internal herniation after GBP surgery: (1) through the mesocolon (retrocolic Roux limb only), (2) through the divided mesenteric leaves of the enteroenterostomy, or (3) internal hernia of the biliopancreatic limb under the Roux limb (Petersen hernia).

Internal hernia, of any kind, is the most common and elusive cause of small bowel obstruction after GBP. The incidence of this complication is 2% to 5% (42). In our series, small bowel obstruction has occurred in 1% and 3% of our open and laparoscopic cases, respectively. Internal hernia can occur immediately or years following surgery. Patients may present with a spectrum ranging from mild intermittent abdominal bloating to intermittent crampy abdominal pain and nausea to severe refractory abdominal pain, retching, and/or vomiting. A high index of suspicion is often necessary to prompt abdominal exploration or diagnostic laparoscopy, as clinical presentation and diagnostic testing (upper GI with small-bowel follow-through) are often non-specific. A unique quality of internal hernias is that they can result in potentially life-threatening closed-loop obstructions particularly if the biliopancreatic limb is obstructed. After GBP, the fundus is excluded. Obstruction of the biliopancreatic limb has no mechanism for decompression. The fundus is at risk for necrosis and perforation which would be highly likely to be fatal.

Marginal Ulceration

Marginal ulceration (stomal ulcer) refers to the development of a mucosal erosion on the intestinal side of the anastomosis. Intestinal mucosa is normally exposed to gastric acid that has been neutralized by biliopancreatic secretions. After GBP or BPD, the intestinal mucosa at the anastomosis is exposed to un-neutralized acid placing it at risk for ulceration.

Marginal ulceration occurs in 5% to 15% and 3% to 5% of patients who undergo undivided and divided GBP, respectively (43–45). The majority of stomal ulcers that occur in the undivided operation occur in conjunction with a disrupted vertical staple line (gastrogastric fistula) (43). The acid produced in the excluded fundus can enter the pouch via the gastrogastric fistula and ulcerate the gastrojejunostomy. The etiology of marginal ulcer in divided GBP is less clear. Acid output by parietal cells in the standard 30 cc gastric pouch is said to be minimal but may vary from patient to patient. Other potential causes include use of non-steroidal anti-inflammatory agents, *Helicobacter pylori*, smoking, or anastomotic ischemia (45).

Marginal ulceration is also seen after BDP. The incidence has been reported to be 2.8% (2). The gastric pouch of the BPD is typically 200 cc in capacity and contains gastric tissue rich in parietal cells. It is surprising that the incidence isn't, in fact, even higher. With the BPD+/−DS, the incidence of an ulceration is reduced by the preservation of the pylorus and proximal duodenum (5).

Marginal ulcer typically occurs within three months of GBP (42). Patients most commonly present with symptoms of mid-epigastric abdominal pain that may radiate to the back. Sub-sternal chest pain can also occur. Patients may also complain of food intolerance and vomiting. Patients who present with symptoms suggestive of ulceration should undergo endoscopy. If an ulcer is found the treatment includes removal of irritants such as tobacco or NSAIDs and either a histamine-receptor antagonist or proton pump inhibitor. Intractability or ulcers thought to be ischemic in origin may require surgery. To decrease the incidence of marginal ulceration, many programs maintain their patients on histamine-receptor antagonists for a period of time after surgery.

Weight-Loss Failure

Weight-loss failure occurs in approximately 20% to 25% of patients (46). Few failures can be traced to technical errors. In most cases, dietary non-compliance or behavioral changes are to be blamed. In these cases, patients chronically overeat and/or abuse calorie-dense foods, candies, or sweets. Patients may present with chronic vomiting, increasing appetite, increasing meal capacity, and gradual weight gain. Most will also have abandoned exercise. The treatment for someone who "fails" a bariatric procedure is controversial. Revision is an option but carries a higher morbidity than the original procedure. Many surgeons would opt to revise to a more radical operation. However, there are no publications to support that shrinking a dilated pouch or revising a dilated anastomosis will lead to renewed weight loss. Limb lengthening is also poorly studied. While dramatically decreasing the common channel will likely succeed in achieving weight loss, it may do so at increased nutritional risks. Re-stapling after gastro-gastric fistula would also be likely to succeed in renewed weight loss. However, since most failures are behavioral and no procedure guarantees success, the decision to revise should be individualized.

CONCLUSIONS

The current group of bariatric procedures achieves a high likelihood of weight-loss success at relatively low peri-operative risk. However, the reduction in dietary intake, changes in eating habits, possible dysfunctional eating, vomiting, and/or nutrient malabsorption can lead to both macro- and micro-nutrient deficiencies. These deficiencies may present years after the surgery and be initially insidious, but could result in severe consequences. Additionally, these procedures are unique and have their own specific complications that may develop and require prompt recognition and treatment. Therefore all bariatric surgeons, including those just entering the field, must be familiar with the potential consequences of the procedures that they perform and be prepared to provide long-term surveillance.

REFERENCES

1. Das SK, Roberts SB, McCrory MA, Hsu LKG, Shikora SA, Kehayias JJ, Dallal GE, Saltzman E. Long–term changes in energy expenditure and body composition after massive weight loss induced by gastric bypass surgery. Am J Clin Nutr 2003; 78:22–30.
2. Bothe A, Bistrian BR, Greenberg I. Energy regulation in morbid obesity by multidisciplinary therapy. Surg Clin North Am 1979; 59:1017–1031.
3. Scopinaro N, Gianetta E, Adami GF, Friedman D, Traverso E, Marinari GM, Cuneo S, Vitale B, Ballari F, Colombini M, Baschieri G, Bachi V. Biliopancreatic diversion for obesity at eighteen years. Surgery 1996; 119:261–268.
4. Tacchino RM, Mancini A, Perrelli M, Bianchi A, Giampietro A, Milardi D, Vezzosi C, Sacco E, De Marinis L. Body composition and energy expenditure: relationship and changes in obese subjects before and after biliopancreatic diversion. Metabolism 2003; 52:552–558.
5. Hess DS, Hess DW. Biliopancreatic diversion with a duodenal switch. Obes Surg 1998; 8:267–282.
6. Pories WJ, Swanson MS, MacDonald KG, Long SB, Morris PG, Brown BM, Barakat HA, deRamon RA, Israel G, Dolezal JM. Who would have thought it? An operation proves to be the most effective therapy for adult-onset diabetes mellitus. Ann Surg 1995; 222:339–352.
7. Avinoah E, Ovnat A, Charuzi I. Nutritional status seven years after Roux-en-Y gastric bypass surgery. Surgery 1992; 111:137–142.
8. Halverson JD. Micronutrient deficiencies after gastric bypass for morbid obesity. Am Surg 1986; 52:594–598.
9. Amaral JF, Thompson WR, Caldwell MD, Martin HF, Randall HT. Prospective hematologic evaluation of gastric exclusion surgery for morbid obesity. Ann Surg 1985; 201:186–192.
10. Rhode BM, Arseneau P, Cooper BA, Katz M, Gilfix BM, MacLean LD. Vitamin B-12 deficiency after gastric bypass surgery for obesity. Am J Clin Nutr 1996; 63:103–109.
11. Printen KJ, Halverson JD. Hemic micronutrients following vertical banded gastroplasty. Am Surg 1988; 54:267–268.
12. Smith CD, Herkes SB, Behrns KE, Fairbanks VF, Kelly KA, Sarr MG. Gastric acid secretion and vitamin B_{12} absorption after vertical Roux-en-Y gastric bypass for morbid obesity. Ann Surg 1993; 218:91–96.
13. Sugarman HJ. Bariatric surgery for severe obesity. J Assoc Acad Minor Phys 2001; 12:129–136.
14. Elliot K. Nutritional considerations after bariatric surgery. Crit Care Nurs Q 2003; 26:133–138.
15. Slater GH, Ren CJ, Siegel N, Williams T, Barr D, Wolfe B, Dolan K, Fielding GA. Serum fat-soluble vitamin deficiency and abnormal calcium metabolism after malabsorptive bariatric surgery. J Gastrointest Surg 2004; 8:48–55.
16. Brolin RE, La Marca LB, Kenler HA, Cody RP. Malabsorptive gastric bypass in patients with superobesity. J Gastrointest Surg 2002; 6:195–203.
17. Skroubis G, Sakellaropoulos G, Pouggouras K, Meda N, Nikiforidis G, Kalfarentzos F. Comparison of nutritional deficiencies after Roux-en-Y gastric bypass and after biliopancreatic diversion with Roux-en-Y gastric bypass. Obes Surg 2002; 12:551–558.
18. Goldner WS, O'Dorisio TM, Dillon JS, Mason EE. Severe metabolic bone disease as a long-term complication of obesity surgery. Obes Surg 2002; 12:685–692.
19. Kushner R. Managing the obese patient after bariatric surgery: a case report of severe malnutrition and review of the literature. J Parenter Enteral Nutr 2000; 24:126–132.

20. Marceau P, Biron S, Lebel S, Marceau S, Hould FS, Simard S, Dumont M, Fitzpatrick LA. Does bone change after biliopancreatic diversion?. J Gastrointest Surg 2002; 6:690–698.

21. Brolin RE, Leung M. Survey of vitamin and mineral supplementation after gastric bypass and biliopancreatic diversion for morbid obesity. Obes Surg 1999; 9:150–154.

22. Hatizifotis M, Dolan K, Newbury L, Fielding G. Symptomatic vitamin A deficiency following biliopancreatic diversion. Obes Surg 2003; 13:655–657.

23. Newbury L, Dolan K, Hatzifotis M, Low N, Fielding G. Calcium and vitamin D depletion and elevated parathyroid hormone following biliopancreatic diversion. Obes Surg 2003; 13:893–895.

24. Papini-Berto SJ, Burini RC. Causes of malnutrition in post-gastrectomy patient. Arq Gastroenterol 2001; 38:272–275.

25. Rhode BM, Shustik C, Christou NV, MacLean LD. Iron absorption and therapy after gastric bypass. Obes Surg 1999; 9:17–21.

26. Mahmud K, Ripley D, Dolscherholmen A. Vitamin B12 absorption tests: their unreliability in postgastrectomy states. JAMA 1971; 216:1167–1171.

27. Crowley LV, Olson RW. Megaloblastic anemia after gastric bypass for obesity. Am J Gastroenterol 1984; 79:850–860.

28. Marcuard SP, Sinar DR, Swanson MS, Silverman JF, Levine JS. Absence of luminal intrinsic factor after gastric bypass surgery for morbid obesity. Dig Dis Sci 1989; 34:1238–1242.

29. Sola E, Morillas C, Garzon S, Ferrer JM, Martin J, Hernandez-Mijares A. Rapid onset of Wernicke's encephalopathy following gastric restrictive surgery. Obes Surg 2003; 13:661–662.

30. Salas-Salvado J, Garcia-Lorda P, Cuatrecasas G, Bonada A, Formiguera X, Del Castillo D, Hernandez M, Olive JM. Wernicke's syndrome after bariatric surgery. Clin Nutr 2000; 19:371–373.

31. Chaves LC, Faintuch J, Kahwage S, Alencar Fde A. A cluster of polyneuropathy and Wernicke–Korsakoff Syndrome in a bariatric unit. Obes Surg 2002; 12:328–334.

32. Sugerman HJ, Kellum JM Jr, Reines HD, DeMaria EJ, Newsome HH, Lowry JW. Greater risk of incisional hernia with severe morbid obesity than steroid dependant patients and a low recurrence with prefasical polypropelene mesh. Am J Surg 1996; 171:80–84.

33. Everhart JE. Contributions of obesity and weight loss to gallstone disease. Ann Intern Med 1993; 119:1029–1035.

34. Kamrath RO, Plummer LJ, Sadur CN, Adler MA, Strader WJ, Young RL, Weinstein RL. Cholelithiasis in patients with a very-low calorie diet. Am J Clin Nutr 1992; 56:255s–257s.

35. Wattchow DA, Hall JC, Whiting MJ, Bradley B, Iannos J, Watts JM. Prevalence and treatment of gallstones after gastric bypass surgery for morbid obesity. Br Med J 1983; 286:763.

36. Deitel M, Petrov I. Incidence of symptomatic gallstones after bariatric operations. Surg Gynecol Obstet 1987; 164:549–552.

37. Shiffman ML, Sugerman HJ, Kellum JM, Brewer WH, Moore EW. Gallstone formation after rapid weight loss: a prospective study in patients undergoing gastric bypass surgery for treatment of morbid obesity. Am J Gastroenterol 1991; 86:1000–1005.

38. Schmidt JH, Hocking MP, Rout WR, Woodward ER. The case for prophylactic cholecystectomy concomitant with gastric restriction for morbid obesity. Am Surg 1988; 54:269–272.

39. Ahmad SA, Schuricht AL, Azurin DJ, Arroyo LR, Paskin DL, Bar AH, Kirkland ML. Complications of laparoscopic cholecystectomy: the experience of a university-affiliated teaching hospital. J Laparoendosc Adv Surg Tech 1997; 7:29–35.

40. Mason EE, Renquist KE. Gallbladder management in obesity surgery. Obes Surg 2002; 12:222–229.

41. Sugerman HJ, Brewer WH, Shiffman ML, Brolin RE, Fobi MA, Linner JH, MacDonald KG, MacGregor AM, Martin LF, Oram-Smith JC. A multicenter, placebo-controlled, randomized, double-blind, prospective trial of prophylactic Ursodiol for the prevention of gallstone formation following gastric-bypass-induced rapid weight loss. Am J Surg 1995; 169:91–97.

42. Byrne TK. Complications of surgery for obesity. Surg Clin North Am 2001; 81:1181–1193.

43. MacLean LD, Rhode BM, Nohr C, Katz S, MacLean AP. Stomal ulcer after gastric bypass. J Am Coll Surg 1997; 185:342–348.

44. Sanyal AJ, Sugerman HJ, Kellum JM, et al. Stomal complications after gastric bypass. Incidence and outcome of therapy. Am J Gastroenterol 1992; 87:1165–1169.

45. Sapala JA, Wood MH, Scapala MA, Flake TM Jr. Marginal ulcer after gastric bypass. A prospective 3 year study of 173 patients. Obes Surg 1998; 5:509–516.

46. Maclean LD, Rhode BM, Sampalis J, Forse RA. Results of the surgical treatment of obesity. Am J Surg 1993; 165:155–162.

Index

Adenoma, 12
Adjustable gastric bands, 142
Amino acids, 3, 80, 86
  see also proteins
Anastomosis, 140–143
  leaks, 140–143, 150
Anemia, 83, 162, 163
Apnea, 14
Appetite, 1, 4, 155
Appetite suppressant, 41, 42, 171
Arthritis, 9, 19

Bacterial overgrowth, outcomes of, 163,
  164
Bariatric operation, 207, 212
  gallstones, treatment of, 212, 213
  importance of patient positioning, 214
  risk factors for DVT, 212
Bariatric operations, 6, 7
Bariatric patients, incidence of liver
    diseases in, 54
Bariatric patients, nutrition education
    of, 78
  hospital facilities for, 71
  information dissemination, 70
    preoperative educational workshops,
      70
    support groups, 70
Bariatric procedure *see also* bariatric surgery
  enteric leak,
    assessment of, 208
    clinical finding of, 208
    diagnosis of, 209
    treatment of, 209
  surgeon knowledge, 207
Bariatric procedure, cardiac risk assessment
    in, 51
Bariatric procedure, characteristics of, 193,
    196–198

Bariatric procedures *see also* bariatric
    surgery, 181, 182
  calorie deficiency, treatment of, 222
  commonly performed, 219
  follow-up, 220
  nutrient deficiencies, 223
  postoperative dehydration, 222
    effects of, 222
    signs of, 223
  postoperative folic acid deficiency, 225
    cause of, 225
  postoperative food intolerance, 227, 229
  postoperative iron deficiency, 225
    etiology of, 225
    treatment of, 225
  postoperative nutrient deficiencies, 223
  postoperative ulceration, 228, 229
  postoperative vitamin deficiency, 223
  protein intake, 223
  protein malnutrition, 221, 222
  risk of iron deficiency, 221, 225
Bariatric psychiatrist, role of, 51
Bariatric surgery, 11, 15, 17, 63, 101, 153,
    154, 156, 164, 181, 182, 186, 188
Bariatric surgery *see also* obesity treatment
  components of, 63
  effects of, 182, 186
  eligibility for, 61, 70
  for adolescents, 62
  hospital requirements, 71
  postoperative care, 62, 65
  postoperative problems, 66
  prevalence in US, 181, 187
  prevention of malnutrition, 63
  psychological assessment tool, 65, 67
  role of physicians, 70
  role of psychologist, 66
  role of websites, 72
  unsuitable patients, 63
Bariatric surgery, effect on mortality, 121

Bariatric surgery, laparoscopic, 94
Bariatric surgery, postoperative diet, 79
  and cardiac patients, 51
  enteric leak, 208
    complications of, 208
    incidence of, 208
    locations of, 208
    signs of, 208
  evaluation of failed surgery, 50, 56
  facility recommendations, 215
  gallstone treatment, 54
  gallstones, occurrence of, 227
  indicators for revisional surgery, 55
  laparoscopic
    pulmonary changes, 103
    renal changes, 104
  marginal ulcer, 213
  patients not recommended for, 51, 56
  postoperative abdominal pain, 226
    causes of, 226
    evaluation of, 226
  postoperative intestinal obstruction, 228
    causes of, 228
  postoperative nutritional derangements,
      219
    and gastrointestinal complications, 219
    etiology of, 219
    thiamine deficiency, 226
    vitamin B12 malabsorption, 224
  preoperative evaluation, 49
  psychological patients not considered in, 51
  role of surgeon, 49
  survival of, 215
  US guidelines, 215
Bariatrician role of, 50
Biliopancreatic diversion, 81, 156–162, 164,
      207, 220
  and bacterial growth, 163, 164
  and bone loss, 163
  and calcium absorption, 163
  and intestinal bypass, 154
  and protein absorption, 163
  and syndrome X, 159–161
  benefits of, 158
  comorbidity resolution, 159
  components of, 160
  decreased lipid absorption, 160
  effect on pregnancy, 162, 164
  effect on syndrome X, 159–161
  effects on liver function, 161, 162
  experimental conclusions, 164
  mortality in, 158
  nutrient deficiencies in, 162, 163
  side effect of, 156–159, 162

[Biliopancreatic diversion]
  technique of
    weight loss in, 220
Blind loop, 156
Blood glucose, 3, 53
Blood pressure, 12
Blood, oxygen in, 3
BMI see body mass index
BMI, 33, 140–142, 144, 154, 158,
      159, 162
Body mass index, 9, 49, 55, 76, 93,
      168, 195
Bowel resection, 5
BPD see biliopancreatic diversion
  postoperative ulceration, 228, 229
  weight loss in, 229
Brain
  evolution of, 5
  function of, 2
  role of carbohydrate for, 3
Breast cancer, 12

Caloric intake, 80
Calories, 10, 34, 37
Cancer
  of breast, 12
  of colon and rectum, 12
  of endometrium, 12
  of multiple sites, 12
  of prostate, 12
Carbohydrate, 3, 10
Cardiopulmonary, 49, 53
Cardiovascular disease, 15, 21
Carpal tunnel syndrome, 19
Cholelithiasis see gallstones
Cholelithiasis see also gallstones
Colon cancer, 12
Comorbid conditions, 11
Comorbid diseases, 9
Comorbidity resolution, RYGB vs gastric
      banding, 202, 203
Consumption, 79
Continuous positive airway pressure, 14,
      117, 170
CPAP see continuous positive airway
      pressure
CPAP, 53

Deep vein thrombosis, 212
Deep venous thrombosis, 19, 49, 55, 109, 111,
      116, 117, 121
Depression, 22, 34, 36, 187

Diabetes, 42, 153, 154, 159, 195, 197, 202, 203
  cure of, 153, 155, 161
  patients, preparation for bariatric surgery, 53
Diabetes management, 79
Diabetes mellitus, 3, 15, 18, 173, 178
  fetal risk in, 18
  prevalence in obese, 10, 13
Diabetic nephropathy, 20
Diet change, 77, 79
  patients' readiness, evaluation of, 78
Diet, 10, 50, 51
Diet, habits, 219, 227
Dietary intake, 75, 77, 80
  and behavior therapy, 36
  and weight loss, 36
  assessment of, 75, 77
  questionnaire, 77
Digestive system, 2
Dopamine, 2, 3
Dopaminergic receptors, 5
Dumping syndrome, 64, 168, 223
Dumping syndrome, treatment of, 85
Duodenal switch, 16, 80, 156–158
DVT see also deep vein thrombosis
  prophylaxis, 212
Dyslipidemia, 13

Eating behavior, 192, 195
EBW see excess body weight
Ectodermal stoma, 2
Endoderm, 2
Endodermal gut, 2
Endometrial cancer, 12
Energy balance, 3, 67
Energy expenditure, 1
Energy intake, 10, 75
Epworth sleepiness scale, 53
Evolution, 1, 7
Excess body weight, 140
  definition of, 75
Excess weight loss, 141, 147
Exercise sessions, 39

Fat, 153
Fat intake, 37
Fat, visceral, 113, 115–117, 120–122
Fatty acid, 3, 4
  absorption of, 162
  synthetase inhibitors, 4
    effect on food intake, 4, 6
Fibrosis, 161, 162

[Fibrosis]
  effect of surgery on, 161
  factors influencing, 155
Fitness, 39
  and obesity, 40
  level of, 39
  relationship with cardiovascular disease mortality, 40
Food, 154–157, 163
  absorption of, 162
  detection and evaluation of, 2
  intake, 4, 6, 153–155
  -motivated behavior, 4
  restriction of, 154, 156, 159
Food diaries see also food record
Food record see food diaries, 34

Gallstones, 54, 113, 227
  formation of, 227
  risk factors for, 212
  treatment approach, 227
    controversy in, 227
    gallbladder removal, effects of, 227, 228
  treatment of, 212
Gastric band, adjustable, 80, 212
Gastric banding, 154, 155
  negative aspects of, 155
  limitations of, 155
Gastric banding, adjustable, 191–94, 197, 199, 201, 203
  adjustable, 167
    adjustability in, 167
    benefits of, 167
    weight loss after, 168, 171
  and weight loss, 167, 178
  related complications, 173
Gastric bypass, 5, 49, 54, 103, 113, 114, 117, 118, 120–122, 139–147, 148, 150, 154, 155, 156, 159, 168, 178, 182, 183, 191–193, 197, 198, 201–203, 209–213, 220, 222, 224
  dumping syndrome in, 85
  gastrojejunal stenosis, diagnosis of, 211
  internal herniation, 228
  intra-abdominal pressure during, 110, 113–115, 117–120
  iron deficiency in, 83
  laparoscopic, 129
  laparoscopic and gastric, 130–145
    complications in, 140
    Nguyen et al.'s study, 141, 144, 146, 147
  laparoscopic and open, 209, 211

[Gastric bypass]
    complication rate, 214
    effect on femoral peak systolic
        velocity, 104
   marginal ulcer
    incidence of, 213
    symptoms of, 213
    treatment of, 213
   nutrient deficiencies in, 80
    cause of, 80
   nutrient deficiencies, 223
    postoperative iron malabsorption, 225
   open and laparoscopic, strictures in, 211,
      214
   open vs laparoscopic, 194
   operative costs for, 144
   postoperative gastrointestinal bleeding,
      treatment of, 210
   postoperative intra-abdominal bleeding,
      210, 211
   postoperative nutrition, 79, 81
    monitoring, 78
   postoperative small bowel obstruction,
      220, 228
   postoperative stricture formation
    causes of, 211
    incidence of, 211
    sites of, 211
   postoperative ulceration, 227
    symptoms of, 227, 229
    treatment of, 229
   postoperative vitamin B12 deficiency,
      treatment of, 225
   resolution of diabetes in
Gastric prolapse, 174
   diagnosis of, 174
   radiographic findings of, 174
   symptoms of, 174–176
   treatment of, 175
   types of, 174
Gastric restriction
   introduction of, 91
Gastric restrictive procedure, 122, 221, 224
   postoperative micronutrient
       deficiency, 223
   weight loss in, 221, 227
Gastric restrictive surgery, 67, 223
   postoperative nausea, causes of, 223
Gastric surgery complications, effect on
      food, 80
Gastric surgery, respiratory insufficiency,
      116, 118
Gastric tubes, 85
Gastroenterostomy, 139, 155

Gastroesophageal reflux disease, 110, 115,
      116, 187
   in morbid obesity, 54
   prevalence in morbid, 16
Gastrointestinal consequences, 219
Gastrointestinal operations, 4
Gastrointestinal resective operations, 5
Gastrojejunal anastomosis, 141
Gastrojejunostomy, 139, 140, 142, 143
Gastroplasty, 154, 155
Gastrostomy, 85
GBP *see* gastric bypass
GERD *see also* gastroesophageal reflux
      disease
   in morbid obesity, 114, 115
   resolution of, 117–119
Ghrelin, 6
Glomerulopathy, 20
   etiology of, 21
   incidence in obesity, 20
Glucose, 3
   homeostasis, 3,14
   level in blood, 3
   regulation, 3
Glucose metabolism, 159
Gut, evolutionary development, 2

Health benefits, 186
Health care, 11, 18, 23
Health providers, 70
Heart failure, 13
Hernia, 54, 110, 143, 175
   -space, 209
   effect of, 228
   hiatal, diagnosis of, 174, 175
   incisional, prevalence in gastric bypass,
      214
   internal, 209
    sites of, 209
    source of, 210
    symptoms of, 209
    treatment of, 209, 210
   treatment of, 210
Hormones, 5
Hunger, 4, 51
   and appetite, 4
   definition of, 4
Hyperparathyroidism, 16
Hypertension, 12, 15, 20, 197, 202, 203
   intracranial, 20
    origins, 20, 22
    symptoms of, 19, 21
Hypertension, intracranial, 110

[Hypertension, intracranial]
  see also pseudotumor cerebri
  management of, 52
Hypopnea, 14, 15
  and apnea, 14
Hypoxia, 3

Ideal body weight, 9, 15
  determination of, 75
Ingestive behavior, 3, 4
Insulin, 85, 117, 159, 160, 187
  resistance of, 117, 187
  sensitivity, 187
Insulin resistance, 12, 14, 15
  relationship to diabetes, 20
Insulin treatment, 53
Intestinal absorption, 153, 154, 156, 164
Intestinal absorptive capacity, 153
Intestinal adaptation, 81
Intestinal bypass, 154
Intestinal flora, 163
Intestinal malabsorption, reason for
  failure, 156
Intra-abdominal bleeding, 211
Intra-abdominal pressure, 14, 19, 102, 103,
  113, 114
Intracranial pressure, 119

Jejuno-ileal bypass, 6
Jejunoilial bypass see intestinal bypass
Jejunojejunostomy, 142, 143, 144
Joint pain, incidence in morbid obesity, 18, 19

LAGB see laparoscopic adjustable gastric
  banding
  adjustability in, 183, 184, 186, 188
  attributes of, 182, 183, 188
  effect of laparoscopic placement, 183,
    184, 185, 188
  effect on diabetes, 181, 187
  incidence of complications, 185
  pattern of weight loss, 186
  reversibility, 184, 188
LAGB, 168, 191, 194–202, 214
  A-trial, 198
  adjustability of, 200
  B-trial, 198
  complication rate in, 191
  conversion to gastric bypass,
    complications in, 198
  conversion to RYGB, complications in,
    199
  device-related complications, 195

[LAGB]
  evaluation of, 195, 196
  incidence of esophageal dilatation, 198,
    203
  international studies of, 195, 197
  marketability of, 200
  mechanism of, 194
  perioperative complications, 199
  preoperative comorbidities, 197
  re-operations in, 202
  reasons for band removal, 196
  related complications, in FDA
    trial, 195
  resolution of comorbidities, 197,
    200, 203
  resolution of diabetes, 202
  studies, 197, 200
    by Angrisani, 195
    by Chevallier, 196
    by Favretti, 195
    by O'Brien, 195
    by Szold, 196
  vs RYGB, 201
  weight loss data, 200
  weight loss failure, 202
    causes of
  weight loss in, 198, 201, 202
    and gastric bypass, 168
    band adjustment in, 171
      office-based, 172
      radiographic-guided, 173
    benefit for super-obese, 168
    comparison with VBG and RYGB, 173
    diagnosis of erosion, 175
    eroded band removal, 176
    excess weight loss in, 172
    food ingestion in, 171
    impact on diabetes, 178
    incisional hernia in, 214
    internal hernia in, 209
    need for band adjustments, 172
    nutrition counseling, 171
    operative technique, 169
    placement of, 175
    postoperative care, 170
    postoperative diet, 171
    postoperative obstruction, 176
      factors contributing to, 177
      patient outcomes in, 177
      prevention of, 170, 177
      treatment of, 175, 176
    postoperative pain management, 170
    reasons for band removal, 177
    related complications, 173

[LAGB]
    strategies to band adjustment, 171
    symptoms of erosion, 175, 176
    techniques of device placement, 169, 177
        pars flaccida approach, 169
    treatment of erosion, 176
    weight loss, 168, 178
    in diabetics, 178
Lap-Band, 183–188, 198, 199
    cohort, 199
    placement, related complications, 198
    placement, 185–188
    effect of
Laparoscopic adjustable gastric banding,
        191, 194, 219
    technique of, 219, 220
    weight loss in, 220
Laparoscopic cholecystectomy, 101, 103,
        141
Laparoscopic gastric bypass, 129, 136, 139,
        141, 142, 210, 214
    anastomotic leaks in, 140, 141, 147
    benefits of, 147
    comorbidity resolution, 143, 150
    complications in, 140
    conversion rates, 140, 142, 143
    dissection and creation of the mesocolic
        window, 131, 135
    first report of, 139
    Lonroth and Dalen's technique, 146–148
    mortality in, 140–142, 146
    outcomes of, 144
    patient positioning, 129
    port placement, 130
    port sites, 130
    reoperative, 142
    Wittgrove and Clark's technique,
        146, 147
    wound complication rate in, 150
Laparoscopic gastroplasty, 102
Laparoscopic operations, 69
Laparoscopic procedures see
        laparoscopic surgery.
Laparoscopic Roux-en-Y gastric bypass,
        140, 143
    comorbity resolution in
    complications in, 140
    de la Torre and Scott's technique, 140,
        146–148
    DeMaria et al.'s study, 146, 147, 150
    Matthews et al.'s technique, 140, 146
    outcomes of, 144
    Schauer et al.'s technique, 141, 146, 150
    Teixeira et al.'s technique, 140

Laparoscopic RYGB, 208, 210, 211
    gastrojejunal narrowing in, 211
    stricture formation in, 211
Laparoscopic RYGB, pioneers of, 194,
        195, 201
Laparoscopic SAGB, 197
    weight loss in, 198, 201
Laparoscopic surgery, 143, 145, 209, 227
    outcomes in, 144
Laparoscopic surgery, effects of, 196
Laparoscopy, 191, 192, 194–196
Laparoscopy, effect on incisional hernia,
        113, 120
    effects of using sequential compression
        devices, 104
    venous stasis, 104
LapBand system, 168, 177
Learning curve, 144, 145, 147
Lifestyle modification programs, 40
Lipids, 3
    components of, 3
Liver disease, prevalence in morbid
        obesity, 16
Liver failure, 121
Liver, 2
    evolutionary development, 2
    function of, 2
Loop reconstruction, 142
Low calorie diet, 37, 79

Macronutrients, 3, 10
Malabsorption, 56
    of fat, 76, 81
Malabsorptive procedures, 80, 154,
        222, 224
    malnutrition in, 221
    postoperative nutritional deficiency,
        221
Malnutrition, 63, 76
Mesoderm, 2
Metabolic syndrome, 181
    prevalence of, 13
Micronutrient deficiencies, 56, 81, 223
Mini-gastric bypass, 142
    complications in, 140
    outcomes of, 144
    Rutledge's technique, 142, 147
Moorehead-Ardelt questionnaire, 66
Morbid obesity, 61, 114, 115, 119, 120,
        153–155, 164
    and depression, 34
    and joint disease, 118
    and weight gain, 154, 158

[Morbid obesity]
associated cardiac changes, 114
associated infectious problems, 120
associated medical conditions, 67
associated medical problems, 33
associated psychological problems, 66
associated renal problems, 20
associated venous stasis, 109, 113, 117
chronic inflammation, 21
effect of respiratory insufficiency,
    115, 116
effect on society, 11
immune alterations, 21
incidence of cancers, 120
incidence of gallstones, 16
menstrual irregularities in, 17
mortality in, 103, 121
patho-physiologic consequences, 67
  importance of consultants, 67
prevalence of, 62
psychological disorders in, 33
psychosocial effects of, 110
surgical need, 154, 158, 161
Morbidly obese, intra-abdominal pressure
    in, 102
Morbidly obese, stereotypes in US, 22
Mortality predictors, 40
Myocardial infarction, 13

NASH see non-alcoholic steatohepatitis
  diagnosis of, 54
Neoplasia, 12
Nimiety, 4
Non-alcoholic steatohepatitis,
    16, 54, 111
Nutrient absorption, 221
  of iron, 221
Nutrient deficiency, reduction of, 65
Nutrients processing of, 2
  signaling, 3
Nutristats, 3
Nutritional counseling, 37, 65
  counselors, role of, 65
Nutritional deficiencies see
    micronutrient deficiencies
Nutritionist
  role of, 50
  assessment of, 75
  education, 78
  impact of threats to, 1, 7
  markers, 76
  postoperative, 79
  status changes, 82

Obese patients, 222
fluid need, 222
guide for fluid intake, 222
medical management of, 33
weight loss expectations, 35
Obesity, 1–7, 9, 10, 182, 184, 186–188
and depression, 187
prevalence of, 181
surgery, 181, 182, 184, 186–188
  characteristics of ideal procedure, 182
  mortality rates, 185
Obesity comorbidities, 207
Obesity research, 159
Obesity surgery, 227
Obesity surgery, patient eligibility, 94
first attempt, 154
indications for, 154
NIH guidelines for, 77
point of reference for, 154
preoperative nutrition assessment, 75
strategies of, 154
Obesity treatment, 61, 67
importance of anesthesiologists, 69
preoperative evaluation, 70
psychological intervention, 67
requirement of, 65
resolution of comorbidities, 61
surgery see also bariatric surgery
Obesity, treatment for younger patients,
    168
abdominal, 12
and depression, 22
and diabetes, 116
and female sexual hormone dysfunction,
    119
and ingestive behavior, 3, 4
and long-chain fatty acids, 3
and nonepileptic seizures, 21
and pulmonary problems, 116
and satiety, 4
and self-esteem, 22
and urinary bladder pressure, 113, 114,
    119
associated hypertension, 114
associated hypertension, pathophysiology
    of, 114, 115, 121
central, associated complications, 113,
    115, 116, 118
children's perception of, 22
classification of, 33
comorbidities, 39
comorbidity
  psychological, 51
consequences of, 10

[Obesity, treatment for younger patients]
  difficult airway management, 56
    risk factors, 57
  effect of intra-abdominal pressure, 110,
    113, 114, 117
  effect on cardiac events, 52
  emotional suffering in, 23
  epidemiology of, 9
  evolution of, 5
  gastric bypass for, 5
  hypoventilation syndrome, effects of, 110,
    113, 115
  hypoventilation, 109, 111, 113, 115, 116
  in children, 10
  incidence of urinary incontinence, 18
  medication and behavior modification,
    37
  mortality-associated problems, 109, 121
  postoperative complications, 49
  pregnancy-related complications in, 17,
    119
  prevalence of psychiatric disorders, 22
  prevalence of, 33
  related problems, 109
  respiratory changes in, 14
  risks in pregnancy, 17
  role of lipids in, 3
  skin problems in, 21
  social consequences of, 11
  stigma attached to
  stigmatization of, 22
  surgery, 42, 114–121
    associated risks, 40
    effects on diabetes and hypertension,
      114, 117
    incidence of hernias, 110, 113, 120
    reduction in comorbidities, 39
  treatment, 5
    appetitive peptides in, 2, 5
    cognitive restructuring, 35
    self-monitoring, 34
    stimulus control, 35
    surgical, 5
    very low calorie diet, 38
Obstructive sleep apnea, 14, 49, 52, 109, 110,
    111, 115, 116, 122, 170, 178, 187
  contributors to, 14
  diagnosis of, 53
  prevalence of, 14
  symptoms of, 14
Obstructive sleep hypopnea, 52
OSA see obstructive sleep apnea
OSH see obstructive sleep hypopnea
Overeating, 36

Overeating, surgical treatment of, 5
  risk situations for, 36
Overweight, 39, 40
Oxygen, in blood

Pancreas, evolutionary development, 2
Peptides, 2, 5
  appetitive, 2, 5
  orexigenic, 5
  satiating, 6
Peterson space, 209
Physical activity, 9, 10, 34, 39
Pickwickian syndrome, 110, 115
Pituitary, 2
Pneumoperitoneum, 57, 69, 130
  cardiac changes in, 102
  CO_2 absorption in, 102
  diminished urine output, 104
  effects of, 102
  factors influencing cardiac function, 103
  hepatic changes, 103
  quantification of CO_2 absorption, 102
  renal function, 104
  ventilatory changes, 101, 102
Polycystic ovarian syndrome, 18
  diagnosis and treatment of, 18
Polycystic ovary syndrome, 110, 112, 117,
    119
Prader-Willi syndrome, 188
PRCT see prospective randomized clinic
    trials
Prospective randomized clinic trials,
    139, 143
  coagulation and fibrinolytic studies, 145
  complications in, 140
  conversions in, 139, 144, 146
  Nguyen et al.'s study, 141, 144, 146, 147
  postoperative pulmonary functions, 140
  Westling and Gustavsson's study, 143,
    146, 147
Prostate cancer, 12
Protein, 2, 3, 65, 163
  see also amino acids
  and body mass, 3
  absorption, 154, 156, 158–160
  deficiency of, 82, 162–164
  highest quality of, 80
  stores of, 82
Protein malnutrition, 221, 222
Pseudotumor cerebri, 109, 110, 117,119
  symptoms of, 109
Psychological instruments, 51
Pulmonary artery pressures, 9

Pulmonary artery vasoconstriction, 115, 118
Pulmonary atelectasis, 56
Pulmonary embolism, 55, 109, 110, 112,
          115–119, 212
    incidence in bariatric patients, 55
    incidence in gastric bypass, 209
Pulmonary hypertension, 52

Quality of life, 18, 33, 67, 141, 154

Respiratory failure, 53
Respiratory mechanics, 56
Restrictive procedures, 154
Roux limb, 140–144
    obstruction of, 144
Roux-en-Y gastric bypass, 49, 75, 140, 143,
          191, 207, 220
    factors for postoperative complications, 49
    Higa et al.'s study, 142, 146
    incidence of gallstones, 54
    outcomes of, 144
    technique of, 220
    vitamin B12 deficiency in, 82
    weight loss in, 220
RYGB see also Roux-en-Y gastric bypass
    introduction of, 191
    reasons for weight gain, 201
    resolution of comorbidities, 197
    superiority of, 192
    superiority over VBG, 200
    vs VBG, mortality, 193
    vs VBG, weight loss, 192
    weight loss in, 191, 192
RYGB, excessive weight loss, 186, 187

SAGB see Swedish Adjustable Gastric Band
    vs RYGB, 201
        complication rates, 197
        mortality rate, 201
        weight loss
Satiety, 4, 51, 155, 171
Set-point theory, 3
SF-36 assessment tool, 144
Skin manifestations, 21
Sleep apnea, 14, 61, 67, 109, 111, 115
    symptoms of, 109
    treatment of, 119
Sleeve gastrectomy, 157
Social isolation, 22
Species, survival of, 2
Steatosis, 161
Stress incontinence, 18

Stress management, 36
Stress testing, 51
Superobesity, 10
Surgery, objectives of, 5
Survival, 2, 3
Swedish adjustable band, 167
Swedish adjustable gastric band,
          197, 201
Syndrome X, 159–161

T2DM see diabetes mellitus
Tongue, 2
Toxicity, recognition of, 2

VBG see also vertical banded gastroplasty
    and BMI, 93, 94
    comparison between open and
          laparoscopic, 98
    laparoscopic, 94
    Mason, postoperative infections, 91, 97
    outcomes for, 97
    patients with poor outcomes, 94
    postoperative care, 96
    postoperative complications, incidences
          of, 97
    postoperative diet, 97
    postoperative monitoring, 98
    staple line disruption, 99
    wedge technique
        benefits of, 98
    weight loss and gain in, 94, 98
VBG and LAGB, comparison of, 200
Venous stasis ulcers, treatment of, 55, 109,
          110, 113, 117
Venous thrombosis, 117, 119
Vertical banded gastroplasty, 91–100, 114,
          118, 142
Very low calorie diet, 38
Visual analog scale, 145
Vitamin B12, 82
    absorption of, 83, 225
    deficiency of, 82, 83, 225
        assays for, 83
    prevention of, 82
Vitamin deficiencies, 168 see also nutrient
          deficiency
Vitamin deficiency, postoperative, 81
VLCD see very low calorie diet

Weight loss failure, 229
    causes of, 229
    treatment of, 229

Weight loss surgery patient education, 67, 70
Weight loss, 13, 75, 77, 109, 114–117,
        140, 141, 143, 153–158, 162, 164,
        191–193
    effect on joint disease, 118
        effect on urinary incontinence, 110,
            113, 117–119
        effects of, 109
    maintenance of
        self-monitoring, 78
    pre-surgical
        procedures of, 75
    surgery, 114–121
Weight loss, effect on diabetes, 53
    in RYGB, 193
    operations, effective, 191

[Weight loss, effect on diabetes]
    RYGB vs VBG, 193
    surgery, 192
    loss of, 38, 41
        and gain, 35
        attempt, problem solving, 34
        dietary counseling, 38
        drug, 34, 41
        goal setting, 35
        goal, realistic, 35
        patient expectations, 35
        surgical treatment, 42
    management of, 35, 36, 43
    scales, 34
    social support, 36
Wernicke-Korsakoff syndrome, 226